AF293910

Current Perinatology

Manohar Rathi
Editor

Current Perinatology

With 31 Illustrations in 36 Parts

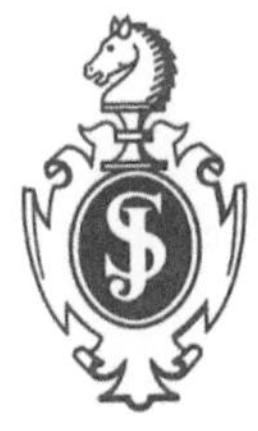

Springer-Verlag
New York Berlin Heidelberg
London Paris Tokyo

Manohar Rathi, M.D.
Director, Perinatal Medicine
Christ Hospital and Medical Center
Oak Lawn, IL
Associate Professor of Pediatrics
Rush Medical College
Chicago, IL, U.S.A.

LIBRARY OF CONGRESS
Library of Congress Cataloging-in-Publication Data
Current perinatology / Manohar Rathi, editor.
    p.   cm.
    Includes bibliographies and index.

    ISBN-13: 978-1-4613-8796-1   e-ISBN-13: 978-1-4613-8794-7
    DOI: 10.1007/978-1-4613-8794-7

    1. Fetus—Diseases.   2. Infants (Newborn)—Diseases.
  3. Pregnancy, Complications of.   I. Rathi, Manohar.
    [DNLM: 1. Fetal Diseases.   2. Infant, Newborn, Diseases.
  3. Pregnancy Complications.   WQ 211 C976]
  RG626.C87   1988
  618.3'2—dc19
  DNLM/DLC
  for Library of Congress   88-20038
Printed on acid-free paper

Typeset by David Seham Associates, Metuchen, New Jersey.

9 8 7 6 5 4 3 2 1

Preface

Perinatal medicine, which is concerned with the problems of the fetus and newborn, has rapidly developed in the last two decades as an important and challenging specialty. Rapid advances in the field, coupled with technological advances, now are making survival of infants with weights as low as 500 grams possible. Ventilator care for severe respiratory problems is on the verge of being replaced by surfactant replacement therapy; on the other hand, development of such technologies as extracorporeal membrane oxygenation and jet ventilation has revolutionized the care of these sick infants.

The advances taking place today in the field of perinatal medicine make periodic updates, like the one provided by this volume, a virtual necessity for clinicians and paramedical personnel alike. A distinguished group of specialists in various aspects of perinatal medicine has contributed to this book. Their wide-ranging experience and points of view should make this book a valuable reference for all physicians and allied health personnel involved in the care of the high-risk fetus and newborn.

MANOHAR RATHI, M.D.

Acknowledgements. I am grateful to the contributors for their cooperation in preparing the manuscripts, to my associates for their help and support, and to the publishers for their continued interest in this work. Above all, I thank Ms. Rose Aiello-Lech and Ms. MaryAnn Cichowski for their hard work in making this publication possible.

M.R.

Contents

Contributors

ROBERT M. ARENSMAN, M.D.
Clinical Associate Professor of Surgery, Louisiana State University School of Medicine, Chief, Division of Pediatric Surgery, Ochsner Clinic, New Orleans, Louisiana

IRA J. CHASNOFF, M.D.
Associate Professor, Departments of Pediatrics and Psychiatry, Northwestern University Medical School, Chicago, Illinois

SUSAN E. DENSON, M.D.
Associate Professor, Department of Pediatrics, The University of Texas Medical School at Houston; Associate Director of Nurseries, University Children's Hospital at Herman and Director of High Risk Clinic, University of Texas Medical School at Houston, Houston, Texas

LEIGH G. DONOWITZ, M.D.
Associate Professor, Department of Pediatrics, University of Virginia School of Medicine, Charlottesville, Virginia

VIVEK GHAI, M.D.
Fellow in Neonatology, University of Illinois Hospital Medical Center, Chicago, Illinois

JAY P. GOLDSMITH, M.D.
Chairman, Department of Pediatrics, Head, Division of Neonatology, Ochsner Clinic and Alton Medical Foundation Hospital, New Orleans, Louisiana; Clinical Associate Professor, Tulane University School of Medicine, New Orleans, Louisiana

MARY HAIRE, R.N., M.S.N.
Clinical Nurse Specialist, Maternal-Fetal Nursing, Vanderbilt University, Nashville, Tennessee

KATHLEEN CONVERY HANOLD, R.N., M.S.
Divisional Coordinator, Parent/Child Health, University of Illinois, Chicago, Illinois

BRUCE A. HARRIS, JR., M.D.
Charles E. Flowers Professor of Obstetrics and Gynecology, University of Alabama at Birmingham, Birmingham, Alabama

PATRICIA A. HOLOBAUGH, M.S.
Microbiologist, Department of Experimental Hematology, Armed Forces Radiobiology Research Institute, Bethesda, Maryland

MAHMOUD A. ISMAIL, M.D.
Associate Professor, Department of Obstetrics and Gynecology, Section of Maternal-Fetal Medicine, University of Chicago, Chicago, Illinois

LUCKY JAIN, M.D.
Fellow, Department of Pediatrics, Neonatology Division, University of Illinois at Chicago, Chicago, Illinois

MICHAEL KATZ, M.D.
Associate Professor of Obstetrics, Gynecology and Reproductive Sciences, University of California San Francisco, Chief, Perinatal Services, Children's Hospital of San Francisco, San Francisco, California

AMY LEMKE, M.S.
Genetic Counselor, Lutheran General Perinatal Center, Lutheran General Hospital, Chicago, Illinois

CHIN-CHU LIN, M.D.
Professor, Division of Maternal-Fetal Medicine, Department of Obstetrics and Gynecology, Pritzker School of Medicine, The University of Chicago, Chicago, Illinois

KATHLEEN MALLIN, PH.D.
Illinois Cancer Council, Chicago, Illinois

MARTHA D. MULLETT, M.D.
Associate Professor, Department of Pediatrics, West Virginia University School of Medicine, Morgantown, West Virginia

KENRAD E. NELSON, M.D.
Professor, Department of Epidemiology, Johns Hopkins University School of Hygiene and Public Health, Baltimore, Maryland

ROGER B. NEWMAN, M.D.
Assistant Professor, Department of Obstetrics and Gynecology, Medical University of South Carolina, Charleston, South Carolina

PATRICE KLEIN PEREZ, R.N., M.S.
Perinatal Outreach Education Coordinator, University of Illinois, Chicago, Illinois

MANOHAR RATHI, M.D.
Director, Perinatal Medicine, Christ Hospital and Medical Center, Oak Lawn, Illinois; Associate Professor of Pediatrics, Rush Medical College, Chicago, Illinois

LOUISE RIFF, M.D.
Associate Professor, Department of Medicine, University of Illinois College of Medicine, Chicago, Illinois

CHARLES ROSENFELD, M.D.
Professor of Pediatrics and Obstetrics/Gynecology, Department of Pediatrics, University of Texas Health Science Center at Dallas/Southwestern Medical School, Dallas, Texas

VICTORIA SCHAUF, M.D.
Professor of Pediatrics, SUNY Stony Brook, Chairman of Pediatrics, Nassau County Medical Center, East Meadow, New York

RODNEY B. STEINER, M.D.
Surgical Resident, Division of Pediatric Surgery, Ochsner Clinic and Alton Ochsner Medical Foundation, New Orleans, Louisiana

ARTHUR A. STRAUSS, M.D.
Assistant Professor of Pediatrics, University of California at Irvine; Associate Neonatologist, Miller Children's Hospital, Long Beach, California.

RABI F. SULAYMAN, M.D.
Chairman, Department of Pediatrics, Christ Hospital and Medical Center; Oak Lawn, Illinois; Associate Professor of Pediatrics, Rush University, Chicago, Illinois

DHARMAPURI VIDYASAGAR, M.D.
Professor, Department of Pediatrics, Neonatology Division, University of Illinois at Chicago, Chicago, Illinois

1
Perinatal Hypoxia in the Growth-Retarded Fetus: Basic Pathophysiology and Clinical Management

CHIN-CHU LIN

Current knowledge of fetal growth and fetal respiratory physiology is based on experimental animal data and on clinical observations that have been developed largely during the past three decades. The majority of studies in this field have occurred primarily in the area of characterization of fetal growth parameters, especially the factor of uteroplacental blood flow in relation to fetal oxygenation. Thus the purpose of this chapter is to describe (1) basic knowledge of fetal oxygenation and placental respiratory gas exchange, (2) fetal adaptation to the hypoxic intrauterine environment, (3) perinatal hypoxia in the fetus associated with intrauterine growth retardation, and (4) its management.

Uterine and Placental Blood Flow in Pregnancy

Before any discussion of fetal oxygenation, fetal metabolism, and fetal growth, it is essential to consider the changes in uterine and placental blood flow that occur during pregnancy. At the present time, our knowledge of uteroplacental blood flow is primarily descriptive for a variety of mammalian species with differing placentations. However, the basic circulatory characteristics in human and subhuman primates appear to be similar to those in lower animals. In ovine pregnancy [1], uterine blood flow patterns cannot be distinguished from those in nonpregnant animals until between days 17 and 20 of gestation. At this time, uterine blood flow begins to increase rapidly, reaching about 600 ml/kg/min at 30 to 35 days; it gradually falls to 280 ml/kg/min at 60 days of gestation. After day 60, the same level of uterine blood flow is maintained until term. The relative proportion of uterine blood flow distributed to the placental cotyledons is approximately 20 to 30% in early pregnancy, 60% at 60 days of gestation, and 85% at term [2–4]. These rapid shifts of uterine blood flow to increase placental blood flow permit sufficient maternal-fetal transfer of metabolic gases and substrates to and from the fetus to assure normal fetal growth and development. In the pregnant rhesus monkey at term, uterine blood flow has been reported to be approximately 170 ml/kg/min, of which 80 to 90% flows through the placenta [5]. In human studies [6,7], uterine blood flow in pregnant women has been determined to lie between 89 and 151 ml/kg/min.

The uteroplacental circulation has been described by Greiss [8] as having three characteristic responses: (1) dramatic vasodilatory capacities enabling it to increase uterine blood flow 100- to 200-fold (from a nonpregnant level of 10–20 ml/min to 2,000 ml/min in ovine twin pregnancy at term), (2) the ability to contribute 80 to 90% of total uterine blood flow to the placental circulation in late pregnancy, and (3) minimal vascular resistance, which permits a progressive increase in placental blood flow throughout pregnancy. In pregnant sheep and in the rhesus monkey, the placental vasculature is widely dilated, responding only minimally to further vasodilator stimuli [9,10]. If placentation is normal, placental blood flow can develop more than adequately to meet the homeostasis of placental transfer as well as the challenge of the stress of labor on the fetoplacental unit. If placentation is abnormal, however, placental blood flow cannot develop adequately, which may lead to the development of pregnancy-induced hypertension, intrauterine growth retardation, or intrauterine fetal death [8].

Transport of Oxygen to the Fetus

The supply of both nutritional substrates and oxygen from the mother to the fetus, and the excretion of carbon dioxide from the fetus to the mother, are closely dependent upon the uteroplacental and umbilical blood circulation [11]. The fetus must maintain an adequate uptake of oxygen in the presence of very low oxygen tension (Po_2 of 25 mm Hg) in the umbilical circulation, in contrast to the high oxygen tension in the maternal arterial blood (Po_2 of 95 mm Hg) [12]. This condition is illustrated in Figure 1.1.

In addition, umbilical uptake of oxygen and glucose constitutes approximately 55 and 28%, respectively, of the total uterine uptake. The discrepancy between uterine and umbilical uptake is due primarily to a high utilization rate for oxygen and glucose by the placenta. The data shown in Table 1.1 were obtained from chronic sheep preparations by simultaneous drawing of blood samples from the fetal abdominal aorta, the common umbilical vein, a uterine vein, and a maternal femoral artery [13].

Despite its low Po_2, fetal blood is capable of transporting large amounts of O_2 from the placenta to the fetal organs. Two adaptations make this possible. First, the hemoglobin of fetal red cells has a high affinity for oxygen. For example, at pH 7.4, human fetal blood is 80% saturated with oxygen at a Po_2 of 34 mm Hg. Second, the rate of perfusion of fetal organs is high in comparison to O_2 requirements. For example, the cerebral blood

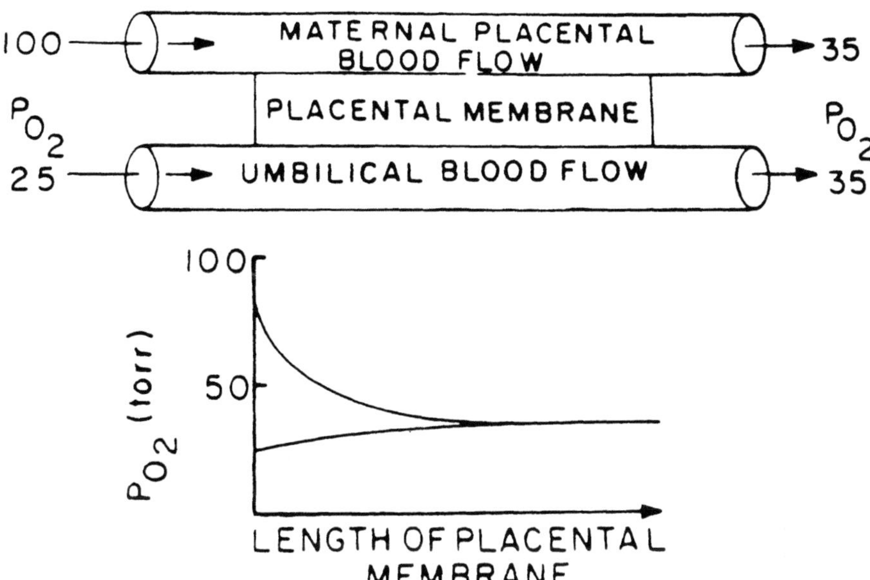

FIGURE 1.1. Concurrent model of transplacental oxygen diffusion. From Meschia G [12], used with permission from WB Saunders.

flow/O_2 consumption ratio is 2.4 times higher in the fetal lamb than in the adult [12].

Mechanisms of Decreased Oxygen Transport in Intrauterine Growth Retardation

Intrauterine fetal growth can be viewed as an incremental change in both the size of the fetus and the function of various organ systems throughout the entire period of pregnancy. These changes can be influenced by both

TABLE 1.1. Simultaneously measured uterine and umbilical oxygen and glucose uptake in ewes.*

	Fetal weight (kg)	Uterine uptake (m mol/min)	Umbilical uptake (m mol/min)	Uteroplacental utilization (m mol/min)
Oxygen	4.03 ± 0.29 (n = 9)	2.16 ± 0.15	1.18 ± 0.06 (55%)	0.98 ± 0.13 (45%)
Glucose	4.53 ± 0.38 (n = 12)	0.29 ± 0.02	0.082 ± 0.008 (28%)	0.206 ± 0.016 (72%)

*All values expressed as mean ± standard error.
Source: Meschia G, Battaglia FC, Hay WW, Sparks JW [13]. Used with permission from the Federation of the American Society for Experimental Biology.

genetic and environmental factors, which interact with cell proliferation, organ differentiation, and metabolic development in the process of fetal growth. These influences in the growth retarded fetus may be associated with decreased growth potential of the fetus or with the actual restriction of the supply of oxygen and nutrients from the mother to the fetus.

Possible causes of IUGR are many, but they can be divided into "intrinsic" and "extrinsic" factors as far as fetal growth and development are concerned. Examples of intrinsic causes of IUGR include chromosomal abnormalities, such as trisomy 18 and Turner's syndrome. The most common extrinsic factors, which affect primarily the placenta during the second half of pregnancy, are related to reduced uteroplacental blood flow, or so-called uteroplacental insufficiency. In experimental animal models, IUGR fetuses are produced by ligation of the uterine vessels [14,15], embolization of the placental vascular bed [16], or prolonged maternal hypoxia [17]. In all of these experiments, oxygen transport from the mother to the fetus is decreased. A similar situation can occur in human pregnancies. Hypertension, preeclampsia, severe anemia, cigarette smoking, and multifetal pregnancy are considered the major causes of IUGR. In a hypertensive milieu, the placental vessels begin to show intimal thickening, and consequently vascular thrombosis and placental infarcts become more common [18]. This reduction in the functional capacity of the placenta will obviously interfere with blood flow and decrease the supply of oxygen and nutrients to the fetus. "Vasospasm" in preeclampsia can greatly reduce uteroplacental blood flow. From 10 to 50% of hemoglobin sickle cell cases are associated with preterm infants, small-for-gestational-age (SGA) infants, or preterm growth-retarded infants [19,20]. The poor fetal outcome in hemoglobin sickle cell patients seems to be caused by a combination of poor fetal oxygenation, poor nutrition, and possibly, placental infarction. Cigarette smoking has been found to cause fetal hypoxia through two independent mechanisms: (1) an acute effect caused by nicotine activation of catecholamine release, resulting in vasoconstriction and a decrease in uteroplacental perfusion, and (2) a prolonged reduction of fetal oxygenation secondary to an increase in maternal carboxyhemoglobin level [21]. Many investigators agree that twinning is a prominent cause of both prematurity and IUGR. The incidence of SGA infants among twin births is reported to be approximately 20% [22,23], versus 4% in singleton pregnancy [24]. McKeown and Record [25] have suggested that in multifetal pregnancy, the normal supply line can adequately support a total fetal weight of close to 3,000 g; beyond that point there is retardation of growth. The more fetuses present, the earlier this limit is reached and growth retardation begins. With this mechanism of competition in the supply of oxygen and nutrients, one of the two fetuses may be growth retarded. This is particularly true when one fetus has an inadequate placental blood supply, as a result of velamentous insertion of the umbilical cord, connection to a smaller placental lobe located at the lower uterine segment, or twin transfusion syndrome.

Fetal Hypoxia and Intrauterine Fetal Adaptation

Fetal hypoxia refers to a decrease in the level of fetal oxygenation below a normal limit. Since fetal oxygenation is dependent on placental inter-villous space blood flow, any factor that interrupts the maternal utero-placental circulation will cause some degree of fetal hypoxia. Similarly, any long-standing decrease in maternal uteroplacental blood flow will in-hibit the supply of substrate to the fetus. Therefore, chronic reductions in uterine blood flow, as seen for instance in cases of maternal hyperten-sion, result not only in a persistently low Po_2 in the fetus, but also in reduced fetal glycogen stores [26]. The fetus adapts to this condition through the following mechanisms, either to conserve energy or to avoid a hypoxic-acidotic effect: (1) decrease or cessation of fetal growth, (2) decrease in fetal activity, (3) redistribution of cardiac output by diversion of blood flow to vital organs, such as brain, heart, and adrenal glands, and (4) increase in the number of circulatory red blood cells, resulting in polycythemia or hyperviscosity syndrome (60% of SGA vs. only 5% of appropriate for gestational age [AGA] infants have a central hematocrit value >65%) [27]. Table 1.2 demonstrates the step-by-step adaptations the fetus makes to conserve energy and lower metabolic requirements in an hypoxic environment.

The fetal response to acute maternal hypoxemia has been demonstrated by Block et al [28] using a chronic sheep preparation. Fetal growth re-tardation was induced following chronic embolization of the placental bed by microspheres. Acute hypoxemia was created in the maternal sheep by decreasing the maternal inspired oxygen content (10% O_2, 2% CO_2, 88% N_2). Fetal lambs with IUGR secondary to uteroplacental embolization undergo a decrease in umbilical blood flow and a redistribution of their combined ventricular cardiac output that favors the brain, heart, and ad-renal glands. As a consequence, the blood flow to other organs, such as the spleen, kidneys, and lungs, decreases (Fig. 1.2). If this blood flow redistribution is prolonged, it can lead to the brain-sparing phenomenon frequently seen in type II IUGR fetuses. Furthermore, fetal hypoxia can cause hyperperistalsis of the fetal intestines, decreased muscle tone in

TABLE 1.2. Demonstration of step-by-step adaptations fetus undergoes to conserve energy and lower metabolic requirements in hypoxic environment.

1. Cessation of growth
2. Decrease in fetal activity
3. Redistribution of blood supply to vital organs (brain, heart, adrenal glands)
4. Increase in number of circulating red blood cells
5. Development of anaerobic metabolism, metabolic acidosis
6. Death

Source: Lin CC. In Maeda K. et al (Eds): *Recent Advances in Perinatology 1986* [89]. Used with permission from Elsevier Science Publishers B.V.

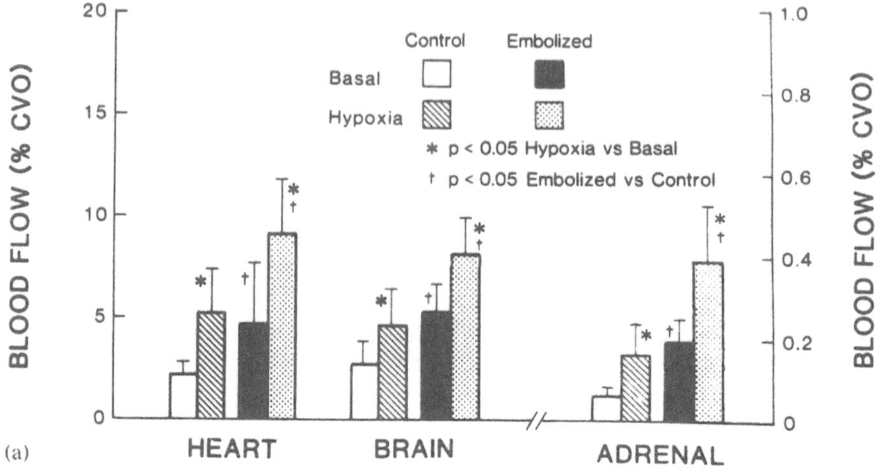

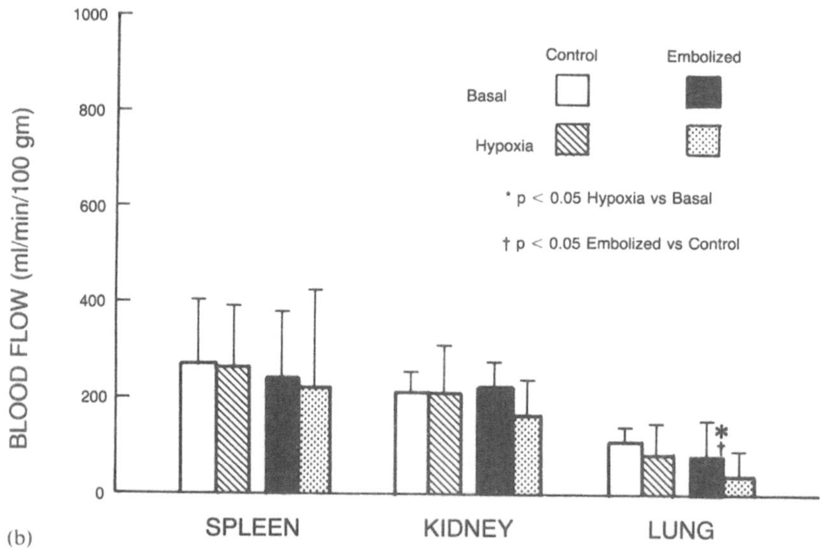

FIGURE 1.2. Comparison of specific organ blood flow expressed in mean percent (± standard deviation) of combined left and right ventricular output under normal conditions and during hypoxemia and embolization.(a) Organ blood flow to heart, brain, and adrenal glands,(b) Organ blood flow expressed in ml/min/100 gm (mean ± standard deviation) to the kidneys, spleen, and lungs. Adapted from Block BS, et al [28], with permission from CV Mosby.

the anal sphincter, and pathologic gasping-type respiratory movements, which may lead to fetal meconium passage and intrauterine meconium aspiration [29].

Antepartum Management of IUGR

CLINICAL DIAGNOSIS

Early diagnosis of IUGR begins with the clinician's ability to recognize the high-risk factors associated with the development of IUGR. These high-risk factors include historical factors and abnormal physical findings during early pregnancy. Galbraith et al [22] reported that two-thirds of IUGR infants come from the population with risk factors. Bakketeig and Hoffman [30] summarized the risk of recurrence of SGA births based on a large population in Norway, as shown in Table 1.3. The risk of SGA increases to 2.5 to 3 times greater than normal if there is one previous SGA birth; the risk of SGA becomes 5 times greater if there are two or more previous SGA births.

Maternal medical diseases that are commonly associated with IUGR are shown in Table 1.4. They include (1) diseases that affect nutritional intake and absorption, (2) diseases of the kidneys that involve protein-losing nephropathy, (3) diseases that cause maternal hypoxia or anemia, and (4) diseases associated with hypertension. The incidence of IUGR associated with these maternal medical complications ranges between 20 and 50%. Women with pregnancies that are complicated by medical disorders should be carefully monitored throughout the gestation both for fetal growth and for possible deterioration of the disease process. This same principle also applies to women with low prepregnancy weight and low weight gains during pregnancy.

TABLE 1.3. Risk of small-for-gestational age (SGA) infant in subsequent births.*

First birth	Second birth	Number of mothers	Subsequent SGA births	
			Percent	Relative risk
Not SGA	—	23,300	8.8	1.0
SGA	—	2,862	28.7	3.3
Not SGA	Not SGA	21,260	6.0	0.7
SGA	Not SGA	2,042	18.6	2.1
Not SGA	SGA	2,040	23.7	2.7
SGA	SGA	820	44.4	5.0

*Based on all 26,162 mothers having their first three singleton births in Norway during a 9-year period. 1967–1976.
Source: Bakketeig LS, Hoffman HJ [30]. Used with permission from Scandinavian Association of Obstetrics and Gynecology.

TABLE 1.4. Maternal diseases that cause risk of intrauterine growth retardation.

Diseases that affect nutritional intake and absorption: ulcerative colitis, pancreatitis, chronic hepatitis

Diseases that affect the kidneys (protein-losing nephropathy): preeclampsia, glomerulonephritis, lupus nephritis, nephrotic syndrome

Diseases that cause maternal hypoxia or anemia: cyanotic heart disease, sickle cell anemia

Diseases associated with hypertension: Chronic hypertension, preeclampsia, systemic lupus erythematosus

Source: Lowensohn RI, Devoe LD [31]. Used with permission from McGraw-Hill.

EVALUATION BY ULTRASONOGRAPHY

Ultrasound is the most reliable diagnostic tool for evaluating fetal size and growth rate as well as fetal well being. Table 1.5 lists the various functions of ultrasound in the IUGR pregnancy [32]. These functions include (1) assessment of gestational age, (2) assessment of fetal size and fetal growth rate, (3) diagnosis of anatomic abnormalities, (4) evaluation of fetal activities and functions as the signs of fetal well being, and (5) direct visualization for many diagnostic procedures.

For accurate diagnosis of IUGR, the precise determination of gestational

TABLE 1.5. Ultrasonic evaluation of intrauterine growth retardation (IUGR).

Assessment of gestational age
  Size of gestational sac
  Crown-rump length
  Femur length
  Biparietal diameter (BPD)
Assessment of fetal size and fetal growth rate in relation to prenatal diagnosis of IUGR
  Serial BPD growth pattern
  Growth-adjusted sonographic age
  Head/abdomen circumference ratios
  Total intrauterine volume
  Quantitative amniotic fluid volume
  Placental maturation grading
  Estimated fetal weight
Diagnosis of anatomic abnormalities of the fetus
Evaluation of fetal activities and fetal functions
  Fetal echocardiography
  Fetal breathing movements and other activities
  Fetal urine production rate
Assistance with other procedures
  Amniocentesis
  Percutaneous umbilical fetal blood sampling
  Intrauterine fetal transfusion

Source: Modified from Lin CC [32], with permission from Appleton-Century-Crofts.

age is a crucial factor. Measurements of the gestational sac and of the crown-rump length in early pregnancy, and measurements of the biparietal diameter of the fetal head and of femur length in the early second trimester, are quite reliable for the assessment of gestational age. Serial biparietal diameter [33] and serial femur length [34] measurements appear to be useful in monitoring the fetal growth rate, while fetal abdominal circumference [35], fetal head/abdominal circumference ratios [36], total intrauterine volume [37], quantitative amniotic fluid volume [38], and even placental maturation grading [39] have been used to diagnose IUGR pregnancies. Campbell and Dewhurst [33] suggested that different biparietal diameter growth patterns can be used to distinguish different types of IUGR, namely, the low growth-profile pattern of the type I versus the late-flattening pattern of the type II IUGR fetus. From a study of 1,457 serial biparietal diameter measurements on 643 pregnant women, Sabbagha [40] found that the incidence of IUGR in fetuses with large initial diameters (>75th percentile) was only 3.5%, compared with 10% in fetuses with average diameters (25th–75th percentile), and 52.1% in those with small initial diameters (<25th percentile). He suggested that all fetuses with biparietal diameters falling below the 25th percentile require intensive prenatal surveillance for the detection of IUGR.

For prenatal diagnosis of IUGR with known gestational age, estimation of fetal weight is, of course, the most practical step. The abdominal circumference measurement has proven to be a better predictor of fetal weight than the biparietal diameter. It becomes apparent that because the fetal mass is obtained mostly in the head and trunk, accurate measurement of fetal weight has to involve measurement of both parameters. Using the sophisticated ultrasound machines that are currently available, it is possible to estimate fetal weight with a greater accuracy than ever before. Table 1.6 summarizes the different formulas for the ultrasonic estimation of fetal weight developed by several investigators [41–44], with an error as low

TABLE 1.6. Accuracy of estimation of fetal weight (EFW) by ultrasound.

Author(s)	Formula for EFW	r	Mean error (%)
Warsof et al [41]	$\mathrm{Log}_{10}(BW) = 1.599 + 0.144(BPD) + 0.032(AC) - 0.111(BPD^2 \times AC)/1000$		11.0
Shepard et al [42]	$\mathrm{Log}_{10}(BW) = 1.7492 + 0.166(BPD) + 0.046(AC) - 2.646(AC \times BPD)/1000$		16.4
Ott [43]	Warsof's formula	0.92	8.2
Thurnau et al [44]	$EFW = (BPD \times AC \times 9.337) - 299$	0.96	7.0

BW, body weight
BPD, biparietal diameter; AC, abdominal circumference.
Source: Lin CC [32], used with permission from Appleton-Century-Crofts.

as 7 to 8%. A good correlation between ultrasonic estimation and actual birth weight has been demonstrated [43].

EVALUATION BY BIOPHYSICAL METHODS

Historically, serial hormonal monitoring by means of substances such as estriol and human placental lactogen were important for evaluating fetal well-being. Recently, evaluations of gross fetal movements, fetal breathing, and fetal heart rate have become increasingly important in assessing fetal health. Manning and co-workers [45] have proposed the use of a biophysical profile that evaluates fetal heart rate nonstress test (NST) results, fetal tone assessment, fetal breathing, gross fetal body movement, and quantitative amniotic fluid volume to predict fetal outcome. At the present time, most medical centers in the United States use the NST as a screening test, backed up by either the contraction stress test (CST) or the biophysical profile scoring system (Table 1.7).

In our own experience, IUGR pregnancies exhibit two times as many nonreactive NSTs and a three times higher incidence of positive CSTs

TABLE 1.7. Fetal biophysical profile scoring system.

Variable	Each variable scores 2	Each variable scores 0
Fetal breathing movements (FBM)	Presence of at least 30 of sustained FBM in 30 min of observation	Less than 30 of FBM in 30 min of observation
Fetal movements	3 or more gross body movements in 30 min of observation (simultaneous limb and trunk movements counted as single movement)	2 or fewer gross body movements in 30 min of observation
Fetal tone	At least 1 episode of motion of limb from position of flexion to extension and rapid return to flexion	Fetus in position of semi- or full-limb extension with no return to flexion with movement (absence of fetal movement counted as absent tone)
Fetal reactivity	Presence of 2 or more fetal heart rate accelerations of at least 15 bpm, lasting at least 15 and associated with fetal movement in 40 min of observation	No acceleration or <2 accelerations of fetal heart rate in 40 min of observation
Qualitative amniotic volume	Pocket of amniotic fluid measures at least 1 cm in 2 perpendicular planes	Largest pocket of amniotic fluid measures <1 cm in 2 perpendicular planes
Maximal score	10	—
Minimal score	—	0

Source: Manning FA, Platt LD, Sipas L [45]. Used with permission from CV Mosby.

TABLE 1.8. Predictive value of nonstress test-contraction stress test results on perinatal morbidity in intrauterine growth retardation.

Nonstress test	Contraction stress test	Perinatal morbidity*
Nonreactive, 20 (39%)	Positive, 13 (65%)	12/13 (92%)†
	Negative, 7 (35%)	2/7 (29%)
Reactive, 32 (61%)	Positive, 5 (16%)	2/5 (40%)
	Negative, 27 (84%)	5/27 (18%)

*Combination of intrapartum fetal distress, low 1-min Apgar score, neonatal complication, and perinatal death.
†Statistical significance $P < 0.001$ between the nonreactive positive group and the combination of the other three groups.
Source: Lin CC. et al [47]. Used with permission from CV Mosby.

than, the incidence seen in the general high-risk population [46,47]. The majority of perinatal deaths in IUGR pregnancy (75%) are associated with a positive nonreactive fetal heart rate pattern, while the remainder occur in the group with a negative nonreactive pattern. Therefore, an adverse fetal prognosis is most accurately predicted by the joint occurrence of a nonreactive NST and a positive CST. Table 1.8 shows the predictive value of the two tests jointly on perinatal morbidity in IUGR.

Recently, umbilical velocity waveforms (Fig. 1-3a) and calculated systolic/diastolic ratios appear to offer promise for the clinical assessment of placental function [48–51]. In IUGR pregnancies, the systolic/diastolic ratio (S/D ratio) markedly increases after 24 weeks of gestation compared with that of normal pregnancies. The mean S/D ratio in AGA pregnancies between 31 and 39 weeks of gestation is 2.5, while for SGA infants under the 10th percentile for gestational age the mean S/D ratio is 3.8 [49]. An abnormal test (S/D $\geq$ 3.0) has proved to be a good predictor of IUGR. The S/D ratio is a reflection of placental resistance to umbilical circulation; its value may be inversely related to umbilical blood flow. Simultaneous evaluation of arterial blood flow velocity waveforms of both umbilical artery and uterine artery may indicate compromised fetoplacental function in IUGR pregnancies, long before the abnormality can be detected by NST-CST evaluation. Furthermore, the most extreme waveform abnormality is the absence of end-diastolic velocity (Fig. 1.3b). This waveform is associated with a higher incidence of IUGR, intrapartum fetal distress, low Apgar scores, congenital anomalies, and perinatal death [50,52]. Absent end-diastolic velocity represents a unique method for diagnosis of a severe fetal condition that may not be identified by present surveillance methods such as the NST, CST, or biophysical profile.

Percutaneous umbilical blood sampling is a newly available technique for studying fetal blood gas abnormalities and other pathologic conditions, such as hemoglobinopathy, thrombocytopenia, Rh-isoimmunization, T-

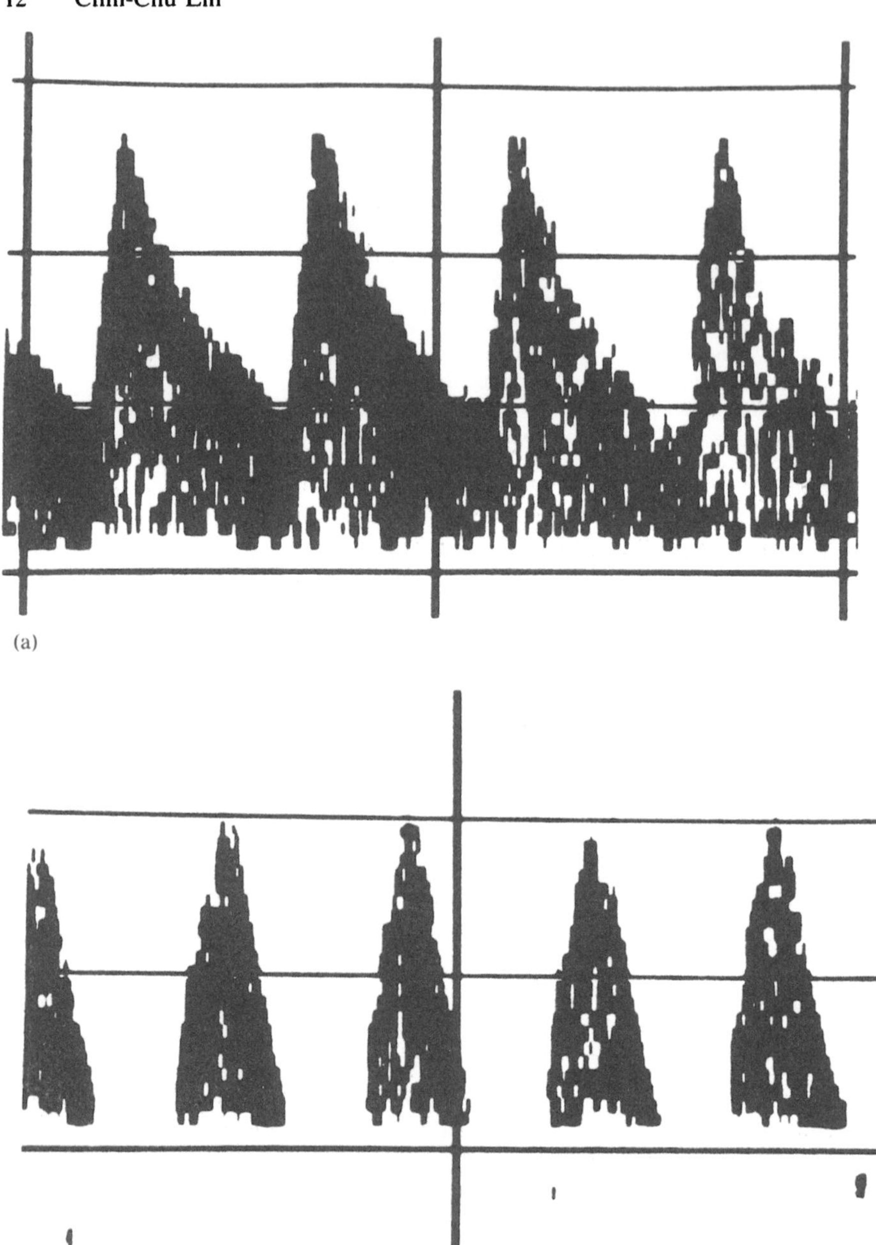

FIGURE 1.3. Umbilical artery blood flow velocity waveforms recorded by Doppler ultrasound (a). Normal waveform (b). Abnormal waveforms from a growth-retarded fetus at 29 weeks of gestation, showing absence of end-diastolic flow. From Erskine RLA, and Ritche JWK [50], used with permission from Blackwell Scientific Publications.

cell deficiency, and hemophilia [53–55]. It is also useful for rapid prenatal diagnosis of various genetic defects [55]. This technique involves the ultrasonographically guided insertion of a needle into the umbilical vein with direct control by the obstetrician performing the procedure. Direct access to fetal blood during the second and third trimester of pregnancy opens new fields of prenatal diagnosis and intrauterine fetal treatment. In view of the high frequency of fetal hypoxia, genetic defects, and hematologic abnormalities associated with the IUGR fetus, this technique offers tremendous promise for antepartum management of IUGR.

TIMING OF DELIVERY

One crucial question frequently asked is when to deliver an IUGR baby. During the past decade, efforts to provide antepartum therapy to improve fetal growth and prolong pregnancy have met with only partial success. Bed rest, reducing the hazard of maternal risk factors (such as the limiting of smoking and alcohol intake, and the medical treatment of hypertension, severe anemia, systemic lupus erythematosis, etc.) and nutritional supplementation (oral and parenteral) are common approaches that are thought to be beneficial. No specific pharmacologic agent has been proven to be absolutely useful in the antenatal treatment of IUGR. On the other hand, with high-quality nursery care, the prognosis for type II IUGR infants delivered between 33 and 35 weeks of gestation appears to be equal to that for those born at term. This is due in part to the fact that various conditions that complicate pregnancy and that may cause IUGR are frequently associated with accelerated fetal lung maturity [56]. These conditions include hypertension; preeclampsia; renal disease; narcotic addiction; classes D, F, and R diabetes; and certain types of placental dysfunction. If such a condition is present, L/S ratio measurements may be initiated as early as the 32nd week of gestation. An IUGR pregnancy may be terminated as soon as fetal lung maturity is documented. Furthermore, the presence of amniotic fluid phosphatidyl glycerol gives added confirmation of fetal lung maturity and is not affected by the presence of blood in the amniotic fluid specimen [57]. Phosphatidyl glycerol in the amniotic fluid has been reported to be the single most useful criterion for predicting an IUGR birth, especially in combination with a small biparietal diameter for the gestational age [58].

The following management guidelines address the question of when to deliver the IUGR fetus [32].

1. If weekly NST-CST results are consistently reactive and negative, or if weekly NST is reactive and a biophysical profile score is normal, the patient should be tested weekly and the pregnancy allowed to continue to 38 weeks. Then, upon documentation of fetal maturity, the patient should be delivered because of the possible risk of placental

deterioration and the increased rate of perinatal mortality beyond that point.

2. If the fetus repeatedly exhibits a nonreactive NST, but a negative CST is obtained, or if the fetus exhibits a nonreactive NST and a biophysical profile score of 4 to 6, the decision regarding delivery depends upon the fetal maturity study. If the fetus is mature, the patient should undergo delivery immediately. If the fetus is not mature, the patient should be hospitalized and the nonstress test repeated daily or every other day. In our experience, the test results of most patients will improve after bed rest and hydration in the hospital.

3. The most serious fetal outcome is encountered in the IUGR patient associated with a positive nonreactive NST-CST pattern, or a biophysical profile score of 4 or less. In addition, diminished amniotic fluid volume and cessation of fetal growth for more than 3 weeks may be observed. The combination of these conditions almost always indicates impending intrauterine fetal death. Immediate delivery regardless of fetal maturity provides a better fetal prognosis than delayed delivery.

4. In case of a progressive deterioration of the maternal condition in a preterm gestation, immediate termination of the pregnancy regardless of fetal maturity should be the management of choice.

Intrapartum Fetal Hypoxia and Acidosis

Labor represents a serious challenge to the IUGR fetus. When the uterus is quiescent the IUGR fetus may exhibit reduced activity but rarely will show acute deterioration. When labor contractions increase in frequency, however, blood flow within the intervillous space decreases, with a concomitant decrease in maternal-fetal transfer of oxygen [59]. At some point the fetus will become hypoxic, which will lead to myocardial depression and the appearance of late decelerations on fetal heart rate tracings [60]. This phenomenon was evident in our study of the oxytocin challenge test in IUGR pregnancies; IUGR fetuses exhibited a threefold increase in the incidence of a positive test compared with the incidence in the general high-risk population [47].

With progressive fetal hypoxia, a state of metabolic acidosis gradually develops through the accumulation of lactate, a product of the anaerobic metabolism of glucose. This condition is followed by an enlarged base deficit and then by a drop in the fetal blood pH [61,62]. This hypoxic-acidotic insult may lead to intrauterine meconium aspiration or fetal death.

IUGR fetuses demonstrate an increased risk of abnormal heart rate patterns and acidosis during labor and delivery, with an increased frequency and severity of late decelerations [61,63,64], decreased baseline heart rate variability [65], and tachycardia [66]. Variable decelerations are also frequently associated with IUGR [67,68]. The high incidence of oligohydramnios in IUGR pregnancy is probably responsible for this "cord compression" pattern. Moreover, fetal bradycardia, occasionally noted during the process of an antepartum nonstress test, is reported to be associated with oligohydramnios [69]. For these reasons, every IUGR fetus should undergo intensive continuous fetal monitoring throughout the course of labor and delivery.

We have studied cord blood lactate, pH, and blood gas values in 37 IUGR and 108 AGA infants at the time of delivery to compare differences in response to the stress of labor [70]. In the absence of intrapartum fetal heart rate decelerations, IUGR fetuses showed no difference in umbilical arterial lactate, pH, and blood gas values compared with AGA infants. When intrapartum fetal heart rate decelerations were present, IUGR fetuses demonstrated a significantly higher lactate level than that of AGA fetuses (Fig. 1.4).

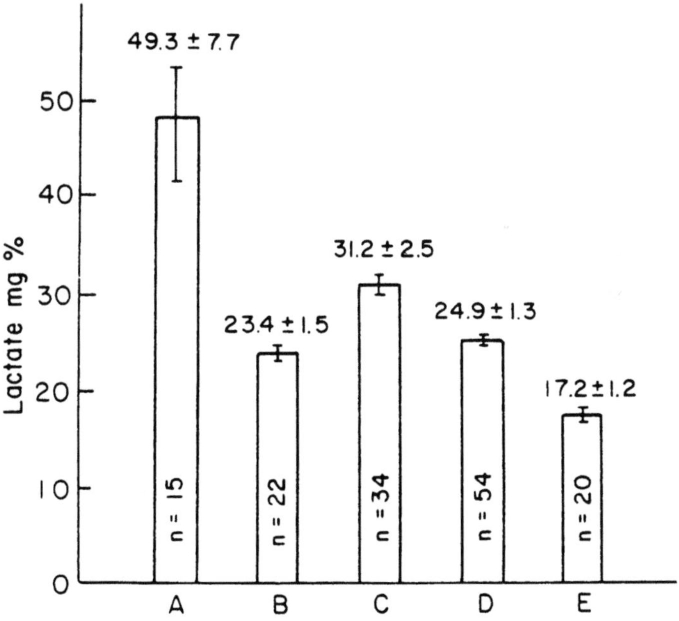

FIGURE 1.4. Comparision of umbilical artery lactate levels in various groups (mean ± SEM). Group A: IUGR with intrapartum fetal heart rate deceleration. Group B: IUGR without intrapartum deceleration. Group C: AGA with intrapartum fetal heart rate deceleration. Group D: AGA without intrapartum deceleration. Group E: AGA delivered by elective cesarean section to serve as a group of prelabor controls. From Lin CC, et al [70], used with permission from CV Mosby.

TABLE 1.9. Comparison of umbilical arterial lactate, pH, and base deficit values according to mode of delivery and fetal heart rate (FHR) pattern in 37 infants with intrauterine growth retardation.

| | | | Fetal blood values (mean ± SD)* | | |
Mode of delivery	Pattern of FHR deceleration	Number of patients	Lactate (mg/100 ml)	pH	Base Excess (MEQ/Li)
Cesarean section, early labor	Late, moderate to severe	5	21.1 ± 9.5	7.26 ± 0.04	−5.0 ± 3.6
Cesarean section, late labor	Late, moderate to severe	5	71.5 ± 42.4	7.07 ± 0.22	−14.6±6.9
Vaginal	Late, mild	2	36.8 ± 19.3	7.24 ± 0.06	−7.0 ± 4.2
Vaginal	Variable, severe	1	48.9	7.20	−10.0
Vaginal	Variable, mild to moderate	2	34.0 ± 9.1	7.28 ± 0.06	−7.3 ± 4.0
Vaginal	None	22	23.4 ± 6.7	7.28 ± 0.01	−4.8 ± 2.0

*Note significant differences ($P < 0.05$) in lactate, pH, and base deficit values between early and late cesarean section groups. On the other hand, values in early group are very similar to values in nondeceleration group.
Source: Lin CC, et al [70]. Used with permission from CV Mosby.

Table 1.9 shows evidence that early surgical intervention in IUGR cases associated with late decelerations can prevent the development of severe fetal metabolic acidosis. Infants who were delivered by cesarean section shortly after the appearance of late decelerations had blood gas and lactate values comparable to those seen in the control group (without intrapartum fetal heart rate decelerations). However, infants who exhibited late decelerations for a longer period of time had severe metabolic acidosis and extremely high levels of lactate, even though they too were delivered by cesarean section. Two conclusions may be drawn from this study: (1) IUGR fetuses tolerate the stress of labor less efficiently than AGA fetuses, and (2) early surgical intervention is the key to ensuring a better outcome for the IUGR fetus associated with intrapartum fetal distress [70].

Fetuses with IUGR are more susceptible to intrauterine asphyxia. Acute intrauterine partial and total asphyxia has been induced using animal models in order to study the pathogenesis of perinatal brain damage secondary to intrauterine asphyxia. Total asphyxia in the human fetus can be produced only by complete cord occlusion (true knot of the umbilical cord) or complete separation of the placenta (total abruptio placentae); fetal life ceases very shortly after either of these events. The majority of human fetuses associated with intrauterine asphyxia resemble the experimental model of partial asphyxia developed in the rhesus monkey [71,72]. Figure 1.5 illustrates the sequence of events in a proposed pathogenesis

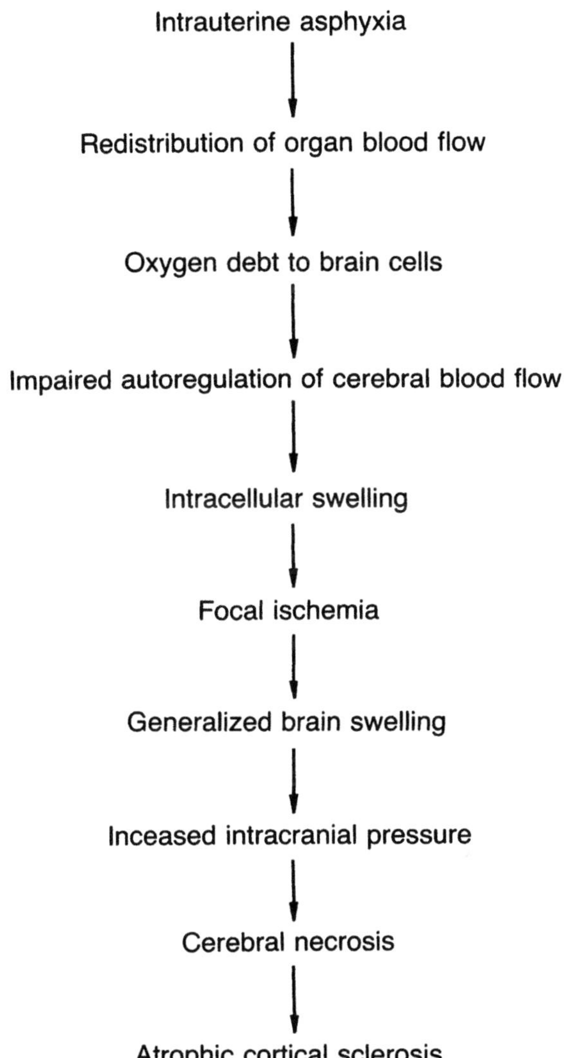

FIGURE 1.5. Illustration of the sequence of events in a proposed pathogenesis of perinatal asphyxia causing permanent brain damage. From Brann AW, and Dykes FD [73], used with permission from WB Saunders.

for perinatal asphyxia causing permanent brain damage in the full-term infant [73].

Currently it is thought that hypoxia-induced brain damage may be related to the lactic acid concentration within fetal brain cells [74]. Cardiac glycogen storage in the IUGR fetus is also markedly decreased from normal. In animal experiments, the ability of the fetus to withstand asphyxia is directly related to the preasphyxial glycogen concentration in the cardiac ventricles [75]. When the cardiac carbohydrate stores are partially depleted by fasting or previous hypoxia, survival time is decreased proportionately. This observation in animals may explain the higher susceptibility to intrauterine asphyxia seen in the human IUGR fetus.

Niswander [76] attempted to relate intrauterine asphyxia and cerebral palsy by a review of the literature, and drew the following conclusions:

1. Fetal asphyxia is a major cause of cerebral palsy, but the asphyxia usually does not occur during the intrapartum period.
2. Case-control studies that have attempted to relate observed cerebral palsy with specific preexisting disease states have contributed little to our understanding of this neurologic abnormality.
3. Most intrapartum asphyxia does not lead to cerebral palsy.
4. Electronic fetal monitoring and fetal blood sampling are poor predictors of brain injury, although they may be the best tools currently available to the obstetrician.
5. Chronic or repeated acute episodes of fetal asphyxia during the prenatal course may cause fetal brain injury that remains undetected until after birth.
6. More randomized clinical trials are needed to determine the usefulness of fetal heart rate monitoring in detecting fetal brain injury.

Nevertheless, careful intrapartum fetal surveillance and prompt active intervention remain important steps to improve the outcome of the IUGR fetus. Clinically, 30% of IUGR fetuses exhibit intrapartum heart rate decelerations, and 20% of them show evidence of either fetal acidosis or low Apgar scores, an incidence three times higher than that for AGA fetuses [77]. It should be noted that perinatal asphyxia is the common denominator for many of the neonatal complications of IUGR that require intensive pediatric management, including postasphyxial seizures, hypoglycemia, hypocalcemia, hyperviscosity syndrome, meconium aspiration, pulmonary hemorrhage, respiratory distress, and hypothermia [78]. Therefore, the prevention of perinatal asphyxia and its sequelae is the most important task in conducting delivery room resuscitation of the IUGR infant.

Perinatal Resuscitation

Perinatal asphyxia is the most serious of all clinical complications in infants with IUGR. As previously described, the IUGR fetus has sustained either acute or chronic stress as a result of the compromised placental transfer of gases and nutritional substrates. Therefore, the IUGR fetus has a greater tendency to develop fetal distress, followed by fetal hypoxia/acidosis. The clinical manifestations of perinatal asphyxia include the appearance of meconium in the amniotic fluid, abnormal fetal heart rate pattern, the presence of fetal acidosis (fetal blood pH < 7.20), and depressed Apgar score at delivery.

Resuscitation of the newborn infant should be considered as requiring the combined efforts of the obstetrician and the pediatrician during labor, delivery, and the immediate neonatal period. The transition from intra-uterine to extrauterine life involves considerable risk to the newborn infant, a risk compounded by profound respiratory and circulatory changes. In addition, the delivery process itself usually leads to progressive increase in fetal hypoxia, hypercapnea, and acidosis. Although only 10% of infants fail to make the transition smoothly in the general obstetric population, the incidence of depressed neonates in IUGR pregnancy is in the range of 20 to 40% [70,79,80].

The resuscitation process should begin with intrauterine resuscitation by the obstetrician. Even after a cesarean section is decided upon in the case of a severe fetal heart rate pattern or evidence of fetal acidosis, several temporary measures including maternal oxygen inhalation, change of maternal position, and the use of uterine tocolytic agents can be instituted immediately to minimize the hypoxic insult to the fetus [81,82]. The obstetrician can also reduce neonatal depression by avoiding the use of analgesic or sedative medications during the late active phase of labor and by seeking alternatives to a difficult mid forceps delivery, shoulder dystocia, or difficult breech extraction. In the presence of thick meconium-stained amniotic fluid, the obstetrician can initiate pharyngeal suctioning with a De Lee catheter just before the delivery of the shoulder, to prevent meconium aspiration [83,84].

The pediatrician should be notified ahead of time by the obstetrician regarding the high-risk condition of the patient as well as the status of the fetus during the process of labor. A pediatrician should be present for the delivery of every IUGR infant. Efforts should be made to prepare for immediate resuscitation for those infants who exhibit any of the signs of fetal distress—meconium-stained fluid, abnormal intrapartum heart rate pattern, or fetal acidosis. The single most important concept in resuscitation of the depressed newborn is the clearing of the airway and inflation of the lungs with oxygen. There are, however, several degrees of the resuscitation, depending upon the condition of the infant, advancing from (1) simple suctioning of the nose, pharynx, and stomach to (2) the use of an oxygen mask, (3) bagging with intermittent positive pressure breathing (IPPB), and (4) endotracheal intubation and cardiac resuscitation. In the severely depressed neonate, the restoration of an umbilical line for chemical resuscitation should also be done as soon as possible [85,86]. In addition, special efforts should be made for resuscitation of the neonate suspected of meconium aspiration at the time of delivery [87,88].

REFERENCES

1. Greiss FC Jr, Anderson SG: Uterine blood flow during early ovine pregnancy. *Am J Obstet Gynecol* **106**:30–38, 1970.
2. Makowski EL, Meschia G, Droegemueller W, et al: Distribution of uterine blood flow in the pregnant sheep. *Am J Obstet Gynecol* **101**:409–412, 1968.
3. Greiss FC Jr, Anderson SG, Still JG: Uterine pressure-flow relationships during early gestation. *Am J Obstet Gynecol* **126**:799–808, 1976.
4. Rosenfeld CR, et al: Circulatory changes in the reproductive tissues of ewes during pregnancy. *Gynecol Invest* **5**:252–268, 1974.
5. Harbert GM Jr, Croft BY, and Spisso KR: Effects of biorhythms on blood flow distribution in the pregnant uterus (Macaca mulatta). *Am J Ostet Gynecol* **135**:828–842, 1979.
6. Metcalfe J, et al: Estimation of uterine blood flow in normal human pregnancy at term. *J Clin Invest* **34**:1632, 1955.
7. Assali NS, Rauramo L, Peltonen T: Measurement of uterine blood flow and uterine metabolism. *Am J Obstet Gynecol* **79**:86–98, 1960.
8. Greiss FC Jr: Uterine blood flow in pregnancy: An overview. In Moawad AH, Lindheimer MD (Eds): *Uterine and Placental Blood Flow*. New York: Masson, 1982, pp. 19–26.
9. Greiss FC Jr: Pressure-flow relationship in the gravid uterine vascular bed. *Am J Obstet Gynecol* **96**:41–47, 1966.
10. Martin CB Jr: Uterine blood flow and uterine contractions in monkeys. In Goldsmith EI, Moor-Janowski J (Eds): *Medical Primatology. Part I*. Basel: S. Karger, 1972, p. 298.
11. Evans MI, Lin C-C: Normal fetal growth. In Lin C-C, Evans MI (Eds): *Intrauterine Growth Retardation: Pathophysiology and Clinical Management*. New York: McGraw-Hill, 1984, pp. 17–53.
12. Meschia G: Placental respiratory gas exchange and fetal oxygenation. In Creasy RK, Resnik R (Eds): *Maternal-Fetal Medicine: Principles and Practice*. Philadelphia: WB Saunders, 1984, pp. 274–285.
13. Meschia G, Battaglia FC, Hay WW, Sparks JW: Utilization of substrates by the ovine placenta in vivo. *Fed Proc* **39**:245–249, 1980.
14. Wigglesworth JS: Experimental growth retardation in the fetal rat. *J Pathol Bacteriol* **88**:1–13, 1964.
15. Hill DE, Myers RE, Holt AB: Fetal growth retardation produced by experimental placental insufficiency in the Rhesus monkey. *Biol Neonat* **19**:68–82, 1971.
16. Creasy RK, Barret CT, De Swiet M, et al: Experimental intrauterine growth retardation in the sheep. *Am J Obstet Gynecol* **112**:566–573, 1972.
17. Van Geijn HP, Kaylor WM, Nicola KR, et al: Induction of severe intrauterine growth retardation in the Sprague-Dawley rat. *Am J Obstet Gynecol* **137**:43–47, 1980.
18. Gruenwald P: Chronic fetal distress and placental insufficiency. *Biol Neonat* **5**:215–265, 1963.
19. Fiakpui EZ, Moran EM: Pregnancy in the sickle hemoglobinopathies. *J Reprod Med* **11**:28–34, 1973.
20. Pritchard JA, Scott DE, Whalley PJ, et al: The effects of maternal sickle cell hemoglobinopathies and sickle cell trait on reproductive performance. *Am J Obstet Gynecol* **117**:662–670, 1973.

21. Quigley ME, Sheehan KL, Wilkes MM, et al: Effects of maternal smoking on circulating catecholamine levels and fetal heart rates. *Am J Obstet Gynecol* **133**:685–690, 1979.
22. Galbraith RS, Karchman EJ, Piercy WN, et al: The clinical prediction of intrauterine growth retardation. *Am J Obstet Gynecol* **133**:281–286, 1979.
23. Miller HC, Merritt TA: Twin pregnancies. In Miller HC, Merritt TA (Eds): *Fetal Growth in Humans*. Chicago Year Book, 1979, pp. 127–141.
24. Tejani N, Mann LI: Diagnosis and management of the small-for-gestational-age fetus. *Clin Obstet Gynecol* **20**:943–955, 1977.
25. McKeown T, Record RG: Observations on fetal growth in multiple pregnancy in man. *J Endocrinol* **8**:386–401, 1952.
26. Nitzan M, Groffman H: Hepatic gluconeogenesis and lipogenesis in experimental intrauterine growth retardation in the rat. *Am J Obstet Gynecol* **109**:623–627, 1971.
27. Humbert JR, Abelson H, Hathaway WE, et al: Polycythemia in small for gestational age infants. *J Pediatr* **75**:812–819, 1969.
28. Block BS, Llanos AJ, Creasy RK: Responses of the growth-retarded fetus to acute hypoxemia. *Am J Obstet Gynecol* **148**:879–885, 1984.
29. Brown BL, Gleicher N: Intrauterine meconium aspiration. *Obstet Gynecol* **57**:26–29, 1981.
30. Bakketeig LS, Hoffman HJ: The tendency to repeat gestational age and birth weight in successive births, related to perinatal survival. *Acta Obstet Gynecol Scand* **62**:385–392, 1983.
31. Lowensohn RI, Devoe LD: Maternal disease. In Lin C-C, Evans MI (Eds): *Intrauterine Growth Retardation: Pathophysiology and Clinical Management*. New York: McGraw-Hill, 1984, pp. 145–150.
32. Lin C-C: Intrauterine growth retardation. In Wynn RM (Ed): *Obstetrics and Gynecology Annual: 1985*. Norwalk, Conn.: Appleton-Century-Crofts, 1985, pp. 127–221.
33. Campbell S, Dewhurst CJ: Diagnosis of the small-for-dates fetus by serial ultrasonic cephalometry. *Lancet* Nov 6: 1002–1006, 1971.
34. O'Brien GD, Queenan JT, Campbell S: Assessment of gestational age in the second trimester by real-time ultrasound measurement of the femur length. *Am J Obstet Gynecol* **139**:540–545, 1981.
35. Campbell S, Wilkins D: Ultrasonic measurement of fetal abdominal circumference in estimation of fetal weight. *Br J Obstet Gynecol* **82**:689–697, 1975.
36. Campbell S, Thomas A: Ultrasound measurement of the fetal head to abdomen circumference ratio in the assessment of growth retardation. *Br J Obstet Gynecol* **84**:165–174, 1977.
37. Gohari P, Berkowitz RL, Hobbins JC: Prediction of intrauterine growth retardation by determination of total intrauterine volume. *Am J Obstet Gynecol* **127**:255–260, 1977.
38. Manning FA, Hill LM, Platt LD: Quantitative amniotic fluid volume determination by ultrasound: Antepartum detection of intrauterine growth retardation. *Am J Obstet Gynecol* **139**:254–258, 1981.
39. Quinlan RW, Cruz AC, Buhi WC, et al: Changes in placental ultrasonic appearance. II. Pathologic significance of Grade III placental changes. *Am J Obstet Gynecol* **144**:471–473, 1982.
40. Sabbagha RE: Intrauterine growth retardation: Antenatal diagnosis by ultrasound. *Obstet Gynecol* **52**:252–256, 1978.

41. Warsof SL, Gohari P, Berkowitz RL, et al: The estimation of fetal weight by computer assisted analysis. *Am J Obstet Gynecol* **128**:881–892, 1977.

42. Shepard MJ, Richards VA, Berkowitz RL, et al: An evaluation of two equations for predicting fetal weight by ultrasound. *Am J Obstet Gynecol* **142**:47–54, 1982.

43. Ott WJ: Clinical application of fetal weight determination by real-time ultrasound. *Obstet Gynecol* **57**:758–762, 1981.

44. Thurnau GR, Tamura RK, Sabbagha R, et al: A simple estimated fetal weight equation based on real-time ultrasound measurements of fetuses less than thirty-four weeks gestation. *Am J Obstet Gynecol* **145**:557–561, 1983.

45. Manning FA, Platt LD, Sipas L: Antepartum fetal evaluation: Development of a fetal biophysical profile. *Am J Obstet Gynecol* **136**:787–795, 1980.

46. Lin C-C, Moawad AH, River P, et al: An OCT reactivity classification to predict the fetal outcome. *Obstet Gynecol* **56**:17–23, 1980.

47. Lin C-C, Devoe LD, River P, et al: Oxytocin challenge test and intrauterine growth retardation. *Am J Obstet Gynecol* **140**:282–288, 1981.

48. Schulman H, Fleischer A, Stern W, et al: Umbilical velocity wave ratios in human pregnancy. *Am J Obstet Gynecol* **148**:985–990, 1984.

49. Fleischer A, Schulman H, Farmakides G, et al: Umbilical artery velocity waveforms and intrauterine growth retardation. *Am J Obstet Gynecol* **151**:502–505, 1985.

50. Erskine RLA, Ritchie JWK: Umbilical artery blood flow characteristics in normal and growth-retarded fetuses. *Br J Obstet Gynaecol* **92**:605–610, 1985.

51. Trudinger BJ, Giles WB, Cook CM: Flow velocity waveforms in the maternal uteroplacental and fetal umbilical placental circulations. *Am J Obstet Gynecol* **152**:155–163, 1985.

52. Rochelson B, Schulman H, Farmakides G, et al: The significance of absent end-diastolic velocity in umbilical artery velocity waveforms. *Am J Obstet Gynecol* **156**:1213–1218, 1987.

53. Ludomirski A, Nemirof R, Johnson A, et al: Percutaneous umbilical blood sampling. *J Reprod Med* **32**:276–279, 1987.

54. Daffos F, Capella-Pavlovsky M, Forestier F: Fetal blood sampling during pregnancy with use of a needle guided by ultrasound: A study of 606 consecutive cases. *Am J Obstet Gynecol* **153**:655–660, 1985.

55. Appleman Z, Golbus MS: Uses of fetal tissue sampling. *Contemp Obstet/Gynecol*, special issue, *Update on Surgery*, pp. 42–49, June, 1987.

56. Gluck L, Kulovich MV: Lecithin/sphingomyelin ratios in amniotic fluid in normal and abnormal pregnancy. *Am J Obstet Gynecol* **115**:539–546, 1973.

57. Strassner HT, Golde SH, Mosley GH, et al: Effect of blood in the detection of phosphatidyl glycerol. *Am J Obstet Gynecol* **138**:697–702, 1980.

58. Gross TL, Sokol RJ, Wilson MV, et al: Using ultrasound and amniotic fluid determinations to diagnose intrauterine growth retardation before birth: A clinical model. *Am J Obstet Gynecol* **143**:265–269, 1982.

59. Greiss FC, Anderson SG: Uterine blood flow during labor. *Clin Obstet Gynecol* **11**:96–109, 1968.

60. Hon EH: The classification of fetal heart rate. *Obstet Gynecol* **22**:137–146, 1963.

61. Low JA, Pancham SR, Worthington D, et al: The acid-base and biochemical characteristics of intrapartum fetal asphyxia. *Am J Obstet Gynecol* **121**:446–451, 1975.

62. Shelley HJ: The metabolic response of the fetus to hypoxia. *Br J Obstet Gynaecol* **76**:1–15, 1969.
63. Lin C-C, Shulman H, Saldana LR: Deceleration/contraction ratios as an index of fetal health during labor. *Obstet Gynecol* **51**:666–670, 1978.
64. Kubli FW, Hon EH, Kahzin AF, et al: Observation on heart rate pH in the human fetus during labor. *Am J Obstet Gynecol* **104**:1190–1206, 1969.
65. Paul RH, Suidan AK, Yeh SY, et al: Clinical fetal monitoring. VII: The evaluation and significance of intrapartum baseline fetal heart rate variability. *Am J Obstet Gynecol* **123**:206–210, 1975.
66. Tejani N, Mann LI, Bhakthavthsalan A, et al: Correlation of fetal heart rate-uterine contraction pattern with fetal scalp blood pH. *Obstet Gynecol* **46**:392–396, 1975.
67. Low JA, Boston RW, Pancham SR: Fetal asphyxia during the intrapartum period in intrauterine growth-retarded infants. *Am J Obstet Gynecol* **113**:351–357, 1972.
68. Odendual H: Fetal heart rate patterns in patients with intrauterine growth retardation. *Obstet Gynecol* **48**:187–190, 1976.
69. Druzin MI, Gratocos J, Kegan KA, et al: Antepartum fetal heart rate testing. VII. The significance of fetal bradycardia. *Am J Obstet Gynecol* **139**:194–198, 1981.
70. Lin C-C, Moawad AH, Rosenow PJ, et al: Acid-base characteristics of fetuses with intrauterine growth retardation during labor and delivery. *Am J Obstet Gynecol* **137**:553–559, 1980.
71. Brann AW, Myers RE: Central nervous system findings in the newborn monkey following severe *in utero* partial asphyxia. *Neurology* **25**:327–338, 1975.
72. Brann AW, Myers RE: Brain swelling and hemorrhagic cortical necrosis following perinatal asphyxia in monkeys. *J Neuropathol Exp Neurol* **28**:1781, 1978.
73. Brann AW, Dykes FD: The effects of intrauterine asphyxia on the full-term neonate. *Clin Perinatol* **4**:149–161, 1977.
74. Myers RE: Experimental models of perinatal brain damage: Relevance to human pathology. In Gluck L (Ed): *Intrauterine Asphyxia and the Developing Fetal Brain*. Chicago: Year Book, 1977.
75. Dawes DA, Mott JC, Shelley HJ: The importance of cardiac glycogen for the maintenance of life in fetal lamb and newborn animals during anoxia. *J Physiol* **146**:516, 1959.
76. Niswander KR: Asphyxia in the fetus and cerebral palsy. In Pitkin RM, Zlatnik FJ (Eds): *The Year Book of Obstetrics and Gynecology*. Chicago: Year Book, 1983, pp. 107–125.
77. Lin C-C, Evans MI: Intrapartum management of IUGR. In Lin C-C, Evans MI (Eds): *Intrauterine Growth Retardation: Pathophysiology and Clinical Management*. New York: McGraw-Hill, 1984, pp. 315–351.
78. Woo D, Gartner LM: The small for gestational age neonate. In Lin C-C, Evan MI (Eds): *Intrauterine Growth Retardation: Pathophysiology and Clinical Management*. New York: McGraw-Hill, 1984, pp. 353–370.
79. Cetrulo CL, Freeman RK: Bioelectric evaluation in intrauterine growth retardation. *Clin Obstet Gynecol* **20**:979–989, 1977.
80. Perry CP, Harris RE, DeLemos RA, et al: Intrauterine growth retarded infants: Correlation of gestational age with maternal factors, mode of delivery, and perinatal survival. *Obstet Gynecol* **48**:182–186, 1976.

81. Lipshitz J: Use of B$_2$-sympathomimetic drug as temporizing measure in the treatment of acute fetal distress. *Am J Obstet Gynecol* **129**:31–36, 1977.
82. Esteban-Altirriba J: Treatment of fetal distress. In *Proceedings of Symposium on Tocolytic Therapy,* Society of Perinatal Obstetricians, New Orleans, 1980, pp. 69–75.
83. Carson BS, Losey RW, Bowes WA, et al: Combined obstetric and pediatric approach to prevent meconium aspiration syndrome. *Am J Obstet Gynecol* **126**:712–715, 1976.
84. Starks GC: Correlation of meconium-stained amniotic fluid, early intrapartum fetal pH, and Apgar scores as predictors of perinatal outcome. *Obstet Gynecol* **56**:604–609, 1980.
85. Clark RB, Arrington RW: Resuscitation of the newborn. In Wynn R (Ed): *Obstetrics and Gynecology Annual.* Norwalk, Conn.: Appleton-Century-Crofts, 1982, pp. 151–173.
86. Levinson G, Shnider SM: Resuscitation of the newborn. In Shnider SM, Levinson G (Eds): *Anesthesia for Obstetrics.* Baltimore: Williams & Wilkins, 1979, pp. 385–401.
87. Gregory GA, Gooding CA, Phibbs RH, et al: Meconium aspiration in infants: A prospective study. *J Pediatr* **85**:848, 1974.
88. Vidyasagar D, Andreou A: Management of meconium aspiration syndrome. In Aladjem S, Brown AK (Eds): *Perinatal Intensive Care.* St. Louis: CV Mosby, 1977, pp. 413–425.
89. Lin CC: Pathophysiology of perinatal hypoxia in fetuses with intrauterine growth retardation. In Maeda K, Okuyama K, Takeda Y (Eds): *Recent Advances in Perinatology,* Excepta Medica, International Congress Series 712. Amsterdam: Elsevier Science Publishers BV, 1986, pp. 55–62.

2
Fetal Asphyxia: Its Impact on the Neonate:
An Approach to Understanding and Anticipating Complications

Susan E. Denson

Asphyxia is a term used frequently in the neonatal period to denote an untoward event, usually occurring during labor or delivery, that results in a compromised neonate. The term comes from a Greek word meaning "a stopping of the pulse," and although not defined in most neonatal textbooks, it is defined in *Dorland's Illustrated Medical Dictionary* as "a condition due to lack of oxygen in respired air, resulting in impending or actual cessation of apparent life" [1]. In utero, the organ of gas exchange that provides "respired air" is the placenta. Asphyxia, then, occurs in situations in which placental function is impaired with subsequent interference with adequate gas exchange. If the situation is not reversed, the fetus will die. When intervention does occur, a surviving neonate often has sequelae as a result of the insult and changes wrought by the fetal compensatory mechanisms.

Normal Placental Function

To understand the impact of asphyxia on the neonate, it is important to understand normal placental function and the chain of events when disruption in this function occurs. The placenta, on which the fetus is dependent, grows rapidly to meet the increasing needs of the developing fetus. The placenta is of dual origin, with two separate circulations. Optimal function is dependent upon normal function of both the maternal and fetal circulations. As there is no direct connection between these two separate circulations, the placenta must in some way be permeable to a variety of substrates. These include nutrients such as glucose, fatty acids, and amino acids and gases such as oxygen and carbon dioxide. Permeation occurs via a variety of active and passive mechanisms, depending upon the substrate to be transported.

Since asphyxia results from interference with gas exchange between the mother and the fetus, the mechanisms whereby it occurs are important. Oxygen transfer across the placenta is by passive diffusion, a fact established for at least 50 years, as noted by Barcroft [2]. Passive diffusion is dependent upon a gradient for the substrate between the two systems. Thus in placental transfer of oxygen, there is a gradient between the maternal or donor stream and the fetal or recipient stream. The exact mechanism is still debated, but as reviewed by Battaglia and Meschia [3], the best explanation is that the placenta corresponds most closely to a nonideal concurrent exchange model. As has been substantiated in a number of animal models, this results in the fetal venous PO_2 being less than the maternal venous PO_2. The fetal PO_2 is then found to be in the range of 30 torr. Since this would be insufficient in postnatal life, the fetus needs to have compensatory mechanisms to tolerate it.

The fetus compensates in three ways:

1. The oxygen-carrying capacity is increased by an increase in hemoglobin. The mean hemoglobin on day 1 of life is 17 g/100 ml compared with the adult female value of 13 g/100 ml [4]. This process is under the control of erythropoietin, produced endogenously by the fetus [5].
2. The second compensatory mechanism is the oxygen dissociation curve for fetal blood, which lies to the left of the curve for maternal blood. This results in the fetal blood's comparatively greater affinity for oxygen at any oxygen tension. This is enhanced by the Bohr effect, which operates as the maternal blood gains CO_2 and acidic products from the fetus. Increased acidity results in a decreased affinity of maternal hemoglobin for oxygen. On the fetal side, the release of CO_2 and acidic products to the mother decreases the acidity of the blood and increases its affinity for oxygen [6].
3. The third compensatory mechanism is related to blood flow patterns in the fetus. Blood that is highly saturated leaves the placenta and passes via the umbilical vein to the inferior vena cava. The fetal circulation is designed so that this blood with the highest saturation attainable in utero crosses the foramen ovale and goes to the left atrium, then to the left ventricle and out the ascending aorta. This highly saturated blood perfuses the myocardium via the coronary arteries and the brain via the carotid arteries before it is mixed with desaturated blood at the level of the patent ductus arteriosus and distributed to the remainder of the fetus [7].

When pregnancy, labor, and delivery progress normally, these compensatory mechanisms allow the fetus to do well; however, when there are alterations, the effects on the fetus may be profound.

Fetal Compensatory Mechanisms During Compromise

The fetus also has compensatory mechanisms to rely upon when hypoxia occurs or when there is impairment in umbilical blood flow. As the human fetus is inaccessible for study, information regarding the effects of asphyxia has come from the laboratory animal. When placental function is impaired and the fetus is not oxygenated, it becomes acidemic. Cardiovascular responses to hypoxemia and acidemia have been studied in fetal lambs using chronically instrumented pregnant sheep who have been made hypoxemic. These studies have shown that during acute hypoxia, fetal heart rate decreases and fetal arterial blood pressure increases. Although cardiac output decreases, this decrease is not significant unless the fetus becomes acidemic. In these studies, umbilical blood flow was maintained, and in fact the percent distribution of cardiac output to the placenta increased from 41 to 48% in the hypoxic group and from 41 to 57% in the group that became acidemic. The blood flow to the brain, heart, and adrenals increased two to three times over control levels in the hypoxic animals at the expense of pulmonary, renal, splenic, gastrointestinal, and carcass blood flow [8]. This compensatory mechanism is successful in the ovine fetus over a wide range of oxygen concentrations, because the product of arterial oxygen content times blood flow to the fetal heart and central nervous system tends to remain constant. The same is presumed to be true in the human fetus as well; however, there is a major difference in that the human fetus, with a brain six to seven times heavier than the brain of the fetal lamb of equal body weight, may develop problems sooner than the lamb. The arterial oxygen content at which the oxygen supply to the human fetal brain becomes inadequate is not known, but it may be considerably higher than the content in the sheep [9]. The clinical correlate to the situation in these animal studies is some form of chronic or acute placental insufficiency. This can occur in many situations including placental infarct, placental edema, or placental abruption.

The other form of compromise to which the fetus may be subjected is umbilical cord compression, occurring through prolapse of the umbilical cord or cord entanglement. Unlike the model of hypoxia in which umbilical venous oxygen content decreases while umbilical blood flow is maintained, cord compression maintains umbilical venous oxygen content while reducing umbilical blood flow. Studies in the ovine fetus have demonstrated that the fetus compensates by increasing oxygen extraction, from a mean of 33% in the control state to 43.8, 52, and 67.7% when umbilical blood flow is reduced by 25, 50, and 75% [10]. Although this mechanism does compensate initially, there comes a point when acidemia develops, the myocardium becomes depressed, cardiac output falls, and no amount of increase in oxygen extraction can compensate for the decline in oxygen delivery.

Effects of Asphyxia on Organ Systems

If the fetus has been subjected to hypoxia or cord compression in utero, at delivery the infant may require resuscitation. During stabilization such an infant requires close attention to many different organ systems, because virtually no organ is spared. Specific problems can be anticipated and managed expectantly.

CARDIOVASCULAR COMPLICATIONS

In looking first at the effects of asphyxia on the cardiovascular system, the differences between adult and fetal myocardium are important. The fetal myocardium has less ability to generate tension, and the extent and velocity of cardiac muscle shortening at any given load are less as well. The reasons are found in differences in microscopic structure and in innervation. Fetal cardiac cells are smaller, and the proportion of the myocardium that is noncontractile is significantly greater. In the adult, 60% of the cardiac muscle is contractile, compared with only 30% [11] in the fetus.

In innervation of the fetal cardiac muscle there is further compromise. As asphyxia depresses the contractility of the heart, one compensatory mechanism is stimulation of the sympathetic nervous system, which in turn stimulates contractility. Histochemical studies on fetal myocardium have demonstrated less sympathetic innervation than in the adult myocardium. Thus the fetal myocardium will be less responsive to sympathetic neurotransmitters, and this compensatory mechanism is not as effective [12].

In addition to these anatomic differences, the glycogen stores that develop during fetal life are rapidly depleted during stress. Depletion results in decreased energy available for the heart, which further contributes to decreased contractility.

As a result of these abnormalities, myocardial dysfunction occurs. Myocardial dysfunction or transient myocardial ischemia following an asphyxial insult can present in several ways: as cardiogenic shock, in which left-sided heart failure results in systemic hypotension [13], as right-sided heart failure secondary to tricuspid valve insufficiency [14], or as heart failure due to global myocardial ischemia [15]. The diagnosis is suggested by the clinical findings of one or more of the following: respiratory distress with cardiomegaly, hepatomegaly, hypotension, or electrocardiogram changes including ST depression or T-wave changes suggestive of myocardial ischemia. A cardiac murmur is also frequently found secondary to tricuspid insufficiency. The diagnosis is substantiated by demonstration of ventricular dysfunction by echocardiography, and low cardiac output can be documented by pulsed Doppler echocardiography [16].

The initial treatment of heart failure as a consequence of asphyxia is supportive. First, the asphyxial insult must be corrected, and thus ventilation is critical to improve oxygenation and acid-base balance. The systemic blood pressure must be maintained to maintain myocardial blood flow. Maintenance of systolic blood pressure may be difficult if the hypotension is due to pump failure, and often an inotropic agent is needed in addition to ventilation. Dopamine is a good choice, as it has a positive inotropic effect on the myocardium through the release of norepinephrine and through stimulation of beta-1 receptors. It has been used with good clinical response [17], and serial echocardiograms obtained after its use have shown improvements in arterial blood pressure, cardiac output, and stroke volume [16].

The outcome of myocardial dysfunction is variable. In some cases it will be severe enough to cause death; in the majority, however, complete recovery to normal cardiac function occurs.

PULMONARY COMPLICATIONS

The effects of asphyxia on the respiratory system are both direct and indirect. An indirect effect is depression of the central nervous system resulting in apnea, which then perpetuates the problems of asphyxia. The direct effect is dependent on gestational age. In the premature infant, asphyxia may increase the risk of respiratory distress syndrome (RDS), which results from surfactant deficiency. Surfactant is the surface-active phospholipid lining in the alveolus, which is important in promoting and maintaining expansion of the lung [18]. It is produced by type II alveolar cells and is involved in a dynamic process of production, secretion, uptake, and reutilization [19].

Although asphyxia has been implicated clinically in the pathogenesis of RDS, the actual mechanism is not clear. Some propose that asphyxia reduces the pulmonary blood flow and thus the nutritional blood supply to the metabolically active type II alveolar cells, resulting in cell death [20] and therefore surfactant deficiency. Others believe there is impairment of surfactant production as a result of alterations in enzyme activity during the asphyxial insult, since the animal model shows recovery after termination of the stress insult [21].

RDS is suspected in a premature infant presenting with respiratory distress (grunting, flaring, and retracting), decreased breath sounds on auscultation, and increasing oxygen requirements and carbon dioxide retention documented by arterial blood gas determinations. The diagnosis is made on the basis of these clinical findings, a chest x-ray that shows decreased lung volume (reticulogranular pattern with air bronchograms), and the clinical course. Management at the current time includes temperature support, nutritional support, and respiratory support including oxygen and mechanical ventilation. Of more potential benefit in the future is the use of specific therapy, or instillation of surfactant into the lung of the premature infant [22]. Various surfactant preparations are currently being studied in clinical trials. Which preparation is optimal must be determined through controlled studies, and the agent must then be standardized and made commercially available.

The full-term, asphyxiated infant is at risk for two forms of respiratory disease: meconium aspiration syndrome and persistent pulmonary hypertension.

Up to 20% of infants will pass meconium in utero, usually as a result of the increase in gastrointestinal motility and relaxation of the anal sphincter that occur during stress. If the meconium is in the oropharynx or nasopharynx after delivery, it can be passively moved into the lungs with the first breath or with manual bagging [23]. The respiratory distress seen in meconium aspiration syndrome has a twofold origin: (1) The bile salts in meconium result in a severe chemical pneumonitis. (2) Particles of meconium and/or secretions can lodge in the airway and cause complete obstruction and atelectasis or can act as a ball valve, allowing air to enter but not to leave, resulting in hyperinflation and its complication of pulmonary air leak.

The diagnosis of meconium aspiration syndrome is suspected in a meconium-stained infant with respiratory distress; it is confirmed by chest x-ray findings consistent with aspiration pneumonia. Treatment is supportive and includes ventilation and pulmonary physical therapy to remove secretions. The mortality rate can be as high as 40% [24].

In view of this, the current approach is prevention. The use of intrapartum pharyngeal suction by the obstetrician to remove meconium before it enters the airway has been demonstrated to significantly reduce the incidence and severity of the meconium aspiration syndrome [25] and should be utilized whenever meconium staining of the amniotic fluid is noted. However, more recent reports still show a substantial incidence of meconium aspiration syndrome in spite of this [24].

The second problem encountered in the asphyxiated term infant is the development of persistent pulmonary hypertension or persistent fetal circulation. This occurs when pulmonary vascular resistance, which is normally high in utero, fails to decrease after birth. This elevated pulmonary vascular resistance can cause right-to-left shunting at the levels of the foramen ovale and the patent ductus arteriosus. The end result is severe hypoxemia as blood bypasses the pulmonary circulation. Pulmonary vascular resistance is inversely related to the size of the pulmonary vascular bed. Certain disorders physically decrease the size of the pulmonary vascular bed, such as disorders with pulmonary hypoplasia. The occurrence of high pulmonary vascular resistance in the asphyxiated neonate, however, is related to vasoconstriction. Lack of oxygen is recognized as an important mediator in vasoconstriction, because hypoxia results in elevation of the pulmonary vascular resistance [26], but the pulmonary vascular bed is under the control of other regulatory mechanisms that are not yet clearly understood [27].

The diagnosis of persistent pulmonary hypertension is suggested by severe hypoxemia in a term or near-term infant. The chest x-ray can be clear in primary persistent pulmonary hypertension or can show evidence of parenchymal disease such as respiratory distress syndrome, meconium aspiration syndrome, or pneumonia if the persistent pulmonary hypertension is secondary to hypoxia in these disorders. The diagnosis can be supported in infants with a right-to-left ductal shunt by demonstrating a difference in arterial saturation in simultaneously obtained arterial blood gases from a preductal vessel (usually the right radial artery) and a post-ductal vessel (usually the umbilical artery or posterior tibial artery). The diagnosis can also be supported by M-mode echocardiography, which shows elevated systolic time intervals. This finding can even precede the clinical diagnosis [28].

Treatment is directed toward supportive care, including ventilation to sustain oxygenation and acid-base status. In the absence of knowledge of the mechanisms underlying elevation of pulmonary vascular resistance, no specific therapy is available.

When supportive care and attempts at pharmacologic management fail, some infants with persistent pulmonary hypertension or meconium aspiration syndrome might be candidates for extracorporeal membrane oxygenators. Survival with this therapy has been reported as 100% in one series of infants with persistent pulmonary hypertension and 84% in another with meconium aspiration; however, it remains experimental at this time [29].

RENAL COMPLICATIONS

The renal complications of asphyxia are primarily ischemic, as might be expected from the redistribution of cardiac output to the brain and myocardium at the expense of the visceral organs including the kidney. Vascular resistance within the kidney, which is high in the fetus, is further increased in the presence of hypoxia and acidosis. This results in the shunting of blood away from the renal cortex and a decrease in the glomerular filtration rate, as shown in the neonatal lamb [30]. The lesion that occurs depends upon the severity of the insult. Direct renal cellular damage occurs first in the tubules, with more severe insults affecting the glomerulus or the entire nephron.

The vulnerability of the renal tubules to insult has been recently demonstrated by measuring urinary beta-2 microglobulin (β_2-M) excretion in a group of infants with meconium-stained amniotic fluid and showing it to be increased. Beta-2M is a protein that in the mature kidney is 99.9% reabsorbed at the level of the proximal tubule. Its presence in the urine is a reflection of renal tubular dysfunction thought to be on the basis of hypoxia [31].

The clinical diagnosis of renal impairment is suggested by findings at the bedside. The decrease in glomerular filtration rate results in oliguria, or in anuria in the more severe case. Disruption of the renal tubule results in impaired electrolyte resorption, hematuria, the presence of red blood cell casts, and proteinuria [32].

During the oliguric phase, the infant is at risk for fluid overload and the metabolic complications of hyponatremia and hyperkalemia. Fluid and electrolyte management is directed toward prevention by providing fluid intake calculated to cover insensible loss plus urine output. Electrolyte levels are followed closely and electrolytes are added as needed.

After a variable period the infant is likely to enter the diuretic phase, at which time the major complications are dehydration and further electrolyte imbalance. Management involves fluid replacement of insensible loss plus urine output and close attention to electrolyte, especially sodium, imbalance [33].

The outcome of renal failure in the neonate is variable. Many will improve within 7 to 10 days [34], while others go on to chronic renal failure. The technology now exists to support these infants with peritoneal dialysis, which may be considered in selected cases.

GASTROINTESTINAL COMPLICATIONS

The gastrointestinal complications of asphyxia are both acute and long-term. The acute complications are related to gestational age and include delay in motility in some full-term infants and the more significant complication of necrotizing enterocolitis in the premature infant.

Necrotizing enterocolitis occurs in 2,000 to 4,000 neonates per year and has a mortality rate of 20 to 40%. It is probably multifactorial in origin. The risk factors include mucosal injury, of which ischemia from asphyxia is one cause; bacterial or viral colonization; and enteral feedings as substrate [35]. The diagnosis is suggested by the nonspecific signs of lethargy, abdominal distention, guaiac-positive stools, and emesis. It is confirmed by an abdominal x-ray showing ileus and pneumatosis intestinalis. Medical management includes supportive measures such as bowel rest, decompression, and intravenous hydration and specific measures such as antibiotics for infection. If the disease progresses, perforation may occur, and surgical intervention will be necessary. The long-term outcome varies. Short-bowel syndrome develops in some infants as a result of bowel resection [36], while strictures develop in some who initially respond to medical management [37]. Overall, outcome is good in most survivors.

A less well-recognized long-term complication of asphyxia is gastroesophageal reflux in infants with neurologic impairment [38]. This must be considered in the infant who has persistent vomiting or in the impaired infant who requires a gastrostomy for nutritional support. The diagnosis is made by radiographic procedures (upper GI series), nuclear medicine procedures (milk scan), or continuous esophageal pH probe monitoring. Treatment may be medical with the use of pharmacologic therapy or surgical with fundoplication.

METABOLIC COMPLICATIONS

Metabolic complications of asphyxia include aberrations in glucose and calcium regulation.

In utero, the fetus receives from the mother a continuous supply of glucose along with fatty acids and amino acids to supply its energy needs. In addition to being used for growth and metabolic needs, some of this energy substrate is stored in the form of glycogen, which will support the infant during labor, delivery, and the first few hours of life. The amount of glycogen is substantial: Studies have shown that glycogen accounts for up to 10% of liver weight at term [39]. After birth, as glucose levels fall, glycogen synthesis becomes depressed and glycogen breakdown accelerates to restore the blood glucose level to normal [40]. Asphyxia in utero, however, may result in depletion of the glycogen store prior to birth. The asphyxiated newborn is then at risk for hypoglycemia.

Symptomatic hypoglycemia should be prevented by prospective management. Intravenous glucose should be started as soon as possible after delivery and the blood glucose level monitored, since some infants will become hypoglycemic in spite of this IV therapy.

Hypocalcemia may occur within 24 hours in asphyxiated infants. Although the mechanisms are poorly understood, it has been proposed that increased phosphorus loads resulting from hypoxia depress the parathyroid gland and lower its responsiveness to the fall in calcium levels [41]. Calcium levels should thus be monitored in the at-risk infant and treated if in the hypocalcemic range.

Hematologic Complications

The most common hematologic complication of asphyxia is bleeding, and the cause is thought to be disseminated intravascular coagulation in most cases. It is hypothesized that the asphyxial event triggers tissue factor release from damaged endothelial cells or leukocytes, thus stimulating the extrinsic pathway and resulting in consumptive coagulopathy. In severe asphyxial insult, decreased factor synthesis by the liver may also play a role [42].

The diagnosis is suspected if an asphyxiated infant is bleeding; it is substantiated by coagulation studies. Results of such studies show a prolonged prothrombin time and partial thromboplastin time, elevated level of fibrin split products, and decreased fibrinogen levels. The platelet count may be only slightly decreased. Treatment is directed toward supportive care, including correction of hypoxemia, acidosis, and hypotension, and specific therapy, including blood component therapy to correct the coagulation abnormalities.

Neurologic Abnormalities

The last complication to be considered is the effect of asphyxia on the central nervous system. This complication has the most impact in postnatal life, since it may result in a variety of problems including mental retardation and motor deficits that impair function. It is also the complication about which we have the least predictive ability. Fetal compensatory attempts to maintain blood flow will sometimes fail, and the infant will be left with hypoxic-ischemic lesions. The types of lesions differ between full-term and premature infants; the reason is felt to be differences in the blood supply to the brain at different gestational ages. Damage in the premature infant is primarily to the germinal matrix in the periventricular region, while damage in the full-term infant occurs primarily in the cerebral cortex [43].

The biochemical mechanisms involved in cell injury and death are complex. They include energy failure within the cell, the effect of elevated concentrations of tissue lactate, extracellular potassium accumulation, intracellular calcium accumulation, and generation of free radicals in the tissue [44]. The exact pathophysiology of brain injury is currently in dispute. In the past, on the basis of animal autopsy studies, cerebral edema resulting in neuronal necrosis was felt to play a prominent role in this injury. Current information, however, suggests that it is more complicated. Selective neuronal injury would suggest other factors as important, including circulatory factors (as previously mentioned), regional metabolic factors, and the role of excitotoxic amino acids in mediating this injury [43].

Although the cellular cause of the injury is still in debate, the clinical findings are not. The findings are dependent upon the severity of the insult and include alterations in state such as hyperexcitability, lethargy, or coma and the presence of seizures [45].

Management includes supportive care to improve oxygenation and maintain blood pressure, and avoidance of hypoglycemia. Specific therapies are controversial. They include phenobarbital to reduce energy demands in the brain and control of cerebral edema with osmotic diuretics. Seizure control is often difficult and requires aggressive intervention.

At the current time, the outcome is variable and good predictors are still lacking. New technology, including magnetic resonance imaging and positron emission tomography, may improve our ability to predict.

Summary

Asphyxia in utero resulting from disruption in placental function is initially compensated. When the compensatory mechanisms fail, however, the fetus is subjected to hypoxic-ischemic insult. This insult leaves no organ system untouched, and the effects on each system depend on the severity of the insult and the vulnerability of the system. Such multisystem damage has effects that are both short-term, such as pulmonary and metabolic abnormalities, and long-term, such as renal failure and neurologic sequelae. The scope of these problems emphasizes the importance of early intervention to minimize the sequelae.

REFERENCES

1. *Dorland's Illustrated Medical Dictionary.* 25th ed. Philadelphia: WB Saunders, 1974.
2. Barcroft Sir Joseph: Researches on Pre-Natal Life. Oxford, England: Blackwell Scientific Publications, 1946.
3. Transplacental diffusion: Basic concepts. Battaglia FC, Meschia G: *An Introduction to Fetal Physiology.* Orlando, Fla.: Academic Press, 1986, pp. 28–48.
4. Dallman PR: Blood and blood-forming tissues. In Rudolph AM, Hoffman JIE, (Eds): *Pediatrics.* 18th ed. Norwalk, Conn.: Appleton & Lange, 1987, pp. 1009–1091.
5. McIntosh S: Erythropoietin excretion in the premature infant. *J Pediatr* 86:202–215, 1975.
6. Pearson JF: Maternal and fetal acid-base balance. In Beard RW, Nathanielsz PW, (Eds): *Fetal Physiology and Medicine.* Philadelphia: WB Saunders, 1976, pp. 492–509.
7. Walsh SZ, Lind J: The fetal circulation and its alteration at birth. In Stave Uwe (Ed): *Perinatal Physiology.* New York: Plenum, 1978, pp. 129–180.
8. Cohn HE, Sacks EJ, Heymann MA, et al: Cardiovascular responses to hypoxemia and acidemia in fetal lambs. *Am J Obstet Gynecol* 120:817–824, 1974.
9. Sheldon RE, Peeters LLH, Jones MD, et al: Redistribution of cardiac output and oxygen delivery in the hypoxemic fetal lamb. *Am J Obstet Gynecol* 135:1071–1078, 1979.
10. Itskovitz J, LaGamma EF, Rudolph AM: The effect of reducing umbilical blood flow on fetal oxygenation. *Am J Obstet Gynecol* 145:813–818, 1983.
11. Friedman WF: The intrinsic physiologic properties of the developing heart. *Prog Cardiovasc Dis* 15:87–111, 1972.
12. Friedman WF, Pool PE, Jacobowitz D, et al: Sympathetic innervation of the developing rabbit heart: Biochemical and histochemical comparisons of fetal, neonatal and adult myocardium. *Circ Res* 23:25–32, 1968.
13. Cabal LA, Devaskar U, Siassi B, et al: Cardiogenic shock associated with perinatal asphyxia in preterm infants. *J Pediatr* 96:705–710, 1980.
14. Bucciarelli RH, Nelson RM, Egan EA, et al: Transient tricuspid insufficiency of the newborn: A form of myocardial dysfunction in stressed newborns. *Pediatrics* 59:330–337, 1977.
15. Rowe RD, Hoffman T: Transient myocardial ischemia of the newborn infant: A form of severe cardiorespiratory distress in full-term infants. *J Pediatr* 81:243–250, 1972.
16. Walther FJ, Siassi B, Ramadan NA, et al: Cardiac output in newborn infants with transient myocardial dysfunction. *J Pediatr* 107:781–785, 1985.
17. DiSessa TG, Leitner M, Ti CC, et al: The cardiovascular effects of dopamine in the severely asphyxiated neonate. *J Pediatr* 99:772–776, 1981.
18. Stark AR, Frantz ID: Respiratory distress syndrome. *Ped Clin N Am* 33:533–544, 1986.
19. Corbet A: Surfactant Replacement: What surfactant does. *Neonatol Gr Rounds* 3:1,2,6, 1986.
20. Stahlman M: Acute respiratory disorders in the newborn. In Avery GB, (Ed): *Neonatology: Pathophysiology and Management of the Newborn.* Philadelphia: JB Lippincott, 1987, pp. 418–445.

21. Brumley GW, Crenshaw C: Fetal lamb lung phosphatidylcholine: Response to asphyxia and recovery. *J Pediatr* **97**:631–637, 1980.
22. Jobe A: Respiratory distress syndrome—new therapeutic approaches to a complex pathophysiology. *Adv Pediatr* **30**:93–130, 1983.
23. Bacsik RD: Meconium aspiration syndrome. *Ped Clin N Am* **24**:463–479, 1977.
24. Davis RD, Philips SB, Harris BA, et al: Fatal meconium aspiration syndrome occurring despite airway management considered appropriate. *Am J Obstet Gynecol* **151**:731–736, 1985.
25. Carson BS, Losey RW, Bowes WA, et al: Combined obstetric and pediatric approach to prevent meconium aspiration syndrome. *Am J Obstet Gynecol* **126**:712–715, 1976.
26. Lock JE, Hamilton F, Olley PM, et al: The effect of alveolar hypoxia on pulmonary vascular responsiveness in the conscious newborn lamb. *Can J Physiol Pharmacol* **58**:153–159, 1980.
27. Drummond WH: Persistent pulmonary hypertension of the neonate: Persistent fetal circulation. *Adv Pediatr* **30**:61–91, 1984.
28. Valdes-Cruz LM, Dudell GG, Ferrara A: Utility of M-mode echocardiography for early identification of infants with persistent pulmonary hypertension of the newborn. *Pediatrics* **68**:515–525, 1981.
29. Barlett RH, Gazzaniga AB, Toomasian J, et al: Extracorporeal membrane oxygenation (ECMO) in neonatal respiratory failure: 100 cases. *Ann Surg* **204**:236–245, 1986.
30. Weisman DN: Influence of hypoxemia associated with normal and decreased arterial blood pH on renal hemodynamics in the neonate lamb. *Pediatr Res* **14**:627, 1980.
31. Cole JW, Portman RJ, Lim Y, et al: Urinary β_2-microglobulin in full-term newborns: Evidence for proximal tubular dysfunction with meconium stained amniotic fluid. *Pediatrics* **76**:958–964, 1985.
32. Brem AS: Neonatal hematuria and proteinuria. *Clin Perinatol* **8**:321–332, 1981.
33. Oh W: Renal functions and clinical disorders in the neonate. *Clin Perinatol* **8**:215–223, 1981.
34. Drago JR, Rohner TJ, Sanford EJ, et al: Perinatal asphyxia and renal failure in neonatal patients. *J Urol* **118**:80–82, 1977.
35. Kliegman RM, Fanaroff AA: Necrotizing enterocolitis. *N Engl J Med* **310**:1093–1103, 1984.
36. Kosloske AM, Martin LW: Surgical complications of neonatal necrotizing enterocolitis. *Arch Surg* **107**:223–228, 1973.
37. Schwartz MZ, Richardson CJ, Hayden CK, et al: Intestinal stenosis following successful medical management of necrotizing enterocolitis. *J Pediatr Surg* **15**:890–899, 1980.
38. Mollitt DL, Golladay ES, Seibert JJ: Symptomatic gastroesophageal reflux following gastrostomy in neurologically impaired patients. *Pediatrics* **75**:1124–1131, 1985.
39. Shelley HJ: Glycogen reserves and their changes at birth and in asphyxia. *Br Med Bull* **17**:137–143, 1961.
40. Ballard FJ: Carbohydrate metabolism and the regulation of blood glucose. In Stave Uwe (Ed): *Perinatal Physiology*. New York: Plenum, 1978, pp. 365–381.
41. Tsang RC, Chen I, Hayes W, et al: Neonatal hypocalcemia in infants with birth asphyxia. *J Pediatr* **84**:428–433, 1974.

42. Hathaway WE, Bonnar J: Bleeding disorders in the newborn infant. In *Perinatal Coagulation*. New York: Grune and Stratton, 1978, pp. 115–169.
43. Volpe JJ: Hypoxic-ischemic encephalopathy—neuropathology and pathogenesis. In *Neurology of the Newborn*. 2nd ed. Philadelphia: WB Saunders, 1987, pp. 209–235.
44. Volpe JJ: Hypoxic-ischemic encephalopathy—biochemical and physiological aspects. In *Neurology of the Newborn*. 2nd ed. Philadelphia: WB Saunders, 1987, pp. 160–195.
45. Volpe JJ: Hypoxic-ischemic encephalopathy: Clinical aspects. In *Neurology of the Newborn*. 2nd ed. Philadelphia: WB Saunders, 1987, pp. 236–279.

3
The Role of External Tocodynamometry in Perinatal Medicine

MICHAEL KATZ AND ROGER B. NEWMAN

Aubry and Pennington [1], more than a decade ago, suggested that only through identification of the high-risk pregnancy could the limited health care manpower, dollars, and technology be appropriately applied to maximize perinatal outcome. Since preterm birth remains the greatest contributor to perinatal morbidity and mortality, these authors further suggested the use of external tocodynamometry to better identify patients at risk for preterm labor and birth. They concluded that "external tocodynamometry appears to be very promising in terms of a clinically useful predictor of impending premature labor."

In this chapter we review some of the work that has been done in pioneering the field of tocodynamometry. We will discuss the technology that allows us to extend external tocodynamometry beyond the labor and delivery suite. In addition, we present the investigations we have been undertaking in an attempt to differentiate physiologic from pathologic uterine contractility among ambulatory patients. Finally, we try to apply these guidelines to a clinical series to test the hypothesis presented by Aubry and Pennington, namely, whether tocodynamometry can improve perinatal outcome.

In the late 1950s and early 1960s, Alvarez and associates performed transabdominal intrauterine pressure measurements in hundreds of pregnant women, and determined what should be considered physiologic uterine activity during normal gestation. They reported that during the first 30 weeks of pregnancy, most contractions generated an intrauterine pressure of 10 to 15 mm Hg and occurred with a frequency of approximately one per hour. The frequency and intensity of this activity increased very gradually until 2 weeks preceding term, when there was a more abrupt increase in uterine activity [2].

Later, Wood et al, who performed tocodynamometry in 26 patients during pregnancy, reported that the six patients who had excessive uterine activity prior to 34 weeks' gestation had subsequently experienced premature labor [3]. In 1968, Turnbull and Anderson [4] reported a comparative study among 28 women who underwent external tocodynamometry at 2-week intervals from 28 weeks' gestation until the onset of labor. These investigators expressed their findings in terms of "uterine activity units." Uterine activity units are the product of contraction intensity and frequency. Turnbull and Anderson did not specifically investigate preterm labor, but they did find a consistently higher uterine activity score among patients delivering prior to their estimated date of confinement compared with women laboring at term. This difference in uterine activity was present as early as 28 weeks' gestation. The gradual increase in uterine contractility demonstrated by these studies during the last 8 to 10 weeks of pregnancy is interesting, but not as intriguing as the finding that "the rate of increase in activity depends on the ultimate time in gestation of the spontaneous onset of labor" [4]. Stimulated by these findings, Aubry and Pennington [1] performed uterine activity monitoring every other week from 20 weeks until term, and also expressed their results in uterine activity units. They established a normal range from 40 control subjects that resembled the findings of Alvarez and Caldeyro-Barcia [2]. When the uterine activity from 10 patients experiencing preterm labor was computed, almost all the recordings exceeded the normal range. This phenomenon was apparent from weeks to months prior to the onset of premature labor.

Schwenzer, Schumann, and Halberstadt [5] performed 24-hour tocograms in 24 patients with uncomplicated pregnancies and compared them with similar tracings from 26 patients hospitalized for observation with threatened preterm labor. The patients with normal pregnancies exhibited fewer than three contractions per hour throughout the study period (25 to 38 weeks' gestation). They also exhibited somewhat of a circadian rhythm, with maximum uterine activity between 2300 and 0300 o'clock, and then after a quiet morning, increased uterine activity between 1100 and 1300 o'clock [5].

A comparison of contraction frequencies throughout gestation was not possible for the patients with threatened preterm labor, because of the acute nature of the studies. However, at least acutely, the tracings among patients threatening to enter preterm labor revealed between three and six contractions per hour and a loss of circadian pattern [5]. This information is extremely useful in that excessive uterine activity may be detected in these women by sampling for 1 or 2 hours at random in any 24-hour period.

Bell [6] performed external tocodynamometry for 1 hour every other week from the 20th week until delivery in a sample of 29 patients, 14 of them "optimal" and low risk for preterm labor and 15 of them very "high risk" for such labor. Bell was concerned mostly with contraction intensity, and discovered that in women entering labor prematurely, an elevation of intrauterine pressure of more than 15 mm Hg was generated significantly earlier in pregnancy (20–28 weeks) than in women laboring at term (>34 weeks) [6]. Bell suggested that this premature synchronization of uterine contractility was present at least 5 and up to 10 weeks prior to the onset of preterm labor.

It is important to note that most of the previously described data on the frequency of prelabor contractions were obtained on an intermittent basis in women either in recumbency or otherwise limited in their activity. Because the majority of women are physically active during pregnancy, the reported data from hospitalized patients may not accurately reflect the true prelabor uterine activity.

Toward this end Zahn [7], in Germany, recorded uterine activity for 1 hour each day in 54 primiparous and multiparous women during the latter half of pregnancy at home. His data suggested that normal uterine contraction frequency prior to 36 weeks' gestation does not exceed four contractions per hour [7]. Zahn found no significant differences in the frequency curves between primiparous and multiparous patients. He also performed 24-hour recordings in a large group of pregnant subjects and described a circadian pattern very similar to that observed by Schwenzer et al [5]. Zahn's findings indicated the presence of a peak in uterine activity between 2230 and 0200 o'clock, and a minimum frequency during the morning hours. This knowledge of circadian patterns is important for interpretation of the day-to-day variations found in the tocographic tracings from the same patient.

Technology

For the past several years we have been actively investigating the use of external tocodynamometry among a referral population of women at high risk for preterm labor.

The tocodynamometer sensor utilized in most of our studies of uterine activity employed a design first described by Smyth in 1957 [8]. The principle underlying this design has been termed the guard-ring principle. Design features include a relatively flattened strain gauge surrounded by an "inert" guard-ring. As the sensor is tightened, there is flattening of the skin, abdominal wall musculature, and underlying uterine wall. This creates an equalization of pressure approximating baseline intrauterine pressure (8–12 mm Hg), thus establishing a continuous flat diaphragm between the amniotic fluid and the sensor. Intrauterine pressure generated by myometrial shortening is transmitted through the uterine and abdominal walls and is recorded by the displacement of a strain gauge. Symth believed that the major advantage of this design was its ability to record uterine activity that correlated well (±1 cm of water) with the information obtained by direct intrauterine pressure monitoring. The accuracy of this external sensor has been independently confirmed by Wood et al (1965) [3], by

Bell (1981) [9], and by Katz and Gill (1985) [10]. All of these studies document the ability of the "guard-ring"-type external tocodynamometer to reliably reflect between 70 and 100% of the absolute elevation of intrauterine pressure. These investigators also noted that the correlation between the guard-ring sensor readings and intrauterine pressures was better for low-intensity contractions, which are most prevalent during the prelabor period. In our own studies of a guard-ring-type external tocodynamometer, we found it to be slightly more reliable than any of three traditional stationary tocodynamometers currently employed in our labor and delivery suite, even when placed in a suboptimal location.

In summary, we have been extremely pleased with the guard-ring-type external tocodynamometer because of its reliability in use, its great sensitivity to even low-level uterine activity, and its accuracy in reflecting the relative change in intrauterine pressures.

Ambulatory Tocodynamometry

Basic Studies

Just as did Zahn in earlier studies, we have emphasized the importance of tocodynamometry at home. However, in contrast to Zahn's work, we felt that it would be valuable to directly compare matched groups of high-risk patients for differences in uterine activity, rather than simply establishing the limits of normality for a sample of low-risk patients.

After referral to our preterm birth prevention program, all patients were given instructions regarding the signs and symptoms of preterm labor and were taught techniques of self-palpation for the detection of uterine activity. Each patient received a tocodynamometer with a sensor design based on the guard-ring principle and was instructed in its use. The particular sensor we utilized weighs only 198 g; it was applied to the abdomen by a strap, allowing the patient to ambulate, drive, or work without difficulty (Termguard, Tokos Medical Corporation, Santa Ana, CA). The sensor was attached to a light-weight (318-g) data storage and transmission unit, which can be carried on a belt or hung from a shoulder strap (Fig. 3.1). If any contractions were perceived by the patient while recording, the patient could press an event marker, which placed an arrow on the tocograph strip. After the monitoring, the stored data were transmitted at a convenient time via the telephone to receiving tocographs located in the study center, with an average transmission time of 6 to 8 minutes per 200 minutes of monitoring. Patients were asked to record their uterine activity four times daily for a cumulative total of at least 200 minutes per day. Included were monitoring periods representative of the morning, afternoon, and evening hours. Additional monitoring sessions could be initiated at the request of either the physician or the patient. The daily

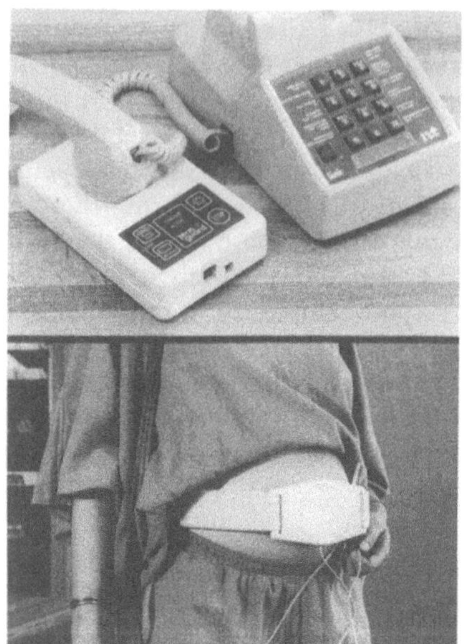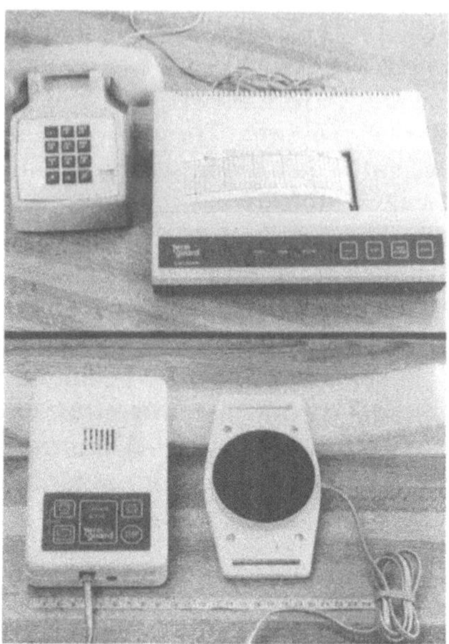

FIGURE 3.1. Patient monitoring by tocodynamometry (right). Ambulatory toco-dynamometer (bottom) and receiving tocograph (top) (left). Patient monitoring (bottom) and data transmission (top). Reprinted with permission from The American College of Obstetricians and Gynecologists. (Obstetrics and Gynecology 1985, 66:273).

records of each patient were comprehensively reviewed for the following characteristics:

1. *Contraction frequency:* Frequency of contractions per hour ($>$ 5 mm amplitude, lasting $>$ than 35 s).
2. *Contraction intensity:* Small ($<$ 11 mm), medium (11–20 mm), or large ($>$20 mm Hg).
3. *Low-amplitude, high-frequency contractions (LAHF):* The percentage of recorded uterine activity data occupied by the repetitive occurrence of uterine contractions of $<$ 5 mm in amplitude and $<$ 35 s in duration (Alvarez waves, "irritability").
4. *Perceptive accuracy:* The percentage of contractions correctly identified (true-positive) as well as the number of marks placed in the absence of any identifiable uterine activity (false-positive).

Only women meeting the following criteria were included in the initial study:

1. At high risk for preterm labor (previous preterm labor and birth, multifetal gestation, uterine anomaly, etc.).
2. Referred during the second trimester for home monitoring.
3. Not receiving tocolytic therapy.
4. Not under any limitation of activity.

The person interpreting the tocodynamometry records was blinded as to the clinical characteristics and pregnancy outcomes of the patients. It is important to note that preterm labor was never diagnosed solely on the basis of uterine contraction frequency, but rather required the additional finding of a change in cervical status. Cervical exams and the diagnosis of preterm labor were not made by the investigators, but by the individual patient's primary physician who did not see the data obtained at home.

Approximately 50% of the patients in our referral population of high-risk women ultimately experienced preterm labor. The clinical characteristics and distribution of risk factors for the group of patients who labored at term and those who labored preterm were very similar. This is important, because certain risk factors may significantly affect the frequency of contractions. By controlling for those differences in uterine contraction frequency that may be attributed to a particular risk factor, a valid assessment of uterine activity in relationship to either term or preterm labor could be carried out.

CONTRACTION FREQUENCY [12,13]

Uterine contractions were counted for each day, summed for each gestational week, and expressed as mean (± SD) frequency contractions per hour at each gestational week. Our results substantiate previous findings that there do appear to be two distinct populations of patients with significantly different baseline patterns of prelabor contractility. Those patients laboring at term (Fig. 3.2, solid circles) never experienced more than two contractions per hour as a weekly average throughout the last half of their pregnancy until 37 weeks' gestation. Conversely, those patients developing preterm labor (Fig. 3.2, solid triangles) averaged two contractions per hour as early as the 22nd week of pregnancy, and this frequency increased progressively until labor.

Because women enter preterm labor at different times in gestation, the uterine activity of our patients was also analyzed for the weeks prior to the occurrence of preterm labor (Fig. 3.3). The data were compared with those observed in patients who reached 37 weeks of gestation without preterm labor. Again, there was a significant difference between the two groups; most important, the differences were apparent up to several weeks before progressive cervical changes appeared. This confirms the findings of Aubry and Pennington and supports the proposal by Hobel et al that preterm labor is not an acute event but rather a cascade in which demonstrable cervical changes and ultimately birth are the terminal sequence of a long chain of events [14].

There were no statistically significant differences in the frequency of uterine contractions recorded from week to week within either group, except for one clinically meaningful situation: the week in which preterm labor was diagnosed. When daily contraction frequency during the 7 days

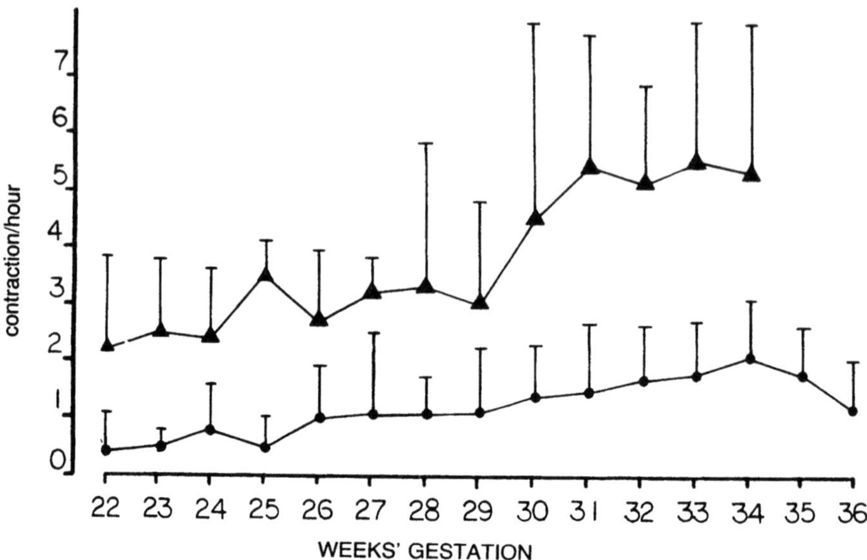

FIGURE 3.2. Frequency of contractions per hour (mean ± SD) in relation to time of gestation in patients who subsequently had preterm labor (triangles) and those who labored at term (circles). Reproduced with permission from the *American Journal of Obstetrics and Gynecology*.

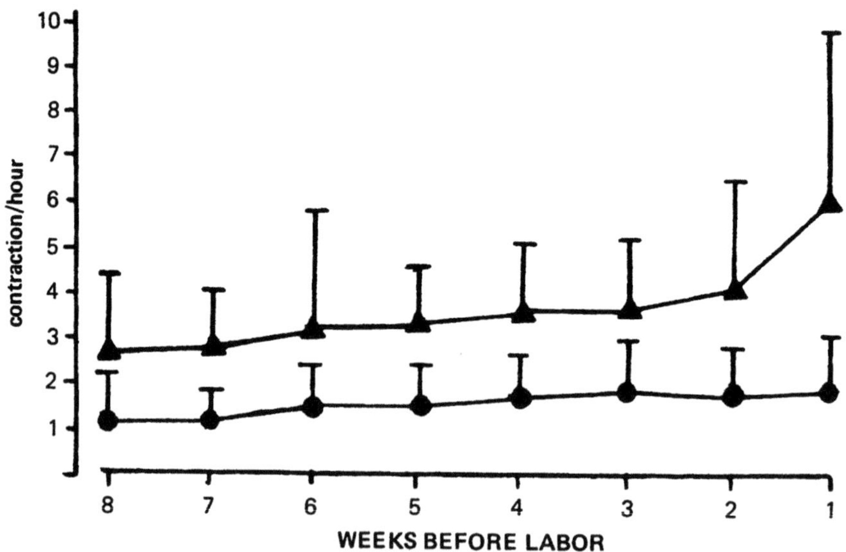

FIGURE 3.3. Frequency of contractions per hour (mean ± SD) during the 8 weeks preceding either onset of preterm labor (triangles) or attainment of 37 weeks' gestation (circles). Reproduced with permission from the *American Journal of Obstetrics and Gynecology*.

preceding the diagnosis of preterm labor was evaluated we found an abrupt and significant rise during the 24 to 48 hours before hospital admission for preterm labor. This rise was superimposed on an already elevated baseline contraction frequency.

On the basis of data provided by these investigations, a normogram was established to provide guidelines as to what should be considered a normal mean weekly contraction frequency for any particular gestational week. A computer-generated line of best fit was utilized to indicate breakpoints for each gestational week, and the individual patient's data were compared with these normal limits to assess their predictive values (Fig. 3.4). None of the patients who maintained weekly per-hour contraction frequencies in the normal range (Fig. 3.4, shaded area) had preterm labor. Of the patients who had a mean contraction frequency above the normal range (Fig. 3.4, clear area), 80% had preterm labor. As more patient data are generated, the accuracy of this division between normal and abnormal contraction frequency in predicting preterm labor should improve. If the prediction with larger numbers remains as accurate as it is now, evaluation of the average hourly contraction frequency over a 7-day period may prove clinically useful.

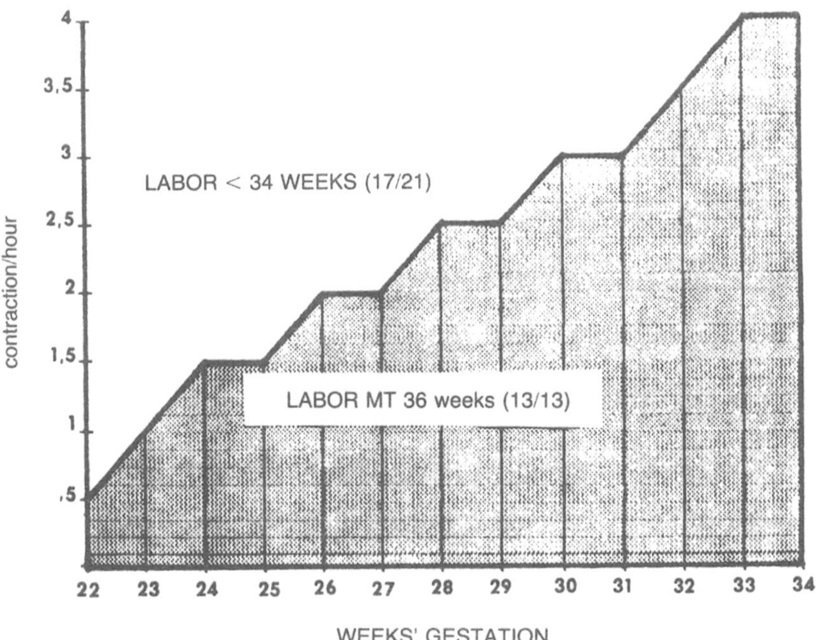

FIGURE 3.4. Calculated mean frequency of contractions per hour separating normal frequency (shaded area) from excessive frequency in relation to weeks of gestation Reproduced with permission from the *American Journal of Obstetrics and Gynecology*.

We decided to determine if hourly contraction frequency had a specific relationship to any one particular risk factor. Our early experience indicated that several patients who had had an excessive amount of uterine activity but did not enter preterm labor shared a common factor, namely, multifetal gestation. To further investigate this, we reviewed ambulatory monitoring strips that had been obtained from 22 high-risk women with a single fetus and 18 women with multifetal gestation, all of them laboring after 36 weeks' gestation. A comparison of the weekly contraction frequencies for these patients has shown that women with multifetal pregnancies have significantly more contractions than their singleton counterparts (Fig. 3.5). Additionally, within the group of patients with multifetal gestation, there was a progressive, significant increase in contraction frequency with advancing gestation. The reason these patients did not have preterm labor despite their high rate of uterine contractility remains spec-

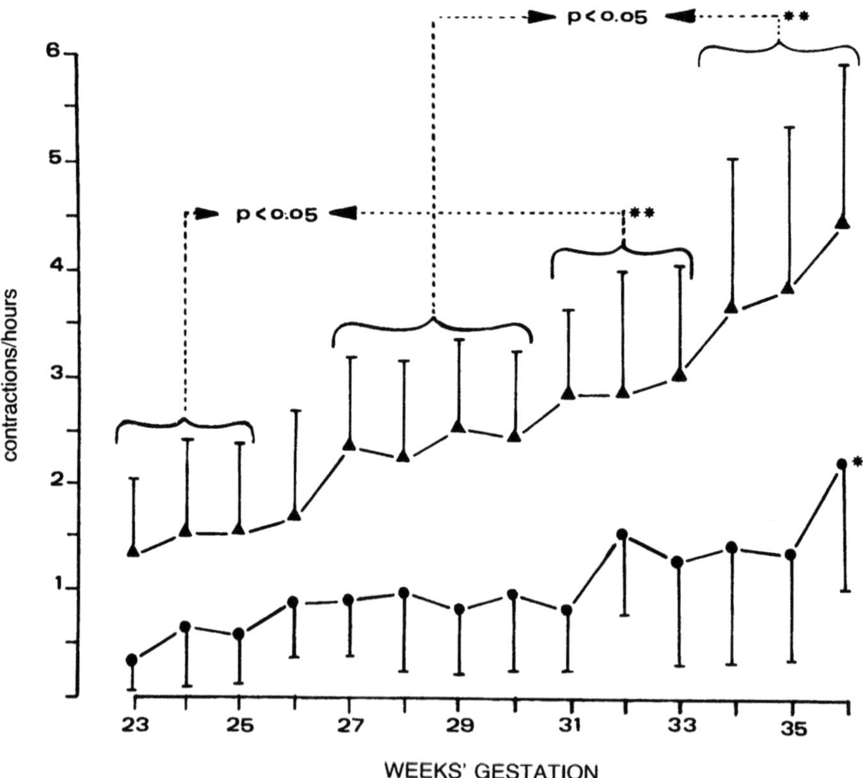

FIGURE 3.5. Frequency of contractions (mean ± SD) during normal term pregnancies among women with single (circles) or multi-fetal (triangles) gestations. Reproduced with permission from the *American Journal of Obstetrics and Gynecology.*

ulative, but possibly relates to lessened intensity of uterine contractility known to be associated with increased uterine volume [2]. No other risk factor was found to be associated with an increase in contraction frequency.

CONTRACTION INTENSITY [15]

Studies by Bell [6,9] suggest that the intensity of prelabor contractions may help identify premature synchronization of the myometrium. In many of the early studies, data were expressed in uterine activity units, which are the product of frequency and intensity. Thus, assessment of intensity seems important in estimating risk of premature labor.

As mentioned previously, external tocodynamometry does not provide an exact measurement of intrauterine pressure, but has been shown consistently to provide a reliable approximation of the generated force. We thus defined the intensity of recorded contractions as small, medium, or large, according to their amplitude.

The vast majority of contractions in the prelabor period were of small intensity. Medium amplitude contractions were present from as early as 21 weeks of gestation; their proportion increased gradually toward term. Large contractions occurred infrequently and were seen only rarely prior to 28 weeks of gestation. Overall, there was a statistically significant increase in the frequency of both medium and large contractions with advancing gestational age. The proportion of contraction intensities was similarly distributed in women who labored prematurely and those who labored at term, with only a modest increase in the frequency of medium and large contractions among the women entering preterm labor. There was, however, a significant increase in the frequency of contractions of greater intensity during the week in which preterm labor was diagnosed. We did note that contractions of medium intensity initially appeared significantly earlier among patients destined to develop preterm labor (25.3 ± 2.9 weeks of gestation) compared with their appearance in women laboring at term (27.9 ± 2.7 weeks). This was also true for large contractions. Women destined to enter preterm labor first experienced contractions of large intensity at a mean gestational age of 27.6 ± 3.3 weeks, while women who labored at term did not experience contractions of that intensity until 31.2 ± 3.8 weeks. This was felt to be consistent with the observations of Bell regarding synchronization of myometrial function [6]. The occurrence of a large contraction prior to 30 weeks' gestation had a sensitivity of 55% in relation to the subsequent occurrence of preterm labor, a specificity of 86%, a positive predictive value of 80%, and a negative predictive value of 64%. Similarly, the occurrence of a contraction of medium intensity prior to the 28th week of gestation had a sensitivity of 91%, a specificity of only 50%, a positive predictive value of 71%, and a negative predictive value of 80%.

As with contraction frequency, these estimations of the predictive values of contractions of a specific intensity at a particular gestational week will need to be further studied and evaluated in a larger sample of patients of both high and low risk. We believe, however, that there is merit to the concept of "premature synchronization" of uterine activity and that antenatal evaluation of prelabor contraction intensities may contribute to the assessment of risk. In addition, a change in the distribution of contraction intensity toward contractions of greater amplitude should, along with contraction frequency, help signal impending clinical preterm labor, when daily evaluations of uterine activity are performed.

Evaluation of the distribution of contraction intensities in women with a singleton gestation and those with a multifetal gestation did not reveal any significant differences. This finding differs from the result of evaluations of contraction frequencies, where multifetal gestations were associated with increased frequency of uterine contractions all along. Additional evaluations of other "traditional" maternal risk factors did not reveal any differences in the distribution of contraction intensities.

Low-Amplitude, High-Frequency Contractions (LAHF) [16]

The clinical significance of this commonly observed pattern of uterine activity or "irritability" (Fig. 3.6) is controversial. It has been said that the presence of LAHF may be associated with preterm labor, but this proposal has never been adequately evaluated. Therefore, we have reviewed more than 7,250 hours of daily external tocodynamometry tracings from 56 women at risk for preterm labor, for the presence of these repetitive low-amplitude contractions. Overall, $8.7 \pm 7.8\%$ of recorded uterine activity data involved this pattern. Between 21 and 31 weeks of gestation, the percentage of time occupied by LAHF was significantly higher in women destined to develop preterm labor compared with matched controls who labored at term ($11.2 \pm 12\%$ vs. $5.7 \pm 7\%$). We found no influence of gestational age or parity on the proportion of time occupied by LAHF pattern. As a predictor of preterm labor, the presence of greater than 10% LAHF on any single tocographic tracing had a sensitivity of 32%, a specificity of 82%, a 49% positive predictive value, and a 69% negative predictive value. While this pattern may be slightly more prevalent among women entering preterm labor, it remains generally ubiquitous, quite variable, and as demonstrated, only marginally helpful in assessing the risk of preterm labor.

Perceptive Accuracy [17]

Investigations by Caldeyro-Barcia and Poseiro [11] demonstrated that women in labor do not effectively perceive their own uterine activity until generated intrauterine pressure exceeded 20 to 30 mm Hg. While elegantly

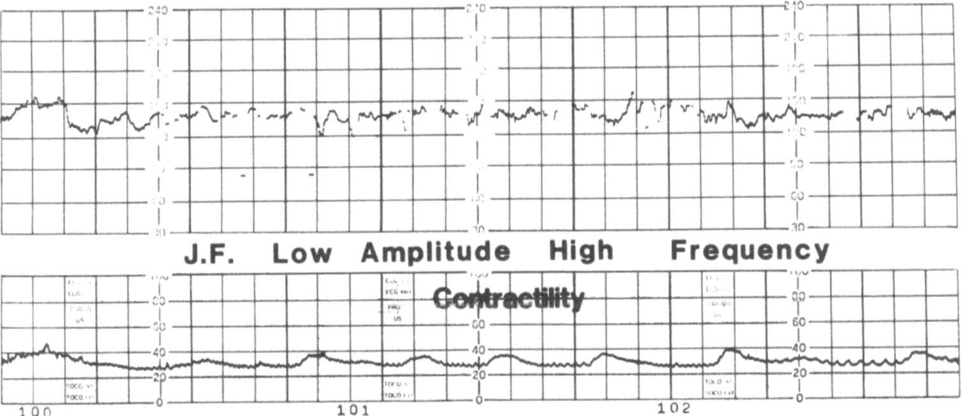

FIGURE 3.6. Low-amplitude, high-frequency contractions, also known as irritability or Alvarez waves.

done, their studies did not include women who had been trained in self-detection techniques, which have now been popularized for patients at risk. Furthermore, the patients in the studies by Caldeyro-Barcia and Poseiro were all in active labor. We believe, and have shown, that the labor patterns characteristic of the earliest stages of preterm labor are more intermittent and much less intense than the patterns characteristic of established labor. Finally, all of the patients studied were in a hospital setting. It is likely that with use of ambulatory home tocodynamometry one would deal more closely with the true mileu in which the pregnant woman could be expected to be aware of her own contractility.

We reviewed tocographic tracings from 44 women at risk for preterm labor who were trained by us in self-palpation. Of over 9,500 prelabor uterine contractions, only 15 ± 21% were correctly perceived. There existed wide variations in individual accuracy—a range of 0 to 69%. Only 11% of the patients correctly identified more than 50% of their contractions, while more than half identified less than 10%.

As would be anticipated from the work of Caldeyro-Barcia, perception improved with contractions of greater intensity. We must emphasize, however, that only 2% of contractions in women with preterm labor were of large intensity, and therefore such contractions are very unlikely to provide adequate warning. The fact that the vast majority of these contractions were less than 11 mm in amplitude was probably responsible for failure of the majority of the women to correctly perceive their own uterine activity.

Perceptive accuracy was evaluated in relation to maternal age, maternal parity, gestational age, maternal risk factors, the occurrence of preterm labor, and the duration of having the home monitoring device itself. None of these variables had any significant effect on perceptive accuracy with the exception of the occurrence of multifetal gestation. It appears that women carrying more than one fetus perceive fewer than half of the prelabor contractions perceived by their counterparts with a single fetus. This difference was statistically significant; we speculate that the existence of a higher resting uterine tone associated with an overdistended uterus, along with a greater number of fetal movements, may be responsible for the diminished accuracy of perception among women with multifetal gestations.

In addition to the fairly low incidence of correct identification of uterine activity, we have observed that for every three contractions that were correctly identified the women placed two marks on the record in the absence of any identifiable uterine activity. Once again we could find no relationship between false-positive marks and the above mentioned obstetrical variables. Of interest was the fact that those women who experienced preterm labor in the current pregnancy did place significantly more false-positive marks than those who labored at term. This may suggest either the influence of anxiety or the presence of other sensations independent of contractions but related to the occurrence of preterm labor. It is also noteworthy that the five patients who correctly identified more than 50% of their contractions were responsible for a disproportionately high percentage of the false-positive marks. In essence, the most accurate were also the most inaccurate—they performed self-monitoring with a "shotgun" approach. This, once again, suggests that prelabor uterine activity must be quite subtle and is easily confused with other common and innocuous symptoms of pregnancy such as pelvic pressure, round ligament pain, low back ache, intestinal peristalsis, bladder fullness, or fetal movements.

In summary, while wide variations exist, the majority of women are unable to identify more than a small percentage of their prelabor uterine activity and seem to be easily confused by other symptomatology of pregnancy. None of the obstetrical variables, including the duration of monitoring itself, had any significant impact on perception, except that women with multifetal gestations were even less accurate in their perceptive accuracy. While perception improved with contractions of greater intensity, we remain concerned that awaiting the repetitive occurrence of contractions of high intensity will not allow the earliest possible diagnosis of preterm labor.

CLINICAL TRIALS [18,19,20]

In one of our early studies we carried out a clinical trial to determine if daily ambulatory external tocodynamometry performed by a group of women at high risk for preterm labor could allow an earlier diagnosis and therefore more effective treatment of preterm labor. The first 76 patients referred for ambulatory monitoring and meeting the criteria outlined earlier were compared with 76 nonrandom contemporary controls matched for risk indicators, maternal age, and parity. The contemporary controls included only those women who started prenatal care at or prior to 12 weeks' gestation, who were cared for by the same group of obstetricians throughout pregnancy, and who were cared for in the same hospital over the same time period as the monitored patients. It did not include any maternal transports.

Patients in both groups were given verbal or written instructions regarding signs and symptoms of preterm labor and performance of self-monitoring by palpation of the uterus. In addition, patients in the monitored group utilized the external tocodynamometer for 200 minutes a day during the late second trimester and the third trimester. All patients were seen for prenatal care every 1 to 3 weeks, and they underwent regular cervical exams for the detection of cervical changes. They were also examined as felt to be necessary on the basis of patient self-perception of uterine activity.

If a patient in the monitored group had more than four contractions in a 1-hour period, she was asked to remonitor while on bed rest. If this level of uterine activity persisted while at rest, she was instructed to come to the hospital for continuous monitoring and evaluation of cervical status. The diagnosis of preterm labor was made when progressive cervical change was noted in association with regular uterine activity.

Approximately half the patients in each group developed preterm labor, attesting to the high-risk nature of these pregnancies and the adequacy of matching (Fig. 3.7). The mean gestational week in which preterm labor was first diagnosed was 28.4 ± 3 weeks for the monitored group and 30.8 ± 2 for matched controls. This difference approached but did not quite achieve statistical significance. However, it suggests that monitoring may have established the diagnosis of preterm labor at an earlier point in the evolution of preterm labor. All the monitored patients who entered preterm labor were suitable candidates for long-term tocolysis (i.e., dilated <3 cm, intact membranes) at the time of hospital admission, which was significantly better than the unmonitored group, in which only 35% with preterm labor were candidates for long-term tocolysis. Even among the candidates for tocolysis, the incidence of failed tocolysis was significantly lower in the monitored group (5% compared with 25% in the unmonitored group, Fig. 3.7). Overall, monitored patients who entered preterm labor gained a mean in utero time of 7.5 ± 3.1 weeks, and delivery occurred after the 36th week of gestation for 88% of them. In contrast, of the women in the unmonitored group who received tocolysis, the mean in utero time gained was 4.1 ± 2.1 weeks, and only 59% of them achieved 36 weeks' gestation. Both of these differences were significant and suggest an advantage to be gained by ambulatory tocodynamometry.

We have also performed a clinical trial to study if daily home tocodyn-

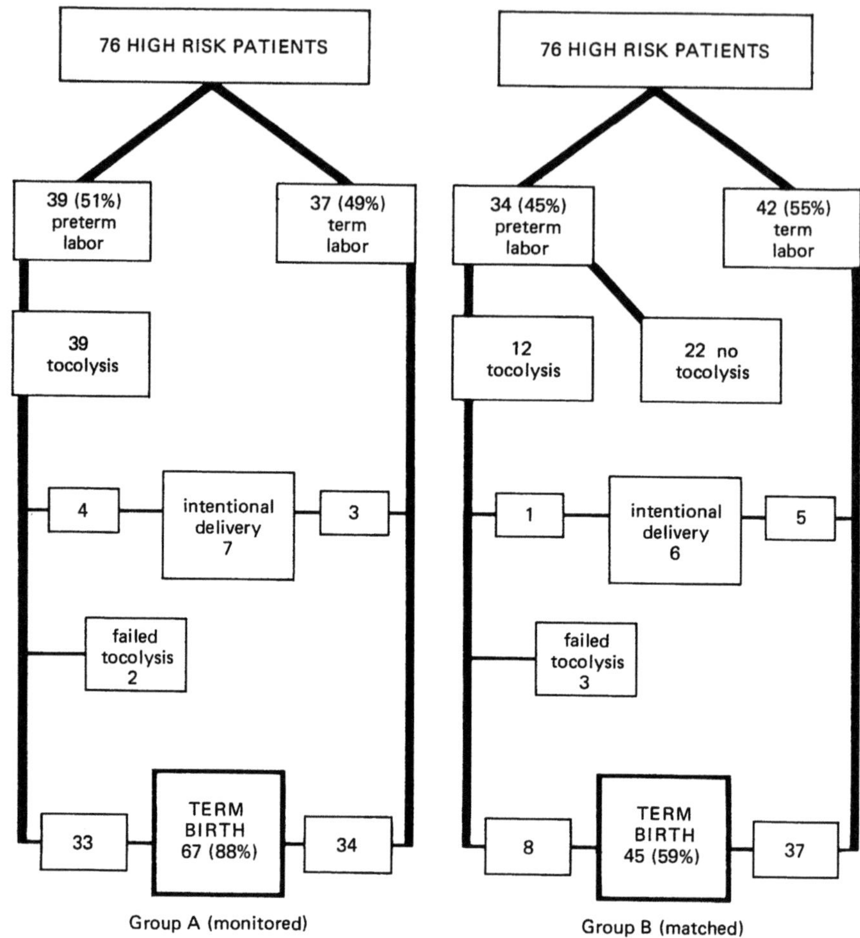

FIGURE 3.7. Schematic representation of perinatal events among 76 monitored and 76 matched high-risk patients. Reprinted with permission from the American College of Obstetricians and Gynecologists (*Obstetrics and Gynecology* 1986; 68:773.)

amometry could improve the management of outpatient tocolytic therapy for the prevention of recurrent preterm labor. Ambulatory tocodynamometry was used for 60 patients released from the hospital with oral tocolytic medications after their initial event of preterm labor was controlled by parenteral tocolysis. This group was compared with 60 nonrandom matched contemporary controls. The selection of patients, monitoring protocol, and data evaluation were identical to those just described. In the presence of excessive uterine activity, oral tocolytic dosage, timing of doses, and patient activity were adjusted to maintain uterine activity at a frequency of three or fewer contractions per hour. If contraction frequency remained higher than this despite adjustments or despite a resting tachycardia of 110 beats per minute, patients were instructed to come to the hospital for monitoring and evaluation to rule out recurrent preterm labor. Management of patients in the unmonitored group was identical, except that adjustments in dosage, timing of doses, and activity could only be made on the basis of pulse rate and subjective assessment by the patient herself.

Preterm labor was first diagnosed at 28.2 ± 2.5 weeks' gestation in the monitored group and at 29.5 ± 2.7 weeks' gestation for the unmonitored matched controls. Oral tocolysis was started approximately 1 week later for each group. Among monitored patients, 77% had 83 episodes of recurrent preterm labor (1.8 ± 1.2 episodes per patient) compared with 67% of the unmonitored patients, who had 59 episodes of recurrent preterm labor (1.4 ± 1.0 episode per patient). Tocolytic therapy failed to control contractions in 22% of unmonitored patients compared with only 7% of women performing home tocodynamometry. As a result, the proportion of preterm births was significantly smaller for patients in the monitored group (15% compared with 34% in the unmonitored group). In addition, the mean in utero time gained from the time preterm labor was initially treated was significantly longer among the monitored patients (7.4 ± 3 weeks) than among unmonitored controls (4.0 ± 1.2 weeks).

The clinical data provided by both studies would seem to suggest that outpatient tocodynamometry allows making the diagnosis of preterm labor earlier than can be expected from relying on the patient's perception of her own uterine activity. This early diagnosis of preterm labor translates directly into patients being candidates for long-term tocolytic therapy, a low failure rate for such therapy, a relatively long mean in utero time gained, and ultimately a high rate of term births.

Conclusions

There appears to be an increasing body of work supporting the utility of external tocodynamometry for the surveillance of patients at risk for preterm labor. In our continuing studies, we hope to better define the individual elements of prelabor uterine activity that have the greatest prognostic significance and can be best utilized as markers for antenatal risk assessment. In addition to the value of external tocodynamometry as a risk identification technique, we feel that its use in daily monitoring may prove to be a reliable and effective tool for the high-risk patient, allowing an early and accurate diagnosis of preterm labor and thereby maximizing the effectiveness of tocolytic therapy. We hope that the application of this technology to the patient at risk for preterm labor will constitute a significant step in ongoing efforts toward reduction of preterm birth rates.

REFERENCES

1. Aubry RH, Pennington JC: Identification and evaluation of high risk pregnancy: The perinatal concept. *Clin Obstet Gynecol* **16**:3, 1973.
2. Alvarez H, Caldeyro-Barcia R: Contractility of the human uterus recorded by new methods. *Surg Obstet Gynecol* **91**:1, 1950.
3. Wood C, Bannerman RHO, Booth RT, Pinkerton JHM: The prediction of premature labor by observation of the cervix and external tocography. *Am J Obstet Gynecol* **91**:396, 1965.
4. Turnbull AC, Anderson ABM: Uterine contractility and oxytocin sensitivity during human pregnancy in relation to the onset of labor. *J Obstet Gynaecol Br Commonw* **75**:278, 1968.
5. Schwenzer T, Schumann R, Halberstadt E: The importance of 24 hour cardiotocographic monitoring during tocolytic therapy. In Jung H, Lamberti G (Eds): *Beta-Mimetic Drugs in Obstetrics and Perinatology.* New York: Thieme-Stratton, 1982, pp. 60–64.
6. Bell R: The prediction of preterm labor by recording spontaneous uterine activity. *Br J Obstet Gynaecol* **90**:884, 1983.
7. Zahn V: Uterine contractions during pregnancy. *J Perinat Med* **12**:107, 1984.
8. Smyth CN: The guard-ring tocodynamometer: Absolute measurement of intra-amniotic pressure by a new instrument. *J Obstet Gynaecol Br Commonw* **64**:59, 1957.
9. Bell R: Measurement of spontaneous uterine activity in the antenatal patient. *Am J Obstet Gynecol* **140**:713, 1981.
10. Katz M, Gill PJ: Initial evaluation of an ambulatory system for home monitoring and transmission of uterine activity data. *Obstet Gynecol* **66**:273, 1985.
11. Caldeyro-Barcia R, Poseiro JJ: Physiology of the uterine contractions. *Clin Obstet Gynecol* **3**:386, 1960.
12. Katz M, Newman RB, Gill PJ: Assessment of uterine activity in ambulatory patients at high risk of preterm labor and delivery. *Am J Obstet Gynecol* **154**:44, 1986.
13. Newman RB, Gill PJ, Katz M: Uterine activity during pregnancy in ambulatory patients: Comparison of singleton and twin gestations. *Am J Obstet Gynecol* **154**:530, 1986.
14. Hobel CJ: Prevention of prematurity. In Nathanielsz PW, Beard R (Ed): Fetal *Physiology and Medicine,* New York, Marcel Dekker, Inc. 1984, pp. 757–778.
15. Newman RB, Gill PJ, Katz M: Intensity of Braxton-Hicks contractions in the high risk pregnancy. *Clin Res* **34**:378, 1986.
16. Newman RB, Gill PJ, Campion S, et al: Antepartum ambulatory tocodynamometry: The significance of low amplitude high frequency contractions. *Obstet Gynecol* **70**:701, 1987.
17. Newman RB, Gill PJ, Wittreich P, et al: Maternal perception of prelabor uterine activity. *Obstet Gynecol* **68**:765, 1986.
18. Katz M, Gill PJ, Newman RB: Detection of preterm labor by ambulatory monitoring of uterine activity: A preliminary report. *Obstet Gynecol* **68**:773, 1986.
19. Katz M, Gill PJ, Newman RB: Detection of preterm labor by ambulatory monitoring of uterine activity for the management of oral tocolysis. *Am J Obstet Gynecol* **154**:1253, 1986.
20. Gill PJ, Katz M: Early detection of preterm labor: Ambulatory home monitoring of uterine activity. *J. Obstet Gynecol Neonat Nurs* **15**:439, 1986.

4
Substance Abuse: Pregnancy and the Neonate

IRA J. CHASNOFF

The problems of drug abuse during pregnancy have been with us since antiquity. It was not until 1973, however, with the modern description of the fetal alcohol syndrome [1], that public attention in the United States was directed toward the possible teratogenic effects of recreational drugs consumed during pregnancy. Around this time, also, descriptions of withdrawal suffered by neonates exposed in utero to narcotics (heroin or methadone) [2] emphasized the need for further study of the behavioral and neurologic effects of drugs on the developing fetus and child.

It is widely recognized that women of childbearing age are regular users of licit and illicit drugs. In the last decade, the list of substances known to affect the unborn child has broadened. Additionally, our concept of teratology has changed: We now recognize that, although most drugs of use and abuse do not produce congenital malformations, they have definite behavioral and neurologic effects that impair the neonate's, infant's, and child's development.

Drug Use Patterns in Pregnancy

Data on women of childbearing age show that they are frequent users of legal drugs, including alcohol, and of illegal drugs. More specifically, early studies looking at drug use during pregnancy revealed that around 75% of women use some analgesics during pregnancy, and about 25% use sedative drugs. The majority of the women involved in studies such as these were receiving prenatal care and were obtaining many of the medications by prescription from their physicians.

In the last 5 years the number of pregnant women who are using and abusing illicit substances during pregnancy, especially cocaine, has increased. Screening of all women enrolling at Prentice Women's Hospital and Maternity Center for routine prenatal care during a 6-month period in 1982 revealed that 3% had evidence of sedative-hypnotics in their urine at the time of admission to the general maternity clinic [3]. This study was performed before cocaine had become society's drug of choice. Currently, with an estimated 20 million Americans having tried cocaine at least once and 5 million using it on a regular basis [4], the number of primary cocaine users enrolling in our program, the Perinatal Center for Chemical Dependence, has rapidly risen. In a survey conducted by the Child Abuse Prevention Program, Department of Health Services in Los Angeles, California, of a total of 5,973 cases of child abuse reported in 1985, 538 cases (9%) involved neonatal withdrawal due to maternal drug use in pregnancy. In the first 6 months of 1986, 403 of 4,299 cases (9.4%) of child abuse were due to maternal addiction during pregnancy. The pattern of drug use in this population showed a shift toward an even higher frequency of cocaine use among reported cases in the first 6 months of 1986 compared with 1985. With this shift to cocaine as the most common primary drug of abuse, polydrug abuse has also become more common, the majority of cocaine users abusing marijuana and/or alcohol in addition. Thus, evaluation and management of the pregnant cocaine abuser and her newborn must take into consideration the effects of these secondary drugs of abuse.

Pharmacology of Illicit Drugs

It is a common belief that the placenta acts as a barrier, protecting the fetus from various toxic substances. However, this is not so. Numerous reviews of drug use during pregnancy show that the placenta is freely crossed by most drugs taken by the mother during pregnancy. Drugs that act on the central nervous system are usually lipophilic and of relatively low molecular weight, characteristics that facilitate the crossing of the substance from maternal to fetal circulation. For many sedative-hypnotic medications, there is rapid equilibration of free drug between the maternal and fetal circulation. Although the exact distribution of drug between maternal and fetal circulation is difficult to determine, it is reasonable to say that drugs with high abuse potential (opiates, cocaine, sedative-hypnotics, alcohol, and stimulants) are found at significant levels in the fetus if the mother is using or abusing these drugs.

Some drugs that accumulate in the fetus can be metabolized by the fetal liver and the placenta. Frequently, the metabolites are water soluble, which hinders passage of the metabolite back across the placenta to the maternal circulation where it can be excreted. Because the fetal liver is not fully developed, anticipating the exact fate of a specific drug in the fetus is difficult. The majority of drugs that have been studied have a longer half-life in the fetus than in the adult. This is also true in the neonate, since the enzymes involved in the metabolic process of glucuronidation and oxidation are not fully developed in the fetus. In addition, the immature renal function of the newborn may delay the excretion of drugs that have been metabolized to an excretable form.

Neonatal Abstinence

The fact that drugs cross the placenta and reach the fetus creates potential problems of fetal development. These problems can be manifested as congenital abnormalities, fetal growth retardation, neonatal growth retardation, and neurobehavioral problems. In addition, one of the important effects of maternal drug use during pregnancy, especially use of drugs with high potential for abuse, is that dependence develops in the fetus as well as the mother. Thus, the fetus will experience withdrawal along with the mother if she stops drug use during pregnancy, or at term.

Symptoms of neonatal withdrawal from narcotics are usually present at birth but may not reach a peak until 3 to 4 days or as late as 10 to 14 days after birth. Symptoms of withdrawal from narcotics persists in a subacute form for 4 to 6 months after birth, with a peak at around 6 weeks of age [5]. Abstinence symptoms in the neonate exposed to nonnarcotic drugs in utero have been described for phenobarbital, diazepam, marijuana, and alcohol. Although withdrawal from these substances does not appear to result in as severe a syndrome of abstinence as withdrawal from narcotics, the newborn does exhibit the irritability and restlessness, poor feeding behavior, crying, and impaired neurobehavioral abilities that are characteristic of the neonatal abstinence syndrome.

The most common features of the neonatal abstinence syndrome (Table 4.1) mimic aspects of adult withdrawal from narcotics. Most significant for the neonate are the high-pitched cry, sweating, tremulousness, excoriation of the extremities, and gastrointestinal upset. In an effort to reduce the severity of withdrawal for the narcotic-exposed newborn, low-dose methadone maintenance programs for pregnant women have been developed, and it is now the general recommendation to maintain a pregnant woman on as low a dose of methadone as possible.

Treatment of the neonate for narcotic withdrawal should be supportive, since pharmacologic therapy can prolong hospitalization and exposes the infant to additional agents that often are not necessary. Mothers should be taught to swaddle the withdrawing infant closely and tightly in a blanket.

TABLE 4.1. Signs and symptoms of neonatal withdrawal.

Tremors	Nasal stuffiness
Restlessness	Rapid respirations
Hyperactive reflexes	Frequent yawning
Vomiting, diarrhea	Sweating
Increased muscle tone	Excoriation of knees, elbows
High-pitched cry	Mottling of skin
Sneezing	Fever
Voracious sucking	Lacrimation
Sleeplessness	Seizures

Use of a pacifier also soothes the infant's irritability and relieves the increased sucking urge. Frequent small feedings are best tolerated by the infant.

Pharmacologic therapy with paregoric, diazepam, or phenobarbital (Table 4.2) should be based on results of evaluation of the infant by one of the abstinence scoring methods [2]. Excessive weight loss or dehydration due to vomiting and diarrhea, inability of the infant to feed or sleep, fever unrelated to infection, and seizures are the most common clinical indications for drug treatment. Other causes for these symptoms, such as infection, metabolic abnormalities (hypoglycemia, hypocalcemia), hyperthyroidism, central nervous system hemorrhage, and birth anoxia should be considered before therapy is begun.

Infants treated with paregoric have improved and more efficient sucking behavior and exhibit better weight gain than infants treated with diazepam or phenobarbital [6]. A major concern regarding the use of opiate preparations in neonates, however, is the marked respiratory depressant effect, although infants manifesting narcotic withdrawal should be more tolerant of this drug than nondrug-exposed infants.

Diazepam rapidly suppresses narcotic withdrawal symptoms in the neonate. However, the newborn infant has a limited capacity to metabolize this drug. Use of diazepam can be associated with depression of the neonatal sucking reflex, and late-onset seizures have occurred in neonates after cessation of treatment [7].

Phenobarbital will quiet the infant with neonatal withdrawal, but it does little for the gastrointestinal symptoms. Large doses of phenobarbital exert a marked sedative effect on the central nervous system of the infant and impair sucking. Blood levels of phenobarbital should be followed closely and adjusted according to the infant's symptoms and the abstinence score results. After symptoms have stabilized, the daily dose of phenobarbital should be decreased to allow the drug level to decrease by 10 to 20% per day.

TABLE 4.2. Pharmacologic therapy of neonatal abstinence.

Medication	Dosage	Note
Paregoric (anhydrous morphine 0.4 mg/ml)	0.2–0.5 ml every 4 hours	Taper off after symptoms of withdrawal abate for 4 to 5 days
Diazepam	1.0–2.0 mg every 8 hours	Do not use in icteric or premature infant
Phenobarbital	Loading dose: 16 mg/kg/in first 24 hours Maintenance dose: 2–8 mg/kg/24 hours	Follow blood levels to maintain therapeutic levels; decrease daily dose after symptoms stabilized to allow phenobarbital level to decrease by 10 to 20%/day

Pharmacologic therapy for infants with symptoms of abstinence due to exposure to nonopiate drugs is usually not necessary, since these infants rarely require any more than supportive therapy. If an infant in this situation should require pharmacologic intervention, phenobarbital, given in the same manner as for opiate withdrawal described above, would be the medication of choice.

Neonatal Outcome

NARCOTICS

Early studies of infants delivered to heroin-using mothers showed that these infants had a higher rate of perinatal morbidity and mortality than infants in the general population. Common problems associated with heroin use during pregnancy were first trimester spontaneous abortion; premature delivery; neonatal meconium aspiration syndrome; maternal/neonatal infection, including venereal disease; and severe neonatal withdrawal. Attempts to provide better control of these pregnancies were anchored in methadone maintenance programs, in which pregnant women attended prenatal obstetric clinics and received daily methadone to replace street heroin. The initial methadone maintenance programs were successful in that the more consistent medical and nutritional care provided for these women resulted in improved pregnancy outcome. However, the high doses of methadone (80 to 120 mg/day) produced a more severe and prolonged period of abstinence for the newborn, compared with patterns of withdrawal for infants exposed to heroin. These complications are avoided when the pregnant woman is placed on low-dose methadone maintenance, especially if the third trimester dose of methadone is held at less than 20 mg.

Infants delivered to mothers who use narcotics (heroin, methadone, "T's," and "blues") have a significantly lower birth weight and length and a smaller head circumference than nondrug-exposed infants [8]. The inhibitory effects of narcotics on fetal growth, as well as the effects of inadequate maternal caloric and protein intake, can produce this fetal growth failure. However, nutritional intake is closely supervised in all women enrolled in our program, and it appears that the significant reduction in growth parameters that we found in narcotic-addicted infants is a direct result of the narcotic exposure.

Infants exposed to narcotics in utero exhibit significant impairment in their interactive abilities, making them difficult to engage and to console. Narcotic-exposed infants are more tremulous and irritable than drug-free infants, demonstrating significant and unpredictable fluctuations in their emotional responses [9]. These factors not only make these infants very difficult to cuddle and comfort but also interrupt the normal processes of maternal/infant attachment that are so important to the early relationship between infant and mother.

Infants born to mothers maintained on methadone throughout pregnancy continue to be significantly smaller in weight and length compared with drug-free infants through 6 to 9 months of age, but usually catch up by 12 months of age. This early stunting during a prolonged period of subacute withdrawal could be due to the direct effect of methadone on the hypo-thalamic-hypophyseal axis of the newborn. Following a period of slow excretion of the methadone, the plasma and tissue drug levels fall, the endocrinologic effects of the drug subside, and neonatal growth recovers. The one exception is head circumference measurement for the opiate-exposed infants; it does not exhibit catch-up growth [8]. The persistent reduction in head size in these infants is of concern, since small head size in young infants has been reported to be predictive of poor developmental outcome and may be an indicator of the prolonged high-risk status of these infants.

Two-year developmental follow-up of narcotic-exposed infants shows that their development, measured on the Bayley Scales of Infant Development, is within the normal range [8]. Of clinical concern, however, is the fact that the infants demonstrate a downward trend in developmental scores at 18 months to 2 years of age, a phenomenon not uncommon in infants from low socioeconomic groups. This observation suggests that the infants' environment, with a lack of stimulation, has a more direct influence on 2-year development than maternal drug use during pregnancy.

Cocaine

Although the annual number of opiate-addicted women delivering in our program has remained fairly constant over the last 10 years, the number of cocaine-using women presenting to the Perinatal Center for Chemical Dependence has continued to escalate. Recent data from our clinic confirm that cocaine rapidly crosses the placenta. Infants born to mothers who have used cocaine 1 to 2 days prior to delivery excrete unchanged cocaine 12 to 24 hours after delivery and continue to excrete benzoylecgonine, a cocaine metabolite, for up to 5 days [10]. By comparison, cocaine and its metabolites persist in the urine of the adult user for up to 60 hours after intranasal use [11]. The persistence of benzoylecgonine in the neonates' urines for 5 days is evidence for slow metabolism of cocaine by the neonate, probably due to the immaturity or relative deficiency of plasma cholinesterases and hepatic enzymes in the newborn infant.

As in other substance-abusing populations, cocaine-addicted women have a high incidence of infectious disease complications, especially hepatitis and venereal disease. There is an increase in complications of labor and delivery in cocaine-using women, so that precipitous delivery, abruptio placentae (usually occurring shortly after administration of cocaine), evidence of fetal monitor abnormalities, and fetal meconium staining are present in a significant number of pregnancies complicated by cocaine use [12,13]. Gestational age tends to be slightly lower for cocaine-exposed infants, and neonatal birth weight, length, and head circumference are smaller compared with growth parameters for drug-free infants [13]. Newborns who have been exposed to cocaine exhibit a high degree of irritability and tremulousness, with a deficiency in state control [12]. The neurobehavioral changes for cocaine-exposed infants are in some areas more severe than changes noted for methadone-exposed infants.

Cocaine acts peripherally to inhibit nerve conduction and prevent dopamine and norepinephrine reuptake at presynaptic nerve terminals, producing an increase in catecholamine levels with subsequent vasoconstriction and tachycardia and a concomitant abrupt rise in blood pressure. Placental vasoconstriction also occurs, decreasing blood flow to the fetus. With increased norepinephrine levels, an increase in uterine contractility has been reported in human beings [14]. The increased incidence of precipitous labor, abruptio placentae, and premature labor in cocaine-complicated pregnancies in consistent with these pharmacologic actions of cocaine. Intrauterine growth retardation would also be expected to occur in these infants, given the intermittent impairment of placental blood flow due to the vasoconstrictive action of cocaine.

Maternal problems at delivery are reflected in the high rate of fetal distress noted in the cocaine-exposed infants, as manifested by fetal monitor abnormalities and fetal meconium staining. Perinatal cerebral infarctions have occurred in infants whose mothers have used cocaine over the few days prior to delivery [10]. These perinatal cerebral infarctions are a severe example of the morbidity associated with intrauterine exposure to cocaine and are similar to intracerebral insults reported in adults who use cocaine.

ALCOHOL

Multiple case reports and studies have confirmed the existence of the fetal alcohol syndrome (FAS). Unlike other forms of substance abuse, FAS is a clinically observable entity with specific parameters for its diagnosis. Nonetheless, there remain major areas of controversy surrounding the clinical management of pregnant alcoholic women and the precise assessment of the impact of alcohol use during pregnancy on the developing fetus and child.

The reported pattern of anomalies in offspring from alcoholic pregnancies is consistent in three particular parameters. These three parameters make up the primary presentation of the FAS: (1) prenatal growth deficiency in length and weight, (2) microcephaly, and (3) short palpebral fissures.

The facial similarities of infants and children with FAS are due to a cluster of features associated with midfacial hypoplasia. Short palpebral fissures are often due to microophthalmia. Other facial characteristics associated with FAS include epicanthal folds, flat nasal bridge with a short upturned nose, indistinct philtrum, thin vermillion border of the upper lip, hypoplastic maxilla, and flattened midface.

Mild to moderate mental retardation is reported frequently, with average IQ scores being around 68, although the range is quite wide. Delayed motor and language development is recognized in early infancy in most cases, and there is no improvement in developmental abilities as the child matures. Hyperactivity, hyperacusis, hypotonia, and tremulousness are commonly described in young FAS infants, and symptoms of withdrawal similar to those of narcotic abstinence in neonates have also been noted. Evaluation of infants born to alcoholic mothers has revealed that they have lower levels of arousal, have poor habituation, and are more restless and irritable than drug-free infants.

Since the full FAS is seen in only some offspring of chronic alcoholic women, it is reasonable to suspect that a less severe outcome may occur in other children of overtly alcoholic women and in some infants of women who drink moderately as well. In recent years, it has been recognized that some infants of frankly alcoholic mothers escape the stigmata of FAS while others have only a few of the characteristics. Infants with only partial expression are thought to display fetal alcohol effects. A simple alcohol dose/response relationship is thus not the answer to the complex issues surrounding the etiology of FAS.

SECONDARY DRUG USE

The association between drug or alcohol use and cigarette smoking has been repeatedly observed, and the effects of cigarette smoking on the developing fetus must be considered in any consideration of an infant being evaluated for intrauterine exposure to drugs of abuse. Women who smoke have infants with significantly lower birth weights than nonsmoking women; however, no increase in rate of neonatal mortality or occurrence of congenital anomalies has been observed in these infants. Of interest, among the many studies relating smoking and low birth weight, none took into account that smoking itself was associated with heavier alcohol use; this could have contributed a significant portion of the variance in birth weight.

Use of additional drugs, especially marijuana and caffeine, further complicates the evaluation of the effects of drugs on the fetus. Many commonly used liquid preparations, including cough syrups, mouthwashes, and alcohol-based "tonics," contain appreciable amounts of alcohol. Their use and abuse have been associated with changes consistent with FAS. Additionally, alcohol is frequently a secondary drug of abuse among opiate-using women. Among women enrolled in our program, 25% of heroin-using women have evidence of concomitant alcohol use.

Special Problems

A 5- to 10-fold increase in rate of sudden infant death syndrome (SIDS) occurs among children born to heroin-abusing mothers [15]. At the Perinatal Center for Chemical Dependence, we have observed a 4% rate of SIDS deaths among infants delivered to women on low-dose methadone maintenance. However, concomitant with the abrupt rise in the numbers of pregnant cocaine-abusing women enrolling in our program during the past 2 years, increases in the rate of SIDS have also been observed. In a preliminary study of 60 cocaine-exposed infants, 15% of the infants died of SIDS. Thus, all infants delivered to substance-abusing women in our program receive intervention either with assessment of sleep cardiorespiratory status (pneumogram) or with home monitoring. These procedures are utilized as an attempt to prevent SIDS among this high-risk population.

Infants born to IV drug-using mothers have more frequent infections than infants of oral drug-abusing mothers or drug-free infants. In a sample of infants under the age of 1 year enrolled in our program, the proportion of infants with an illness was greater in the offspring of IV-addicted mothers than in those of oral drug abusers or nonaddicted mothers. The number of episodes of illness was also increased among infants of IV-addicted mothers. Some of the illnesses were the clinical manifestations resulting from exposure to specific organisms (*Chlamydia* pneumonia, thrush, *Monilia* diaper rash), while others were caused by a spectrum of microorganisms (bronchiolitis, otitis). Of note is the finding that the thrush in these patients was qualitatively different than the thrush in these patients was qualitatively different than the thrush usually observed in nondrug-exposed infants. It was more severe and persisted for a longer time, despite the use of conventional antifungal therapy. These observations suggest a possible immune defect, although none of these infants has as yet developed severe opportunistic infections or acquired immune deficiency syndrome (AIDS). Immunologic studies, however, have not been performed in a systematic manner.

Long-Term Follow-up

Little reliable information regarding long-term outcome of infants passively exposed to drugs of abuse is available. To best evaluate these children at school age, environmental factors must be taken into account. These environmental factors are not only socioeconomic but should include aspects of the maternal-infant relationship, including maternal psychopathology and personality. One study that did attempt to control for the caretaking environment of substance-exposed children compared these infants with those whose families began to use drugs after the birth of the children [16]. No differences were found between the in-utero-exposed children and the children exposed to the social environment of drug-using caretakers. Further studies are needed before final conclusions can be drawn as to the long-term effects of in utero drug exposure on infant and child development.

The problems involved in evaluating the effects of maternal exposure to substances of abuse on the developing fetus and infant are multiple, not the least of which are the difficulties involved in following these infants over a long period of time. The chaotic and transient nature of the drug-seeking environment impairs the intensive follow-up and early intervention processes necessary to ensure maximum development by each infant. In addition, most women from substance-abusing backgrounds lack a proper model for parenting. These factors, compounded by the early neurobehavioral deficits of the drug-exposed newborns, earmark these infants to be at high risk for continuing developmental and later school problems.

REFERENCES

1. Jones KL, Smith DW, Ulleland CW, et al: Pattern of malformation in offspring of alcoholic mothers. *Lancet* **1**:1267–1271, 1973.
2. Finnegan LP, Connaughton JF, Kron RE, et al: Neonatal abstinence syndrome: Assessment and management. In Harbison RD (Ed): *Perinatal Addiction.* New York: Spectrum, 1975, pp. 141–158.
3. Chasnoff IJ, Schnoll SH, Burns WJ, et al: Maternal nonnarcotic substance abuse during pregnancy: Effects on infant development. *Neurobehav Toxicol Teratol* **6**:277–280, 1984.
4. Fishburne PM: National survey on drug abuse: Main findings 1979. Rockville, Md.: National Institute on Drug Abuse, 1980 (DHHS Publication No. ADM80-976).
5. Chasnoff IJ, Burns WJ: The Moro reaction: A scoring system for neonatal narcotic withdrawal. *Develop Med Child Neurol* **26**:484–489, 1984.
6. Kron RE, Litt M, Phoenix MD, et al: Neonatal narcotic abstinence: Effects of pharmacotherapeutic agents and maternal drug usage on nutrative sucking behavior. *J Pediatr* **88**:637–641, 1976.
7. Kandall SR: Late complications in passively addicted infants. In Rementeria JO (Ed): *Drug Abuse in Pregnancy and the Neonate.* St. Louis: CV Mosby, 1977, p. 116.
8. Chasnoff IJ, Burns KA, Burns WJ, et al: Prenatal drug exposure: Effects on neonatal and infant growth and development. *Neurobehav Toxicol Teratol* **8**:357–362, 1986.
9. Chasnoff IJ, Burns WJ, Hatcher R: Polydrug- and methadone-addicted newborns: A continuum of impairment? *Pediatrics* **70**:210–213, 1982.
10. Chasnoff IJ, Bussey M, Savich R, et al: Perinatal cerebral infarction and maternal cocaine use. *J Pediatr* **108**:456–459, 1986.

11. Ambre J: The urinary excretion of cocaine and metabolites in humans. *J Analyt Toxicol* **9**:241–245, 1985.
12. Chasnoff IJ, Burns WJ, Schnoll SH, et al: Cocaine use in pregnancy. *N Engl J Med* **313**:666–669, 1985.
13. Chasnoff IJ: Cocaine use in pregnancy: Perinatal morbidity and mortality. *Neurotox Teratol* **9**:291–293, 1987.
14. Lederman RP, Lederman E, Work BA Jr, et al: The relationship of maternal anxiety, plasma catecholamines, and plasma cortisol to progress in labor. *Am J Obstet Gynecol* **132**:495–500, 1978.
15. Chavez CJ, Ostrea EM Jr, Stryker JC, et al: Sudden infant death syndrome among infants of drug-dependent mothers. *J Pediatr* **95**:407–409, 1979.
16. Wilson GW, McCreary R, Kean J, et al: The development of preschool children of heroin-addicted mothers: A controlled study. *Pediatrics* **63**:135–141, 1979.

5
The Use of Transcutaneous Nerve Stimulation in the First Stage of Labor

PATRICE KLEIN PEREZ AND
KATHLEEN CONVERY HANOLD

A safe assumption is that women in labor experience pain to some degree. Pain results from cervical dilatation, uterine contractions, and distention and pressure on tissues [1,2]. The stress of the experience and the persistent pain affects the spinal segmental and suprasegmental reflex responses. This results in alteration of bodily functions such as ventilation, circulation, and endocrine activity [2]. Catecholamine release, particularly norepinephrine, is exaggerated and can lead to a 35 to 70% reduction in blood flow to the uterus [2]. Persistent pain in labor, if not alleviated, can contribute to uterine dysfunction, vasoconstriction, fetal hypoxia, and poor perception of the childbirth process [1]. A study of methods that modulate pain in laboring women is therefore indicated.

Historically, pain relief in labor has been multifaceted, ranging from psychoprophylaxis to the utilization of narcotic analgesics, amnesic drugs, and inhalation anesthesia. A multitude of techniques are employed in meeting the unique needs of the woman in labor. Because of the various physical and psychological considerations affecting patient response, different approaches to pain in labor have been examined. With any approach, a balance has to be maintained between humane pain relief and maternal and fetal safety. One method offering this balance is trancutaneous nerve stimulation (TENS). Limited studies have described the efficacy of TENS in the parturient woman, and further investigation is indicated [3–7].

A multitude of factors affect pain in labor. Among them are patient personality, previous experience, availability or lack of support person(s), cultural and educational background, anxiety level, physical response to labor, parity fetal size, and fetus position [1].

The perception of pain in labor is thought to also be influenced by social conditioning. Dick-Read first described the fear-pain-tension cycle in 1933. He believed women anticipate labor with fear and anxiety due to ignorance, prejudice, and misinformation. The resulting emotional tension increases muscle tension, including the lower uterine segment. This can induce pain and may impede cervical dilatation. With arrested cervical dilatation pain continues and labor is prolonged [8]. Many psychoprophylactic strategies to relieve tension have been derived from Dick-Read's beliefs.

Physiologically, the pain of uterine contractions is caused by cervical stretching, distention of the lower uterine segment, ischemia of the muscle fibers, and traction on the ligaments supporting the uterus [9]. Noxious impulses from the cervix and uterus are transmitted to the spinal cord via A delta and C afferent (sympathetic) nerve fibers through the uterine and cervical plexus, lumbar and thoracic sympathetic chains to the white rami [2]. The pain from these impulses is referred to the abdomen and back at spinal segments T-10 to L-1 in the first stage of labor and S-2 to S-4 in the second stage of labor [3].

It is in this area of neural transmission that TENS offers promise in the modulation of pain in labor. TENS is thought to provide a counter-stimulation to "block" the "gate" of neural transmission described by Melzak and Wall's gate control theory of pain [6]. It is hypothesized to stimulate large afferent fibers and to prevent the transmission of small carrying C fibers to the brain [6]. TENS operates by emitting low-frequency pulsed electrical waves that interfere with pain transference through the substantia gelatinosa and stimulate an increase in naturally occurring beta endorphins [10].

TENS is a therapeutic alternative that offers pain relief without systemic pharmaceutical use or restraint of patient mobility. Its use in the laboring woman provides noninvasive pain modulation, optimal maternal and fetal safety, and the opportunity for patient control. The patient can adjust the intensity of the pulsations to maximize her comfort. Other advantages include the possibility of continued ambulation due to the compact size of the TENS unit. The unit may be clipped onto clothing or monitor belts.

The battery-operated TENS unit consists of four parameters. The *pulse width* is the duration of electrical stimulation or "pulses." It is measured in microseconds. The *pulse rate* determines the number of pulses released each second from the unit. It is measured in pulses per second (pps). The *mode* describes the type of stimulus the machine delivers. Examples include standard, the constant steady delivery of stimulation, or cycle burst, an intermittent delivery of stimulation. These parameters are generally preset and unavailable to patient manipulation.

The *intensity* of the stimulus is controlled by the patient. Some units contain two channels, each adjusted separately. Settings used for the relief of acute pain would be indicated for the laboring patient. The electrodes are applied to the back in the areas correlating to T-10 to L-1 for the first stage and S-2 to S-4 for the second stage of labor. The electrodes should be cross-channeled for maximum distribution of the current. This provides for a fairly equal stimulation to both sides, which is more comfortable as well as more effective.

For application of the electrodes, a variety of landmarks are used. The root of the spine of the scapula corresponds to T-3. After locating this by palpation one can count down seven vertebrae to arrive at T-10. The iliac crest corresponds to L-4. L-1 is located by palpating up four vertebrae. The electrodes are then applied with any conducting gel and secured with hypoallergenic tape.

After the electrodes have been secured, the intensity is adjusted so the patient feels a tingling sensation. This should not be uncomfortable or painful. A second unit may be applied if second stage use is desired. The S-2 segment is located at the level of the posterior superior iliac spines or "dimples." S-4 will be located by palpating down two vertebrae. Cross-channeling should also be employed here.

TENS is well recognized for its effectiveness in pain relief [11–14] and has wide applicability outside obstetrics [15]. For many years it has been used successfully in chronic and acute postoperative pain. TENS has been found to have a placebo effect in chronic pain patients. This effect is comparable to that found in double-blind studies of medications [16].

Research with TENS in labor has described pain relief in vague terms such as "minimal or no" relief, "moderate to some" relief, and "good" relief [3,6,7]. In general, the studies available [3–7] are few in number, are poorly controlled, and utilize small numbers of patients.

European clinical trials utilizing TENS in labor were first described by Augustinsson et al in Sweden in 1977 [3]. A convenience sample of 147 women (90 primiparae, 57 multiparae) without selection criteria was used. TENS was applied via thoracic electrodes during the first stage of labor, with sacral stimulation added later. Conventional pain relief measures were available. Patients responded to a questionnaire a few hours post delivery. Sixty-five (44%) of the women reported TENS provided good to very good relief, 65 (44%) reported moderate relief, and 17 (12%) reported no effect. Supplemental anesthesia was administered to 50 to 75% of the women. TENS was not found to be helpful in the second stage of labor. The patients reported that TENS interfered with voluntary expulsive efforts. No material or neonatal complications occurred.

In clinical trials at Oxford, England, Robson [6] studied 35 women (13 primiparae, 22 multiparae) in labor. He reported that for the first stage of labor, 20% of the patients found TENS to be of "great benefit" but required an additional analgesia. The remaining 80% reported obtaining "some" to "considerable" relief. They received supplementary analgesia. "Few" mothers obtained any benefit from TENS in the second stage of labor. TENS was helpful in relieving low backache in 21 of the women.

Stewart [7] reported on TENS use in labor in 54 women in Scotland. Patients were offered TENS for "early labor" (undefined) or if admitted for induction. Of this group, 16 (23–25%) received considerable pain relief, 38 (55–59%) received some help, and of this 5 (7%) required no additional analgesia. Again TENS was not found helpful in the second stage of labor.

Bundsen et al [4] applied TENS to 24 women with induction of labor in a randomized prospective study of pain relief in labor. The control group ($n=9$) used only conventional pain relief measures (nitrous oxide-oxygen; pethidine). The TENS group ($n=5$) also had the option for the use of conventional methods. Low back pain was assessed hourly during the first stage of labor. The subjects rated the intensity of their pain each hour using a 5-point ordinal scale ("no pain" to "almost unbearable pain") and completed a postpartum interview. Pain relief was attributed to TENS on the basis of a decrease in use of nitrous oxide in the TENS group and reports of less low back pain. The TENS group reported minimal or moderate low back pain throughout labor, while the control group felt an increasing intensity of low back pain as labor progressed. The effect of suprapubic pain was insignificant in both groups. The newborns were evaluated on the basis of Apgar score, blood lactate level, plasma hypoxanthine level, cord blood gas analysis, and neurobehavioral assessment.

Bundsen and Erickson [5] applied TENS to 15 laboring women to study its safety aspects. In the absence of an applicable safety standard, they attempted to determine current density that constitutes an adequate safety measure for the fetal heart when used to stimulate tissue. Results of this study indicated current densities should not exceed 0.5 $\mu A/mm^2$ when used with laboring patients and the electrodes applied to the low back/suprapubic regions.

In addition to the analgesic effects of TENS, the literature also reports that TENS may decrease the length of labor. Severe pain and anxiety during human labor causes an increase in catecholamine release [17]. Epinephrine inhibits contractility, diminishing the frequency and amplitude of contractions. Norepinephrine augments uterine activity by increasing the frequency and amplitude of contractions, although these contractions are not well coordinated [18]. Inhibition or modulation of pain diminishes the catecholamine release response. Therefore, TENS is postulated to decrease the length of labor by virtue of its pain-modulating effect.

Bundsen et al [5] reported the interval from 5 cm dilatation to delivery was 2.3 hours ($\pm$ 1.5 hours) in the TENS group compared with 2.7 hours ($\pm$ 2.3 hours) in the control group. These results were not statistically significant. The cervical status of the control group patients was more favorable, as determined by a modified Bishops score, and these patients displayed faster dilatation to 5 cm. The TENS group, however, experienced a more rapid dilatation from 5 to 10 cm and from 10 cm to birth.

Stewart reported shorter labors (undefined) for patients using TENS [7]. Patients not requiring other forms of analgesia were reported to have shorter labors. The need for minimal analgesia could be attributed to the shorter duration of labor rather than or in addition to the effectiveness of TENS.

The literature on TENS research in laboring women reflects a need for further objective evaluation of its pain-modulating effects. Although the studies cited suggest TENS is effective for achieving some pain relief in labor, they lack objective data regarding the nature of psychometric properties of the instruments used to measure pain or pain relief. In addition, evaluation is without exception based on recall and includes this source of error or bias with postpartum interview. No comparable measures of pain assessment were used in these studies, making it difficult to determine overall efficacy of TENS for labor management.

Confounding variables, such as the use of supplemental analgesia/anesthesia, lack of patient selection criteria, and homogeneity of groups, were not objectively evaluated. Other data that are lacking include comparison groups (except Bundsen et al), demographic data, childbirth preparation status, and definition of variables. The literature suggests that TENS is safe for mother and infant, reporting only minor skin irritations from hypersensitivity to the electrode gel or tape as sequelae.

To further evaluate the effect of TENS on laboring women, a prospective experimental study was designed. The study was conducted in the labor and delivery area of a large midwestern perinatal center. This center provides care to a largely indigent, high-risk (85%) population with approximately 4,000 deliveries annually. Twenty-four-hour anesthesia services are available with epidural and paracervical anesthesia and meperedine analgesia available for pain control during labor. Because this population is predominantly high risk, however, minimal supplementary anesthesia/analgesia is administered due to associated maternal and fetal risks. For this reason, TENS research was appropriate and promising as an adjunctive, safe method for pain relief in this setting.

Criteria for selection included confirmation of a low-risk pregnancy and early but established labor (3–4 cm cervical dilatation, uterine contractions every 2–3 minutes with 50–60 second duration). Exclusion criteria included previous cesarean section, evidence of fetal abnormalities (meconium-stained amniotic fluid, variable or late decelerations), prematurity (less than 37 weeks' gestation), advanced labor (cervical dilatation greater than 5–6 cm), and the planned use of epidural anesthesia.

The women approached for the study were offered an explanation and demonstration of the TENS unit. Informed consent for study participation was obtained before active labor ensued. Those consenting were randomly assigned to an experimental TENS, a placebo (the TENS apparatus without batteries), or a control group. The control group received no TENS unit. All three groups agreed to blood pressure and pulse measurements taken 30 minutes prior to the placement of the unit and every 30 minutes thereafter. Patients were informed that supplementary analgesia would be available to them with a physician's order if they so desired. Those requesting epidural anesthesia would be dropped from the study. TENS could be discontinued at any time upon patient request.

TENS application for the experimental group included blocking of segments T-10 to L-1 and S-2 to S-4 with TENS units. Stimulation parameters were set in accordance with acute pain recommendations (pulse rate 50–

100 Hz, pulse width 40–75 μs, cycle burst constant). Intensity was patient controlled, varying with comfort. Data were also collected on all medications (pain and/or any others), gravity and parity, location of pain, length of labor, and infant's Apgar score. TENS was discontinued if indicated by altered maternal status (preeclampsia, chorioamnionitis, decision to deliver by cesarean section) or fetal status (fetal distress or meconium staining).

Blood pressure and pulse were selected as measures for their proven validity and reliability. Physiologic responses accompany the experience of pain as a result of the activation of the autonomic nervous system [8]. Blood pressure and pulse will increase with sympathetic stimulation and the release of norepinephrine. Human studies with nonmedicated primigravidae in labor have demonstrated a 50 to 150% increase in cardiac output with a resultant 20 to 40% increase in blood pressure [17]. Therefore the pain-modulation effects of TENS may be demonstrated by changes in mean arterial pressure.

The sample consisted of 42 women among the TENS, placebo, and control groups ($n = 8$, $n = 12$, $n = 12$, respectively). The groups were found to be homogeneous for race, age, gravidity, length of gestation, childbirth preparation, and location of pain, based on chi-square analysis ($P > 0.05$). Statistics indicated randomness was achieved. Only 26% (11 of 42; $n = 3$, $n = 5$, $n = 3$) required additional analgesia. Pitocin augmentation was utilized by 14% (6 of 42; $n = 2$, $n = 3$, $n = 1$) of the women. Only 4 of 42 (9%) had any childbirth preparation.

Length of labor for the first stage was compared among the three groups using the one-way ANOVA test. Differences were not significant even though the data appeared to indicate a shorter first stage. The relatively small sample size may have influenced this statistic.

Mean arterial pressure and pulse were compared by *T*-test for indications of pain relief. Although individual responses appeared favorable, the results were not statistically significant.

Anecdotally, the patients rated TENS very well overall. Several patients reported TENS helped low back pain and was a pleasant sensation. Two patients felt the stimulation was unpleasant. Those who left the unit on through the second stage of labor (3 of 42) felt the stimulation confused and interfered with expulsive effort.

This study had several limitations. Mean arterial changes, although not significant in this study, might reflect pain relief with a larger sample size. A difficulty in maintaining standardized measures of blood pressure and pulse was experienced. With advancing labor and parturient discomfort, it often becomes difficult to use the same extremity and position for auscultation. This may or may not have confounded the results.

Another variable requiring further research with TENS is childbirth preparation. It may be postulated that with advance preparation, an increasing understanding of the dynamics of the birth process would result, with a concomitant decrease in anxiety. If TENS was introduced prior to labor it might be more effective in decreasing anxiety.

Other TENS research might involve time of application and efficacy. Perhaps TENS might be more effective if applied during the latent phase as opposed to the active phase. Pain modulation could begin before the increasing discomfort of active labor. The patient, being more in control and less apprehensive, might derive more benefit from TENS at this time.

Finally, a greater sample size would benefit further TENS research. The potential is here, and further investigation is both warranted and necessary. TENS could be an alternative treatment if anesthesia services are unavailable. Nurses and nurse midwives can administer and utilize it to support their patients. Parturient women desiring control yet not wanting pain medication would benefit from TENS. It should be stressed that TENS will not stop the pain but rather minimizes the sensation perceived and facilitates control. TENS may alter obstetric pain control in the future.

REFERENCES

1. Roberts JE: Factors influencing distress from pain during labor. *MCN* **8**:62–66, 1983.
2. Bonica JJ: Peripheral mechanisms and pathways of parturient pain. *Br J Anes* **51**:3–85, 1979.
3. Augustinsson LE, Bohlin P, Bundsen P, et al: Pain relief during delivery by transcutaneous electrical nerve stimulation. *Pain* **4**:59–65, 1977.
4. Bundsen P, Peterson LE, Selstam U: Pain relief in labour by transcutaneous electrical nerve stimulation: Evaluation of the newborn. *Acta Obstet Gynecol Scand* **1**:129–136, 1982.
5. Bundsen P, Erickson K: Pain relief in labor by transcutaneous electrical nerve stimulation: Safety aspects. *Acta Obstet Gynecol Scand* **1**:1–5, 1982.
6. Robson J: Transcutaneous nerve stimulation for pain relief in labor. *Anesthesia* **34**:357–360, 1979.
7. Stewart P: Transcutaneous electrical nerve stimulation as a method of analgesia in labour. *Anesthesia* **34**:361–364, 1979.
8. Jacox A: *Pain: A Source Book for Nurses and Other Health Professionals.* Boston: Little, Borwn, 1977.
9. Abouleish E: Pain control in obstetrics. Philadelphia: JB Lippincott, 1977.
10. Solomon RA, Viernstein MC, Long DM: Reduction of postoperative pain and narcotic use by transcutaneous nerve stimulation. *Surgery* **2**:142–146, 1980.
11. Hampe G: Introduction to the use of transcutaneous electrical nerve stimulation. *Phys Ther* **12**:1450–1454, 1978.
12. Melzak R: Prolonged relief of pain by brief, intense, transcutaneous somatic stimulation. *Pain* **1**:357–373, 1975.
13. Taylor AG, West BA, Simon B, et al: How effective is TENS for acute pain? *Am J Nurs* **8**:1171–1178, 1983.
14. Tyler G, Caldwell C, Ghia NJ: Transcutaneous electrical nerve stimulation: An alternative approach to the management of postoperative pain. *Anes Anal* **5**:49–55, 1982.

15. Brucks MD: Nonpharmaceutical methods for relieving pain and discomfort during pregnancy. *MCN* **9**:390–394, 1984.
16. Thorsteinsson G, Stonnington HH, Stillwell GK, et al: The effect of transcutaneous nerve stimulation. *Pain* **5**:31–41, 1978.
17. Bonica JJ: *Principles and Practice of Obstetric Analgesia and Anesthesia.* 2nd ed. Amsterdam: Netherlands World Federation of Societies of Anesthesiology, 1980.
18. Melzak R, Wall PD: Pain mechanisms: A new theory. *Science.*

6
Prolonged Pregnancy

BRUCE A. HARRIS, JR.

Human pregnancy is generally supposed to be approximately 40 weeks in duration, beginning with the first day of the last menstrual period (LMP) [1]. A substantial number of human pregnancies exceed 40 weeks in length [2]. In about 13% of these pregnancies, fetal mortality or morbidity are encountered [3]. The remaining gestations apparently have little difficulty: In fact, they often tend to produce babies who are larger than average size.

The major difficulties encountered during prolonged pregnancy are intrauterine growth retardation (IUGR), meconium aspiration, and oligohydramnios. The latter often results in umbilical cord compromise. Both IUGR and oligohydramnios are believed to be the result of uteroplacental insufficiency, due basically to progressive incompetence of the aging placenta.

Duration of Human Pregnancy

The average duration of human pregnancy is from 38 to 42 weeks after the LMP. This amounts to 280 days, or about 266 days after conception, assuming that the latter takes place 13 to 14 days after the first day of the LMP. Pregnancy is said to extend beyond 42 weeks in 3.5 to 10% of cases, beyond 43 weeks in 4% of cases, and beyond 44 weeks in 0.4% of cases [4]. However, about 70% of "prolonged pregnancies" may be the result of delayed ovulation [5]. Moreover, there is further evidence to show the unreliability of pregnancy dating [6]. To be 90% certain that a patient will produce an infant at 38 weeks by the best pediatric assessment, the following criteria must be fulfilled:

1. The LMP must have occurred 42 weeks ago.
2. The fetal heart tones (using a standard fetoscope) must have been present for 21 weeks.
3. Fetal motions must have been noted by the patient for 25 weeks.

It will be apparent that very strict criteria are required for the dating of the supposedly prolonged pregnancy. At the University of Alabama at Birmingham, a diagnosis of prolonged pregnancy is made according to the following criteria:

1. A reliable menstrual history indicating that 42 gestational weeks have been completed.
2. Performance of a bimanual pelvic examination before 12 weeks' gestation.
3. Performance of ultrasound examination as early as possible, preferably before 20 weeks.
4. Ability to hear the fetal heart tones (with an unamplified stethoscope) for at least 22 weeks.

A reliable menstrual history is defined to mean that the exact date of the last menstrual period is known, the duration and amount of flow have been normal for the particular patient, and oral contraceptives have not been used within 3 months of that last period. If the menstrual history is reliable, one of the other three criteria is necessary for a definite diagnosis. If the menstrual history is unreliable, a diagnosis of prolonged pregnancy requires that at least two other criteria be consistent with 42 or more weeks.

It will thus be apparent that many "prolonged pregnancies" actually do not fulfill the criteria for this diagnosis. Moreover, studies at the University of Alabama show that the increased use of ultrasonic fetal surveillance in early pregnancy has substantially reduced the *supposed* incidence of postdate pregnancy (R. Goldenberg, unpublished data).

Consequences of Prolonged Pregnancy

PERINATAL MORTALITY

Prolonged pregnancy was originally thought to carry little or no increased risk. However, a study by McClure-Browne [7] involving all births in England and Wales for 3 months in 1965 showed perinatal mortality rates twice as high at 44 weeks as at term. (Nevertheless, 95% of babies delivered at 44 weeks survived, at least initially.) Of postdate babies who die, 30% die before the onset of labor, 55% during labor, and 15% following delivery [4], with the death rate being slightly higher in male fetuses. Perinatal death is principally due to meconium aspiration or cord complications, [8] or generalized wasting (IUGR).

PERINATAL MORBIDITY

It has been supposed that gradual placental senescence takes place as pregnancy continues beyond term [4]. The placental growth rate declines with age, although placental growth continues. The fetal growth rate declines. Most important, the amniotic fluid volume declines markedly after 38 weeks' gestation [9]. An infant with the full-blown "postmaturity syndrome" (PMS) shows the stigmata of intrauterine malnutrition [10]. These include wasting, heavy meconium staining, peeling of skin, and inability to maintain body temperature.

These changes are thought to be the result of placental dysfunction. The placenta in postterm patients has been described as showing white "infarcts," fibrin deposition, and calcification [11]. The villi are said to show diminished vascularity and increased fibrosis, and intervillous thrombosis is described. The rate of increase in the nuclei of the aging placenta is diminished [12].

Placental study in the postdate pregnancy has been relatively unrewarding because of the heterogeneity of the organ. All the changes just described may be seen in a normal-term placenta. At present, there do not appear to be any pathognomonic changes in the postterm placenta.

In IUGR the placenta is small, with significantly less surface area for exchange between mother and fetus than the normal-sized placenta. The total number of cells in the placentae of growth-retarded infants in markedly decreased [13]. Studies of a similar nature have not been performed in postdate placentae, but the baby showing PMS frequently exhibits the stigmata of intrauterine growth retardation.

A particular concern in postdate pregnancy is the presence of meconium in the amniotic fluid. This complication occurs in about 22% of term fetuses. The percentage is even larger in the postterm pregnancy. Meconium per se is not a sign of fetal distress unless it is associated with a non-reassuring electronic monitor tracing [3]. Nevertheless, the presence of amniotic fluid meconium poses a constant hazard, because of the possibility of intrapartum fetal meconium aspiration [8]. Fetal death in utero or severe intrapartum fetal distress is thought to be the result of hypoxia consequent to placental insufficiency. Fetal compromise may also result from umbilical cord compression consequent to oligohydramnios. The latter is due primarily to diminution of output of fetal urine and fetal pulmonary fluid, consequent to diminished transfer of water across the aging placenta as well as to fetal renal and pulmonary dysfunction due to hypoxia.

Onset of Human Labor

The exact mechanism of the onset of human labor is unknown. Therefore the etiology of prolonged pregnancy is equally obscure. It appears that the fetus may in some way produce a signal that triggers the contractions of true labor [14]. The route of transfer of this signal may be via the amniotic fluid, which in turn affects the membranes and decidua. It now seems generally agreed that arachidonic acid metabolites, principally prostaglandins, serve importantly in the stimulation of labor [15].

The amnion synthesizes prostaglandin essentially to the exclusion of other prostaglandins. The obligatory precursor of all prostaglandins of the 2-series is arachidonic acid, which in turn appears to be derived from precursors in the amniotic fluid [16]. These precursors are acted upon by phospholipase A_2 and phospholipase C, as well as other substances found in fetal urine; these reactions involve calcium ion.

The decidua synthesizes PGE_2 and PGF_2-alpha; myometrium produces PGI_2 [17]. The latter, contrary to the other prostaglandins, tends to suppress uterine contractions.

Coordinated myometrial action is apparently made possible by the formation of gap junctions, or intercellular bridges, between myometrial muscle cells [18]. Formation of gap junctions is dependent upon the presence of estrogen and PGF_2-alpha.

Production of PGI_2 during pregnancy *may* act as a sedative to the myometrium. Production of large amounts of corticosteroids during labor may block this synthesis, without blocking the release of PGE_2 and PGF_2-alpha from amnion and decidua, which are not corticosteroid sensitive.

What triggers the release of the signal from fetus to mother? The onset of human labor appears related in some way to the fetal adrenal. For example, fetuses with reduced amounts of adrenal tissue are often carried well beyond the expected date of confinement [19]. However, administration of corticoids to the postterm gravida has had an inconsistent effect [20]. Human parturition is preceded by a progressive increase in plasma estradiol concentrations during the final 6 weeks of pregnancy [21]. When placental estrogen production is low, prolongation of gestation is noted [20]. Estrogen and prostaglandins are apparently *both* required for the formation of myometrial gap junctions [18]. Finally, oxytocin appears to be a secondary, not a primary, agent in human labor, since plasma oxytocin levels of both mother and fetus rise only *after* the onset of labor.

In summary, it appears that the myometrium must be primed by increasing estrogen levels. Concurrently, local progesterone withdrawal is accomplished by a progesterone-binding protein that is elaborated by the fetal membranes in late pregnancy [14]. A fetal signal, perhaps from the adrenal, may trigger the release of phospholipases C and A_2, which in the presence of calcium ions may act upon prostaglandin precursors in the amniotic fluid. Estrogen and prostaglandins act to facilitate gap junction formation; this in turn permits coordinated myometrial activity under the influence of prostaglandins.

How and why the fetal signals fails to be transmitted in prolonged pregnancy is a matter of speculation. Perhaps an additional factor is needed. For example, most postterm babies are simply large fetuses. It may be that the smaller fetus fits more easily into the pelvis before labor, and that the consequent distention of the cervix sets up some sort of reflex arc.

On the other hand, the typical wasted baby with PMS does not fit this description. Perhaps corticoid production in these fetuses is in some way deficient.

Dating the Pregnancy

Exact determination of gestational age is desirable. The following criteria apply:

Determinant	Considerations, Pro and Con
Last menstrual period	Frequency of irregular cycles may cause error. Oral contraceptive use may cause amenorrhea
Basal body temperature chart, date of conception	Highly valuable if available
Initial examination	Useful if examiner experienced and findings well recorded
Uterine growth	Highly subjective
Quickening	Highly subjective
Fetal heart tones	Reliable if fetal heart tones have been audible for at least 20 weeks with non amplified stethoscope
Adjusted ultrasonographic age	Highly reliable if observations made sufficiently early in pregnancy

At the University of Alabama the pregnancy is dated by sonography insofar as possible. Some sonographic criteria are as follows:

First trimester	Sac at 4 weeks
	Fetal movements at 7 weeks
	Fetal heart action at 5–7 weeks
	Crown-rump length at 10 weeks (accurate within ± 1 to 3 days)
Second, third trimesters	Biparietal diameter at 20–26 weeks (± 11 days' accuracy)
	Femur length (up to 36 weeks) (± 10 days' accuracy)
	Growth-adjusted sonographic age (± 3 days' accuracy)

Fetal Assessment in Prolonged Pregnancy

It is generally agreed that pregnancy should be regarded as prolonged and worthy of special consideration when 42 weeks of gestation have been completed, according to the very best criteria. Recently several eminent perinatologists have suggested that 41, rather than 42, weeks be used as the guideline (J. Hauth, personal communication).

Estriol production, measured both in maternal urine as the conjugated form and in maternal serum as unconjugated estriol, has been used extensively in fetal evaluation [22]. Maternal estriol production is a measure of the function of the fetal adrenal glands and of the maternal placenta. However, urinary estriol determinations must be done daily. They are clumsy, expensive, and poorly adapted to outpatient care. Finally, a drop in urinary estriol is frequently not observed until the baby's condition has already deteriorated. Kochenour [23] concluded that the measurement of serum unconjugated estriol, rather than urinary estriol, is the most convenient and reliable method of measurement of estrogen metabolites.

Gauthier et al [24] felt that serum unconjugated estriol determinations can be done biweekly. If levels are above 13 ng/ml, the baby usually does well. If levels are below 12 ng/ml, 20% of the fetuses will show distress during labor.

Despite the apparent accuracy of the serum unconjugated estriol measurement, most clinics do not follow postterm patients with estriol determinations alone at this time. The primary usefulness of estrogen assays appears to be to support the decision to postpone delivery until some future date.

In 1974, Hobbins et al [25] proposed measurement of human placental lactogen as a means of monitoring prolonged pregnancy. Subsequent experience has failed to confirm this position. At present, this test is not employed as a measure of fetal well-being in prolonged pregnancy.

Observation of fetal movement has been advocated by Sadovsky et al [26] as a means of evaluating fetal well-being. Diminution of fetal movements has been reported as a response to placental insufficiency. This method may be used as an adjunct to other means of surveillance but appears insufficient in itself; further, it produces marked maternal anxiety.

Manning et al [27,28] pointed out that biophysical monitoring of the fetus has largely replaced older biochemical methods. The availability of high-resolution ultrasound has made close fetal observation possible. Maternal hypoxemia (due to an aging placenta) produces fetal hypoxemia, which in turn produces fetal apnea, diminution in fetal movement, loss of fetal heart rate variability, and diminution of fetal tone. Fetal hypoxemia may also produce diversion of fetal blood supply toward the brain and away from the kidneys, resulting in diminution of fetal urine output and the volume of fetal lung fluid. This, in turn, will be followed by oligohydramnios.

On the basis of these principles, Manning has proposed the fetal biophysical profile. In this profile, results of the nonstress test (NST), fetal breathing movements, fetal tone, fetal movements, and amniotic fluid volume are studied, each variable being scored either 2 or 0. In Manning's series, the probability of abnormal outcome was greatest when all or most tests were abnormal (total score <4). The positive predictive accuracy of a score of 8 or greater was 88.1%.

The criteria used by Manning are as follows:

Fetal breathing movements: At least one episode of 30 seconds' duration in 30 minutes

Movement: At least 3 discrete body/limb movements in 30 minutes

Fetal tone: At least one episode of active extension with return to flexion of fetal limbs(s) or trunk (including opening and closing of hand)

Amniotic fluid volume: At least one pocket of fluid that measures at least 1 cm in two perpendicular planes

Fetal heart reactivity (NST): At least two episodes of acceleration of 15 beats per minute and at least 15 seconds' duration associated with fetal movement in 30 minutes

In a recent study, Manning's group [29] reported 307 postdate pregnancies that were managed using the biophysical profile. There were no stillbirths or perinatal deaths in this group. However, perinatal *morbidity* was by no means elminated.

The presence of meconium in the amniotic fluid has previously been regarded as an ominous sign. However, the presence of meconium per se in the amniotic fluid cannot be reliably correlated with fetal prognosis [3]. Therefore, amniocentesis for meconium presence or amnioscopy for the same purpose probably has no role in the management of prolonged pregnancy.

Contraction stress testing (CST), with the addition of ultrasonic evaluation of amniotic fluid volume, is the principal method of evaluation of the postdate pregnancy at UAB. The following criteria are employed:

Negative:	No late decelerations
Positive:	Late decelerations of at least 5 beats per minute after each contraction in a 10-minute period
Equivocal:	Occasional late decelerations
Hyperstimulation:	Five or more contractions in 10 minutes
Unsatisfactory:	Cannot be interpreted

The last three require repetition within 24 hours.

Disagreement exists as to the type of Electronic Fetal Monitoring to be employed. Freeman and his group have been strong advocates of the CST [30]. In a series of 679 postdate gravidas assessed with weekly CSTs, this group encountered no fetal deaths. Fetal distress occurred in 37% of cases, illustrating that even a negative CST does not guarantee that the fetus will successfully endure the labor process. Further, Pritchard [31] reported a case in which a CST was done three consecutive times during 1 week and was negative each time. However, fetal death in utero ensued.

The NST has also been advocated. In a series by Eden [32], this test was performed twice weekly and supplemented with weekly ultrasonic fetal evaluation. Decelerations of 30 seconds in duration during the NST (whether reactive or nonreactive) and oligohydramnios were indications to effect delivery. A high rate of intervention (24%) and of cesarean delivery (29%) was reported. The authors felt that the reactive NST was at least as good a predictor of immediate normal outcome as a negative CST.

Miyazaki and Miyazaki [33] reported a series of 125 postterm patients with reactive NSTs. They noted a "false reactive" rate of 8%, including four antepartum deaths, one neonatal death, one case of brain damage, and four cases of fetal distress on admission.

If the NST is used as the primary test for following prolonged pregnancies, the importance of variable decelerations must be stressed. Variable decelerations, even in the presence of a reactive NST, are of ominous significance, strongly suggesting oligohydramnios and impending fetal hypoxia due to cord compression.

It is possible that the fetus with oligohydramnios may be subjected to a recurrent series of sublethal, but potentially very damaging, episodes of cord compression. These episodes may pass unnoticed because the mother is not being monitored at the time.

In summary, currently there is no foolproof single method of fetal assessment in the prolonged pregnancy. A combination of biophysical parameters appears to offer the best results, but perinatal morbidity and mortality still occur.

A Suggested Method of Management for Prolonged Pregnancies

The first consideration in dealing with a supposed postdate pregnancy is proper dating. When the pregnancy has reached 42 weeks as computed by the *best possible parameters,* the cervix should be evaluated by the Bishop scoring method [34]. If the Bishop score is 5 or more, induction of labor should be offered to the patient. However, the average Bishop score at 42 weeks is only 3.6 [35]. Moreover, routine weekly attempts at induction, beginning at 42 weeks, do not change the time of delivery [36]. Therefore, induction of labor at 42 weeks is not the answer for most women with prolonged pregnancies.

If the cervix is not favorable for induction (Bishop score of 5 or more), careful ultrasound evaluation is done. A CST should be performed concurrently. If the CST shows variable decelerations, even if negative, delivery should be undertaken. If oligohydramnios is present (defined as no area in which at least 1 cm of amniotic fluid is present), delivery should be undertaken. Induction with oxytocin may be attempted, with very careful monitoring of mother and fetus. Cesarean delivery should be readily available.

If the CST is positive and reactive, delivery should be undertaken. Induction of labor may be attempted, with ready resort to cesarean delivery. If the CST is positive and nonreactive, induction of labor, while feasible, is regarded by many authors as likely to be associated with severe fetal distress. In such a situation elective cesarean section is, in my opinion, the wisest choice.

If a positive nonreactive CST is obtained, the fetus may already be in serious trouble. The patient should be transported immediately to the delivery suite, placed in the left lateral decubitus position, and given oxygen and fluids. If prompt improvement of the tracing does not occur, delivery should be undertaken at once, preferably by C-section.

If the CST is negative, variable decelerations are not noted, and the amniotic fluid volume is satisfactory, the patient may be reevaluated in 1 week's time. However, as time passes, tension grows. At 42 weeks of gestation, the risks and benefits of elective cesarean delivery, versus the risks and benefits of continued pregnancy, should be carefully explained to the patient and her spouse. Every effort should be made to allow the patient to make a fully informed choice between elective delivery and continuation of the pregnancy [37]. No matter how close the surveillance or how skilled the observer, the intricacies of prolonged pregnancy have not yet been entirely solved, and an occasional fetal or neonatal death or injury cannot be completely obviated by any of our current methods of management.

The Conduct of Labor in Prolonged Pregnancy

The fetus who has stayed overlong in the womb is regarded as being at high risk. Labor should be conducted in the left lateral recumbent position—the position in which uterine and renal blood flow are maximal. Leveno and his associates [38] have pointed out that the pathophysiology of intrapartum fetal distress in prolonged pregnancy is related to oligohydramnios and umbilical cord compression. The former is almost certainly the result of placental insufficiency. Accordingly, constant fetal monitoring and ready availability of fluids, oxygen, and skilled nursing care are essential. Cesarean delivery should be possible on very short notice, and skilled neonatal care, as well as intensive-care nursery facilities, should be present in the hospital where labor is conducted. Intrapartum morbidity, according to Freeman [30], is related to episodes of fetal distress and to meconium passage during labor. Meconium passage is very common in postterm fetuses, and per se it does not carry an ominous significance [3]. Nevertheless, the presence of meconium in the amniotic fluid during labor carries the risk of meconium aspiration by the fetus [8]. Any fetus born through meconium, whether vaginally or by cesarean section, should be subjected to careful suctioning of the upper airway as soon as the head is accessible. Directly after birth and clamping of the cord the infant should be handed over to the pediatrician. A laryngoscope should be introduced and the vocal cords visualized. Any meconium above the cords should be removed by careful suctioning; an endotracheal tube should also be introduced and as much meconium sucked out of the pulmonary tree as possible. Successive endotracheal tubes should be passed until no more meconium can be obtained. This may take several tubes. Despite this very thorough airway management, however, fatal meconium aspiration syndrome may still occur, perhaps as the result of aspiration by the fetus in utero. Such aspiration has definitely been proven to occur, both in humans and in experimental animals, if the fetus is sufficiently stressed [8].

A final hazard of labor is the risk of macrosomia. Many postdate babies are simply large babies. This, in turn, raises the specter of shoulder dystocia. The accoucheur who attends a woman in labor with a postdate pregnancy should be well versed in the management of shoulder dystocia and have a plan constantly ready for overcoming this serious complication.

If the postdate infant appears, on good evidence, to exceed 4,000 g in weight, and certainly if it exceeds 4,500 g, cesarean delivery should be very strongly considered.

Care of the Newborn

Delivery of the postdate infant should occur in an institution where skilled neonatal care is readily available. If such care is not present in the primary hospital, transfer of mother and fetus to a level III unit is desirable *prior to delivery.*

The newborn who has been the victim of placental insufficiency, cord compression, and/or meconium aspiration requires expert care. The baby is at risk of dehydration, hypoglycemia, hyperviscosity, acidosis, and cerebral and adrenal hypofunction. All of these are, of course, the stigmata of intrauterine growth retardation—the hallmark of chronic placental insufficiency. Again, skilled neonatal care and a neonatal intensive care unit must be readily available for the treatment of these conditions.

REFERENCES

1. Beischer NA, Evans JM, Townsend L: Studies in prolonged pregnancy. I. The incidence of prolonged pregnancy. *Am J Obstet Gynecol* **103**:476–482, 1968.
2. Resnik R: Post-term pregnancy. In Creasy RK, Resnik I (Eds): *Maternal-Fetal Medicine.* Philadelphia: WB Saunders, 1984, pp. 443–448.
3. Knox GE, Huddleston JF, Flowers CE: Management of prolonged pregnancy: Results of a prospective randomized trial. *Am J Obstet Gynecol* **134**:376–381, 1979.

4. Weingold AB: The management of prolonged pregnancy. In Pitkin RW, Zlatnik FJ (Eds): *Yearbook of Obstetrics and Gynecology, 1982*. Chicago: Year Book Medical Publishers, 1982, pp. 69–86.

5. Stewart HL: Duration of pregnancy and postmaturity. *JAMA* **148**:1079–1083, 1952.

6. Hertz RH, Sokol RJ, Knoke JD, et al: Clinical estimation of gestational age: Rules for avoiding preterm delivery. *Am J Obstet Gynecol* **131**:395–402, 1978.

7. McClure-Browne JC: Postmaturity. *Am J Obstet Gynecol* **85**:573–581, 1963.

8. Davis RO, Philips JB, Harris, Jr BA, et al: Fetal meconium aspiration syndrome occurring despite airway management considered appropriate. *Am J Obstet Gynecol* **151**:721–736, 1985.

9. Vorherr J: Placental insufficiency in relation to pregnancy and fetal postmaturity. *Am J Obstet Gynecol* **123**:67–103, 1975.

10. Clifford S, Postmaturity—with placental dysfunction. *J Pediatr* **44**:1–13, 1954.

11. Siegil P, Raban USW: Die Haufigkeit der sogenannten plazentar Infarkte bei Ubertragungen, Fruhgeburten und schwangerschaftspezifische Erkrangungen. *Zentral Gynakol* **88**:345–350, 1966.

12. Sands J, Dobbing J: Continuing growth and development of the third-trimester human placenta. *Placenta* **6**:13–21, 1985.

13. Teasdale F: Idiopathic intrauterine growth retardation: Histiomorphometry of the human placenta. *Placenta* **5**:83–92, 1984.

14. MacDonald PC, Porter JC, Schwarz GE, et al: Initiation of parturition in the human female. *Semin Perinatol* **2**:273–286, 1978.

15. Casey ML, MacDonald PC: The initiation of labor in women: Regulation of phospholipid and arachidonic acid metabolism and of prostaglandin production. *Semin Perinatol* **10**:270–275, 1986.

16. Okita JR, Johnston JM, MacDonald PC: Source of prostaglandin precursor in human fetal membranes: Arachidonic acid content of amnion and chorion laeve in diamnionic and dichorionic term placentas. *Obstet Gynecol* **147**:477–482, 1983.

17. Abel MH, Kelly RW: Differential production of prostaglandins within the human uterus. *Prostaglandins* **18**:821–828, 1980.

18. Garfield RE, Hayashi RH: Appearance of gap junctions in the myometrium of women during labor. *Am J Obstet Gynecol* **140**:254–260, 1981.

19. Challis JRG, Mitchell BF: Hormonal control of preterm and term parturition. *Semin Perinatol* **5**:192–202, 1981.

20. Liggins GC, Forster CS, Grieves SA, et al: Control of parturition in man. *Biol Reprod* **16**:39–56, 1977.

21. Schwarz BE, Milewich L, Gant NF, et al: Progesterone binding and metabolism in human fetal membranes. *Ann NY Acad Sci* **286**:304–310, 1977.

22. Lundwall F, Staliemann G: The urinary excretion of estriol in postmaturity. *Acta Obstet Gynecol Scand* **45**:301–319, 1966.

23. Kochenour NR: Estrogen assay during pregnancy. *Clin Obstet Gynecol* **25**:659–672, 1983.

24. Gauthier RJ, Griego BD, Goebelsmann LI: Estriol in pregnancy. VII. Unconjugated plasma estriol in prolonged gestation. *Am J Obstet Gynecol* **139**:382–389, 1981.

25. Hobbins JC, Goldstein L, Hofschild J: Value of HCS determination in management of prolonged pregnancy. *Obstet Gynecol* **44**:802–805, 1974.

26. Sadovsky E, Yaffe H, Polishuk ZW: Fetal movement monitoring in normal and pathologic pregnancy. *Int J Gynecol Obstet* **12:**75–80, 1974.
27. Manning FA, Baskett TF, Momson I, et al: Fetal biophysical profile scoring: A prospective study in 1184 high-risk patients. *Am J Obstet Gynecol* **140:**289–294, 1981.
28. Manning FA: Assessment of fetal condition and risk: Analysis of single and combined biophysical variable monitoring. *Semin Perinatol* **9:**168–183, 1985.
29. Johnson JM, Harmon CR, Lange IR, et al: Biophysical profile scoring in the management of the post-term pregnancy. An analysis of 307 patients. *Am J Obstet Gynecol* **154:**269–273, 1986.
30. Freeman RK, Garite TJ, Modanlou H, et al: Postdate pregnancy: Utilization of contraction stress testing for primary fetal surveillance. *Am J Obstet Gynecol* **140:**128–135, 1981.
31. Pritchard JA: In Pritchard JA, MacDonald PC, Gant NR (Eds): *Williams Obstetrics*. 17th ed. Norwalk, Conn.: Appleton-Century-Crofts, 1985, p. 763.
32. Eden RD, Gergely RZ, Schifrin BS, et al: Comparison of antepartum testing schemes for the management of postdate pregnancy. *Am J Obstet Gynecol* **144:**683–692, 1982.
33. Miyazaki FS, Miyazaki BA: False reactive nonstress tests in postterm pregnancies. *Am J Obstet Gynecol* **140:**269–272, 1981.
34. Bishop EH: Pelvic scoring for elective induction. *Obstet Gynecol* **24:**266–268, 1964.
35. Harris BA Jr, Huddleston JF, Sutliff G, et al: The unfavorable cervix in prolonged pregnancy. *Obstet Gynecol* **62:**171–174, 1983.
36. Hauth JC, Goodman MT, Gilstrap LC, et al: Postterm pregnancy. I. *Obstet Gynecol* **56:**467–470, 1980.
37. Feldman GB, Freiman JA: Prophylactic cesarean section at term? *N Engl J Med* **312:**1264–1268, 1985.
38. Leveno KJ, Quirk JG, Cunningham FG, et al: Prolonged pregnancy. I. Observations concerning the causes of fetal distress. *Am J Obstet Gynecol* **150:**465–473, 1984.

7
Hypertension in Pregnancy

Bruce A. Harris, Jr.

Definition

Pregnancy hypertension has been defined in many ways [1,2]. At the University of Alabama at Birmingham, the following criteria are employed:

1. *Blood Pressure:* At least 130/80 mm Hg on two separate occasions, or a rise of 30/15 mm Hg above the previous reading. (Other authors [1] regard 140/90 mm Hg as the upper limit of normal blood pressure in pregnancy. However, many cases of undoubted pregnancy-induced hypertension take place when the maximum blood pressure is below 140/90 mm Hg.)

Hypertension may be the sole necessary criterion for the diagnosis; albuminuria and edema may be present, but not necessarily so. If albuminuria and edema are present, the following criteria apply:

2. *Proteinuria:* 400 mg protein per liter of urine in 24 hours, or more than 1 g/L in two random collections.
3. *Edema:* Must be substantial and must be cephalad to the inguinal ligament.

Classification

Many classifications have been proposed for the hypertension associated with pregnancy. Table 7.1 shows the scheme currently in use at the University of Alabama.

Etiology

The etiology of PIH is uncertain: many theories have been advanced [2]. It is clear that in women afflicted with PIH, sensitivity to vasopressors

TABLE 7.1. Classification of pregnancy hypertension used at the University of Alabama, Birmingham.*

Type	Signs
Pregnancy-induced hypertension (PIH) (also called preeclampsia-eclampsia, acute toxemia)	
Mild	Blood pressure: 30/15 mm Hg rise in blood pressure since last reading Proteinuria (not necessarily present): < 5 g in 24 hours Urine output: > 500 ml in 24 hours Edema: need not be present
Severe	Blood pressure: 160/110 mm Hg (or greater); 60/30 mm Hg rise (or greater) since last reading Proteinuria (usually present): > 5 g in 24 hours Urine output: < 500 ml in 24 hours Evidence of involvement of parenchymatous organs (including blood) Edema: need not be present, but usually is; may reach level of anasarca and/or pulmonary edema
Chronic hypertension† (CH)	Any diastolic blood pressure > 90 mm Hg before 26 weeks of gestation Any diastolic blood pressure ≥ 85 mm Hg before 26 weeks' gestation
PIH Superimposed on CH (also called pregnancy-aggravated hypertension [PAH])	In a patient with known CH, the appearance of albuminuria, signs of parenchymatous organ involvement, or a rise in blood pressure of 30/15 mm Hg or more since last observation

*Another type, "transient" or "gestational hypertension," is often added. We believe this condition represents a manifestation of CH.

†Chronic hypertension may be "essential" or may be due to known pathologic entities such as chronic renal disease of whatever origin.

is markedly increased, while normal pregnant women are resistant to vasopressors [3,4]. This increased sensitivity to vasopressors is noted as early as the 16th week of pregnancy, long before the disease is clinically manifest. It is thus apparent that PIH is actually a chronic disease. If the pregnant patient with PIH is hospitalized, her blood pressure may decline but her sensitivity to pressor agents remains [5].

How is this increased pressor sensitivity mediated? In normal pregnancy, the endothelium, internal elastic lamina, and smooth muscle of the media of the decidual spiral arterioles are replaced by trophoblast and fibrin [6]. These changes extend into the myometrium. This replacement of the muscular coats of the spiral arterioles allows these vessels to dilate and remain dilated under the influence of the maternal blood pressure. In women with PIH, the same changes occur, but to a much more limited extent. The changes are limited to the decidual portions of the spiral arterioles. As a result, the uterine vasculature retains its ability to respond to vasoactive influences.

In PIH, not only do the spiral arterioles retain their ability to respond to vasoactive influences, but they also are reduced in diameter, being only about 40% of the diameter of the corresponding vessels in normal pregnancy [6].

There is no satisfactory animal model for PIH. However, Abitbol et al [7] have produced uterine ischemia in pregnant animals by aortic compression. The lesions produced in the parenchymatous organs of these animals have been said to resemble those seen in the organs of women afflicted with PIH. Other investigators [8] have noted a rise in blood pressure in association with placental ischemia.

The idea that a poorly perfused placenta might produce, or fail to produce, vasoactive substances naturally follows from the preceding considerations. Everett et al [9] have demonstrated that prostaglandin synthetase inhibitors (indomethacin and acetylsalicylic acid) prevent the normal pregnant woman's resistance to vasopressors.

Because of the foregoing considerations, the most commonly held current theory is that PIH represents a state in which an inadequately perfused placenta fails to produce sufficient quantities of vasodilatory prostaglandins, such as (but not limited to) PGE_2. There is some evidence to support this idea: PGE_2 production is diminished in women with preeclampsia [10]. Moreover, PGE_2 infusion diminishes the angiotensin sensitivity of pregnant women.

Prostacyclin, or PGI_2, is a very potent systemic vasodilator. It has been postulated that failure of placental generation of PGI_2 may be involved in the etiology of PIH [11]. Glance et al [12] have shown that injection of angiotensin II into the fetal circulation of isolated human placental cotyledons increases the production of prostaglandin E and 6-keto-prostaglandin F-1-alpha (the stable metabolite of prostacyclin). However, Parisi and Rankin [13], studying ovine placentas, found that prostacyclin not only does not diminish, but actually further *increases* the placental vascular constriction produced by angiotensin II.

Furthermore, Jouppila et al [14] showed that PGI_2 infusion caused significant decreases in blood pressure in women with PIH. However, there was no change in placental and umbilical blood flow during the infusion.

A recent study [15] assessed production of PGI_2 and thromboxane (TXA_2) in perfused placentas derived from hypertensive pregnancies. TXA_2 is the antagonist of PGI_2 and has profound vasoconstrictor and platelet-aggregatory properties. Both sides of the placenta produced about five times more TXA_2 metabolites than PGI_2 metabolites. It is possible that the relative increase of TXA_2 production in the placentae of hypertensive gravidae may contribute to the vasoconstrictive and thrombotic changes seen in the placentae of these individuals.

Thus, a rationale has been made for prophylactic treatment of hypertensive complications of pregnancy with small amounts of prostaglandin synthetase or thromboxane synthetase inhibitors. Such studies are now in progress in many centers.

In summary, it now seems possible that reduction of placental perfusion may cause the production of vasoconstrictor substances or the failure of production of vasodilatory substances. The exact nature of these substances remains obscure at this time.

Incidence and Distribution

The incidence of PIH and PAH has been variously quoted [2] as from 5 to 15% of pregnancies in the United States. PIH and PAH occur more commonly among women with multiple pregnancy, polyhydramnios, primigravidity, hydatidiform mole, diabetes, and fetal hydrops.

Pathologic Physiologic Changes in PIH

Generalized vasospasm is the best-known manifestation of PIH [16]. Associated with this phenomenon is a 30 to 40% reduction in the blood volume [17] (with respect to the volumes encountered in normal pregnancy). Sodium is retained, to the extent of about 900 mEq [18]. Concurrently, there is an increase in concentration of intracellular sodium and a decrease in intracellular potassium; associated with these phenomena is an increase in neuromuscular hyperactivity.

In the chronic hypertensive gravida, there is already a hyperplastic-arteriosclerotic change in the radial arteries of the myometrium and their derivatives, the spiral arterioles of the decidua [9]. Thus, a foundation may be laid for the subsequent development of superimposed PIH, since the possibility of reduced uteroplacental blood flow already exists. It is therefore not surprising that plasma volume fails to increase in CH [19] or that in affected women, pregnancy-derived increases in plasma volume fall short of what would be expected for the normal gravida [20].

During *normal* pregnancy, there are increases in plasma renin activity and in plasma renin, renin substrate, angiotensin II, and aldosterone concentration. In PIH, the level of renin substrate apparently remains elevated. Plasma renin concentration, plasma renin activity, angiotensin II concentration, and aldosterone level have all been reported to be increased, decreased, or unchanged [21].

Pathology

Since PIH is a disease of pregnancy, the placenta might be expected to show fundamental changes. In 1950, Zeek and Assali [22] described a necrotizing arteriolitis, or "acute atherosis," in the walls of the spiral arterioles in PIH. The affected vessels are necrotic: Their walls are infiltrated with fat-laden "foam cells." This lesion may progress to infarction of the corresponding placental lobules. This work has been confirmed by Husten and co-workers [23] using more modern techniques. Similar changes are observed in intrauterine growth retardation. Infarction of areas of the decidua and the overlying placental lobules may cause release of tissue factor III (thromboplastin), initiating the coagulation cascade and producing a tendency to disseminated intravascular coagulation (DIC). Concurrently, decidual necrosis may produce prostaglandin precursors, triggering the prostaglandin cascade and producing uterine irritability.

Light microscopy of the placenta does not show specific lesions. At various times, lesions such as syncytial knotting, intervillous fibrin deposition, intervillous thrombosis, and ischemic necrosis of villi have been described as characteristic of PIH. However, all these conditions can be demonstrated in normal placentae. Moreover, studies of villi from the placentae of women with PIH do not show changes in biochemical activity [24].

The kidney shows swelling of the glomerulus, with diminution of the capillary lumen and thickening of the basement membrane bordering the epithelial cells [16,25,26]. This lesion is reversible after delivery. It is called glomeruloendotheliosis and is thought by some to be pathognomonic of PIH. Associated with these changes is a 25 to 50% reduction of renal plasma flow and glomerular filtration rate.

The liver shows a hemorrhagic necrosis of the peripheral areas of the lobules. This may be so extensive that a massive subcapsular hematoma may result (especially on the right). Spontaneous rupture of the liver may then occur [27].

In the brain [27] hemorrhage may be massive. Cerebral hemorrhage is one of the principal causes of death in PIH. However, cortical petechial hemorrhages are a more common finding. Fresh hemorrhages in the retinae may well reflect similar conditions in the cerebral cortex.

Subendocardial hemorrhages are frequently found [27]. The adrenals also show areas of necrosis and hemorrhage. The retinae show the pervasive arteriolar spasm of PIH; this may be associated with changes characteristic of chronic hypertension. Retinal edema and retinal detachment may occur; scleral edema may be so severe that the eyelids cannot be closed.

The blood frequently shows thrombocytopenia, microangiopathic hemolytic anemia, and a substantial diminution of serum albumin in favor of high-molecular-weight globulin [11]. Hemolysis, elevated liver enzyme levels, and low platelet counts are frequent concomitants of severe PIH, and the acronym of "HELLP syndrome" has been applied to this group of manifestations [28]. The hemolytic anemia is thought to be the result of intense spasm of small vessels, with resulting endothelial damage. A similar explanation might account for platelet deficiency. Hypoalbuminemia may result from selective loss of albumin through damaged glomeruli, while elevated liver enzyme levels are the result of the hemorrhagic necrosis previously described.

Clinical Management

The first step in management is to distinguish PIH from CH. The patient with CH is usually a multipara; often she is older than 35 years. She may show old retinal changes or have a history of having been hypertensive prior to the 20th week of pregnancy. By contrast, the patient with PIH is usually a primigravida, often in her teens, with no antecedent hypertension. Her retinae show arteriolar spasm and her disease (with the exception of hydatidiform mole) has its clinically recognizable onset at or after the 26th week of pregnancy.

The patient with PAH has a history and/or physical findings strongly suggestive of underlying CH; now, late in pregnancy, she develops an acute rise of blood pressure and albuminuria. Blood pressures in PAH are often extremely high: readings of 190/120 mm Hg or higher are by no means uncommon.

CHRONIC HYPERTENSION

If the chronically hypertensive gravida is taking drug therapy, we proceed as follows. All diuretics are gradually discontinued. (Reduction of circulating blood volume is undesirable, since this reduces placental perfusion.) Antihypertensives are cautiously stopped. If they prove to be required (see below), we substitute alpha-l-methyldopa, a drug that has been extensively studied [19] and that has stood the test of time in our clinic. The following protocol constitutes our standard management of CH:

1. Regular diet without added sodium.
2. Cessation of work.
3. Two hours of bed rest every day in the left lateral decubitus position.
4. With a fixed diastolic blood pressure of 100 mm Hg or more, alpha-l-methyldopa (Aldomet) is used, in a dose of 250 mg, from twice daily to four times daily depending on response.
5. If alpha-l-methyldopa does not control the blood pressure, propranolol (10 mg four times daily) may be used. (Propranolol and other beta-

blockers are the subjects of controversy; see the section on drug therapy.)

6. Cessation of smoking (reduction of uterine blood flow is clearly undesirable).
7. Close observation of renal function with serum creatinine determinations.
8. Weekly or biweekly visits, with close attention to blood pressure, proteinuria, and any untoward symptoms.
9. Ultrasound studies, preferably by 20 weeks of pregnancy, for definition of dates and as a baseline to detect intrauterine growth retardation (IUGR) later. Ultrasound is done again at 28 weeks. If IUGR is suspected, ultrasound evaluation is repeated every 2 weeks.
10. Electronic fetal monitoring (contraction stress test [CST]) weekly, beginning at 32 weeks or as early as 30 weeks if hypertension is severe (above 150/100 mm Hg) or if IUGR has been definitely diagnosed.
11. Amniocentesis for lecithin/sphingomyelin ratio and/or phosphatidylglycerol level if disease is severe or CST is positive.
12. Pregnancy not allowed to go beyond term.

However, if there is no PAH, no labor, and the CST is negative, one may await spontaneous labor at term. Labor is induced if untoward manifestations appear.

ACUTE PIH

An otherwise normal patient whose previous diastolic blood pressures were equal to or less than 85 mm Hg, who shows a rise of 15 mm Hg in her diastolic blood pressure *or* acute and persistent blood pressure of 140/90 mm Hg, regardless of other signs and symptoms, is regarded as having acute PIH.

Management steps are as follows:

1. Hospitalize.
2. Give a regular diet without added salt.
3. Place the patient at bed rest in the labor and delivery suite.
4. Give no diuretics.
5. Give no antihypertensives unless the diastolic pressure is regularly 100 mm Hg or more.
6. Do electronic fetal monitoring (contraction stress test) daily.
7. Do ultrasound evaluation of the pregnancy.
8. Perform amniocentesis for lecithin/sphingomyelin ratio and/or phosphatidylglycerol level.

In many cases the symptoms abate, and occasionally the patient may be sent home under carefully guarded conditions. If, however, the condition appreciably worsens despite optimum care, delivery should be seriously considered. If central nervous system hyperactivity is noted, magnesium sulfate should be given as noted below.

SEVERE HYPERTENSION

If the blood pressure reaches 160/100 mm Hg, 5 g or more of protein appears in the urine, less than 500 cc of urine is excreted in a 24-hour period, or evidence of damage to a parenchymatous organ or organs (including the blood) develops, delivery should be undertaken, whether or not the amniotic fluid lipid profile has reached a desirable level. Otherwise, the baby may die or the mother may have a brain hemorrhage, pulmonary edema, eclampsia, or placental abruption.

The following protocol is employed:

1. Four grams of magnesium sulfate is given intravenously over 20 minutes. Thereafter, the infusion is delivered at a rate of 2 to 3 g/hour. Magnesium levels are monitored every 6 hours. A desirable level is 6 to 7 mEq/L.
2. With diastolic blood pressure rise to 100 mm Hg or more, hydralazine is given intravenously in small repeated boluses of 2.5 to 10 mg at intervals of 15 to 30 minutes depending upon response.
3. The severely hypertensive patient should ideally be followed either with a central venous pressure (CVP) monitor or with a flow-directed pulmonary artery catheter. The latter is superior, in our opinion, since in some patients the CVP does not reflect changes in the pulmonary capillary wedge pressure. An arterial line should also be placed for accurate monitoring of blood pressure.
4. Constant fetal monitoring is instituted; rapid delivery may be required in the event of fetal deterioration.
5. An indwelling bladder catheter is placed for recording of urinary intake and output.
6. Oxygen is given at the rate of 7 L/minute by face mask.
7. Delivery is vaginal, if possible. Induction should be carried out, using intravenous oxytocin delivered by a calibrated infusion pump. If satisfactory contractions and progressive cervical dilatation have not occurred within 4 hours, cesarean delivery should be strongly considered. Any evidence of fetal distress is also grounds for consideration of cesarean delivery.
8. Epidural anesthesia may be employed if the anesthesiologist is highly knowledgeable and especially qualified in the field of obstetric complications. In other situations, meperidine for labor sedation and pudendal block supplemented with nitrous oxide inhalation may be used for delivery. The latter may be by easy low forceps, if an easy spontaneous delivery cannot be achieved. If cesarean delivery is required, a general anesthetic is suggested unless the anesthesiologist is specially qualified, as noted above.

Both conduction and general anesthesia pose grave problems. Conduction anesthesia can produce profound peripheral vasodilatation, with severe reductions in uterine blood flow and resultant fetal jeopardy. On the other hand, catastrophic rises in maternal blood pressure may occur during tracheal intubation, which is a necessary part of use of any general anesthetic.

ECLAMPSIA

If convulsive seizures develop, they are controlled with magnesium sulfate, as noted above. If magnesium sulfate does not control convulsions, intravenous pentothal may be administered by an anesthesiologist. Once convulsions have been controlled, an adequate serum level of magnesium (6–7 mEq/L) may be maintained.

The prevention of injury to the tongue and mouth of the patient and protection of the airway to prevent aspiration are of great importance. Appropriate use of obturators to prevent chewing of the tongue, as well as endotracheal intubation, are indicated.

The remainder of the management of eclampsia is similar to the management of severe hypertension, as previously described. Induction is carried out when the patient is oriented as to time and location. Delivery by cesarean section is undertaken in the event of fetal distress or failure of induction. Once convulsions have occurred, delivery is mandatory. It is not uncommon for the patient to look reasonably well on the morning after a convulsion, but failure to effect prompt delivery will result in recurrence of the seizures and frequently cerebral edema, often with the most dire consequences.

DRUG THERAPY

Magnesium Sulfate

This drug has a curarelike action, blocking release of acetylcholine at the myoneural junction. Although neurologists and internists decry its use, magnesium remains the "Rock of Gibraltar" for most American teaching institutions in the care of obstetric hypertension. Magnesium also slows or blocks cardiac conducting system transmission, decreases smooth-muscle contractility, and depresses central nervous system irritability [29]. In all probability [29], magnesium sulfate also exerts an anticonvulsant effect on the cerebral cortex. Magnesium sulfate also causes diminution of uterine contractility, although the mechanism of this process is obscure. The therapeutic level of magnesium ion is 6 to 7 mEq/L. Reflexes tend to be lost at 10 mEq/L. The lethal level is approximately 20 mEq/L. The antidote is calcium gluconate: 10 cc of 10% calcium gluconate can be given intravenously over a period of 3 minutes.

Alpha-Methyldopa

This drug is a centrally acting antihypertensive agent. It operates by favoring the production of methyl-norepinephrine instead of norepinephrine [21]. Alpha-methyldopa does not reduce cardiac output or renal blood flow. For these reasons, obstetricians have long favored this drug for the control of chronic hypertension in pregnancy, especially when the diastolic blood pressure is at a fixed level of 100 mm Hg or more. Alpha-methyldopa has a slow onset of action (12 hours), with its maximum effect being 4 to 6 hours later. The duration of action of this drug is of the order of 8 hours. Alpha-methyldopa may also cause affective disorders, hepatitis, and a positive Coombs' test.

Diazoxide

This drug is related to the thiazide diuretics. It causes relaxation of arterial smooth muscle [30]. It also enhances sodium and water retention, inhibits insulin release, and increases uricemia and serum levels of free fatty acids. Diazoxide is also a powerful inhibitor of uterine contractions. In the usually recommended dose (300 mg intravenously) diazoxide will produce very substantial drops in both systolic and diastolic blood pressure. For this reason, diazoxide should not be used prior to delivery, since blood flow through an already compromised uteroplacental unit would be further reduced.

Sodium Nitroprusside

This drug [30] is the most effective agent available for the immediate treatment of hypertensive emergencies. It is a profound arteriolar dilator and has the advantage of almost immediate action. The effect is very short, so that the action of the drug can be turned on and off almost at will. Sodium nitroprusside should not be used while a living fetus is present in the uterus except during the most profound emergencies. (Occasionally, the anesthesiologist may find this drug useful should induction of general anesthesia be required prior to cesarean delivery in a severely hypertensive patient.) Prolonged use of sodium nitroprusside may lead to cyanide poisoning of both mother and fetus.

Hydralazine

Hydralazine is a direct dilator of arteriolar smooth muscle [31]. It apparently does not reduce uteroplacental blood flow. Hydralazine decreases systemic blood pressure and increases cardiac output. Renal blood flow seems to be unchanged or increased. The maximum effect of this drug, given orally, occurs in 3 to 4 hours. If the drug is given by vein, the maximum effect occurs in about 30 minutes. Hydralazine is used when diastolic pressure reaches levels of 100 to 110 mm Hg or more. At such levels there is danger of cerebral hemorrhage. Hydralazine is given in bolus doses of 2.5 to 10 mg intravenously, with additional boluses being given as needed every 30 minutes or so. The important consideration in hydralazine therapy is to avoid sudden drops in maternal arterial blood pressure, especially if the diastolic pressure drops significantly below 90 mm Hg. Such drops in diastolic blood pressure may diminish uteroplacental blood flow and endanger the fetus.

Oral use of hydralazine is indicated occasionally during pregnancy when maximum doses of alpha-l-methyldopa are not sufficient to reduce dangerous blood pressure levels. An initial dose of 10 mg is given daily. This dosage may be increased to 50 mg daily.

Thiazide Diuretics

From about 1953 to about 1970, American obstetricians administered countless numbers of thiazide pills to pregnant women, in the belief that these drugs would prevent hypertension as well as alleviate disagreeable symptoms, such as edema. The former effect has never been established; the latter effect is often accompanied by fatigue and exhaustion associated with sodium and potassium loss. Thiazides cause a temporary depletion of plasma volume [31]. An antihypertensive effect is also present, and is prolonged. Because the volume depletion is temporary and the antihypertensive effect prolonged, a few obstetricians still advocate limited use of thiazides.

Most obstetricians oppose the use of thiazides in pregnancy hypertension. The blood volume is already reduced, and further reductions are thought to have a negative effect upon uteroplacental blood flow. Thiazides also increase serum glucose and uric acid levels and, like diazoxide, depress uterine contractility. Other side effects of thiazide diuretics include acute hemorrhagic pancreatitis in the mother and thrombocytopenia in the fetus.

Beta-Blockers

The beta-blockers lower blood pressure by reducing myocardial contractility and heart rate. Moreover, renal renin secretion is diminished. Finally, unopposed alpha stimulation acts on the central nervous system to decrease blood pressure [31].

Propranolol has been widely used for the treatment of pregnancy hypertension in Europe, but has not been extensively employed in the United States. Good results [32] have been reported in hypertensive women treated during pregnancy with propranolol.

Oxyprenolol [15] has not been shown to be superior to methyldopa for mild to moderate hypertension.

Metoprolol [33] shows no convincing evidence of good blood pressure control in hypertensive pregnant women. Although this drug has some blood-pressure lowering effect, it does not appear to prevent the development of preeclampsia.

Propranolol and other beta-blockers readily cross the placenta. They increase uterine irritability and may cause fetal cardiac arrhythmias. For these reasons, most American obstetricians feel that drugs of this type are contraindicated during pregnancy. Certainly, further studies [31] are indicated before these drugs can be recommended for hypertensive pregnant patients.

REFERENCES

1. De Voe SJ, O'Shaughnessy R: Clinical manifestations and diagnosis of pregnancy-induced hypertension. *Clin Obstet Gynecol* **27**:836–853, 1984.
2. Chesley LC: Hypertensive disorders in pregnancy. In Hellman LM, Pritchard JA (Eds): *Williams Obstetrics*. 14th ed. New York: Appleton, 1971, p. 716.
3. Gant NF, Daley GL, Chand S, et al: A study of angiotensin-II pressor response throughout primigravid pregnancy. *J Clin Invest* **52**:2682–2689, 1973.
4. Abdul-Karim R, Assali NS: Pressor response to angiotensin in pregnant and non-pregnant women. *Am J Obstet Gynecol* **82**:246–251, 1961.
5. Whalley PJ, Everett RB, Gant NF, et al: Pressor responsiveness to angiotensin II in hospitalized primigravid women with pregnancy-induced hypertension. *Am J Obstet Gynecol* **145**:481–483, 1983.
6. Brosens IA, Robertson WB, Dixon HG: The role of the spiral arteries in the pathogenesis of preeclampsia. *Obstet Gynecol Annu* **1**:177–191, 1972.
7. Abitbol MM, Gallo GR, Pirani CL, et al: Production of experimental toxemia in the pregnant rabbit. *Am J Obstet Gynecol* **124**:460–470, 1976.
8. Bergen M, Cavanagh D: Toxemia of pregnancy: The hypertensive effect of acute experimental placental ischemia. *Am J Obstet Gynecol* **87**:293–305, 1963.
9. Everett RB, Worley RJ, MacDonald PC, et al: Effect of prostaglandin synthetase inhibitors on pressor response to angiotensin II in normal pregnancy. *J Clin Endocrinol Metab* **46**:1007–1010, 1976.
10. Pederson EB, Christensen NJ, Christensen P, et al: Preeclampsia—a state of prostaglandin deficiency? *Hypertension* **5**:105–111, 1983.
11. Worley R: Pathophysiology of pregnancy-induced hypertension. *Clin Obstet Gynecol* **27**:821–835, 1984.
12. Glance DG, Elder MG, Myatt L: Prostaglandin production and stimulation by angiotensin II in the isolated perfused human placental cotyledon. *Am J Obstet Gynecol* **151**:387–391, 1985.
13. Parisi VM, Rankin JHG: The effect of prostacyclin on angiotensin II induced placental vasoconstriction. *Am J Obstet Gynecol* **151**:444–449, 1985.
14. Jouppila P, Kerkinen P, Koivula A, et al: Failure of exogenous prostacyclin to change placental and fetal blood flow in preeclampsia. *Am J Obstet Gynecol* **151**:661–665, 1985.
15. Fidler J, Smith V, Fayers P: Randomized controlled study of methyldopa and oxyprenolol in treatment of hypertension in pregnancy. *Br Med J* **286**: 1927–1930, 1983.

16. Pollak VE, Nettles JB: The kidney in toxemia of pregnancy: A clinical and pathologic study based on renal biopsies. *Medicine* **39**:469–526, 1960.

17. Blekta M, Hlavaty V, Trukova M, et al: Volume of whole blood and absolute amount of serum proteins in the early stage of late toxemia of pregnancy. *Am J Obstet Gynecol* **106**:10–13, 1970.

18. Chesley LC: Sodium retention and preeclampsia. *Am J Obstet Gynecol* **95**:127–132, 1966.

19. Gibson HM: Plasma volume and glomerular filtration rate in pregnancy and their relation to the difference in fetal growth. *J Obstet Gynaecol B Commonw* **80**:1067–1074, 1973.

20. Soffronoff EC, Kaufmann BM, Konnaughton JF: Intravascular volume determinations and fetal outcome in hypertensive disease of pregnancy. *Am J Obstet Gynecol* **127**:4–9, 1977.

21. Roberts JM: Pregnancy-related hypertension. In RK Creasy and R Resnik (Eds): *Maternal-fetal medicine*. Philadelphia: WB Saunders, 1984, pp. 703–752.

22. Zeek P, Assali NS: Vascular changes in the decidua associated with eclamptogenic toxemia of pregnancy. *Am J Clin Pathol* **20**:1099–1109, 1950.

23. Husten J, Foidart JM, Lambotte R: Maternal vascular lesins in preeclampsia and intrauterine growth retardation: Light microscopy and immunofluorescence. *Placenta* **4**:489–498, 1983.

24. Hellman LM, Harris BA, Andrews MC: Studies of the metabolism of the human placenta. *Bull Johns Hopkins Hosp* **87**:203–214, 1950.

25. Spargo BH, McCartney CP, Winemiller R: Glomerular capillary endotheliosis in toxemia of pregnancy. *Arch Pathol* **68**:593–599, 1959.

26. McCartney CP: Pathological anatomy of acute hypertension of pregnancy. *Circulation* **30** (suppl 2):37–42, 1964.

27. Sheehan HL, Lynch JB: *Pathology of Toxemia in Pregnancy*. London: Churchill Livingstone, 1973, pp. 328–331, 524–545.

28. Weinstein L: Syndrome of hemolysis, elevated liver enzymes, and low platelet count: Severe consequence of hypertension in pregnancy. *Am J Obstet Gynecol* **142**:59–167, 1982.

29. Borges LF, Gucer G: Effect of magnesium on epileptic foci. *Epilepsia* **19**:81–91, 1978.

30. Berkowitz RL: The management of hypertensive crises during pregnancy. In RL Berkowitz (Ed): *Critical Care of the Obstetric Patient*. New York: Churchill Livingstone, 1983, p. 299.

31. Holland OB, Kaplan NM: Propranolol in the treatment of hypertension. *N Engl J Med* **294**:930–936, 1976.

32. Makila JM, Viinikka L, Ylikorkala O: Increased thromboxane A_2 production but normal prostacyclin by the placenta in hypertensive pregnancies. *Prostaglandins* **27**:87–95, 1984.

33. Wickman K, Ryden G, Karlberg BE: A placebo controlled trial of metaprolol in the treatment of hypertension. *Scand J Lab Invest* **44** (suppl 169):90–95, 1984.

8
Current Concepts and Practice in Improving Fetal Outcome in Diabetic Pregnancies

Chin-Chu Lin and Judith Hibbard

Maternal diabetes has been known to be a significant cause of perinatal morbidity and mortality for many decades. Although the incidence of diabetes in obstetric populations varies from country to country, the impact of poorly controlled diabetic pregnancies on fetal outcome is always serious.

Gabbe [1] has reviewed the changes in the management of pregnant diabetics and the consequent improvement of fetal outcome over a 6-decade period. Prior to the availability of insulin, the physician's primary concern was maternal survival. At that time, many pregnant diabetic women died from ketoacidosis or diabetic coma. Prior to 1940, the incidence of sudden and unexpected intrauterine fetal death in diabetic pregnancies was reported to be 30%. It became possible to reduce perinatal mortality to 20% between 1940 and 1970 and to 10% or less between 1970 and 1980 (Fig. 8.1). This steadily improved fetal outcome is the result of team care, of identification of high-risk groups by systematic classification, of the use of early delivery to avoid sudden fetal deaths, and of the use of cesarean section to prevent birth trauma from vaginal delivery of the macrosomic fetus.

Most sudden fetal deaths are observed after the third trimester of pregnancy, with the worst prognosis seen in cases complicated by vascular disease, renal disease, hypertension, polyhydramnios, diabetic ketoacidosis, and macrosomic fetus. Therefore, both White's classification [2] and Pedersen et al's "poor prognostic signs" [3] became clinically useful in the prediction of fetal outcome in diabetic pregnancies. However, the strategy of early delivery, that is, women with diabetes class D, F, and R delivering at 35 weeks' gestation and those with class B or C at 37 weeks' gestation, is inevitably associated with a higher incidence of respiratory distress syndrome (RDS).

Revolutionary changes in obstetric care during the 1970s and 1980s have further improved fetal outcome in diabetic pregnancies. Tight maternal blood glucose control, antepartum fetal surveillance, and the use of preconceptional diabetic control to avoid congenital malformations of the

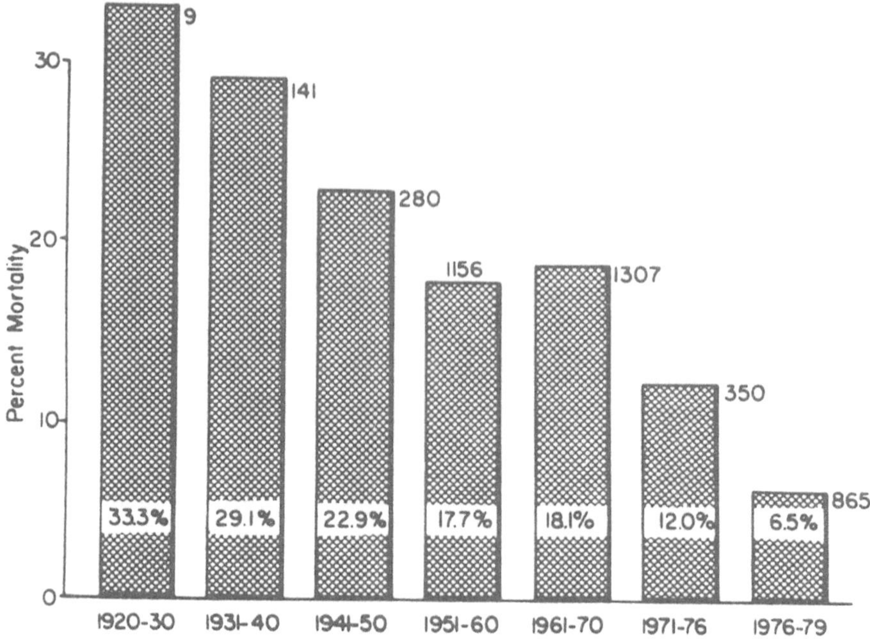

FIGURE 8.1. Perinatal mortality in pregnancies complicated by insulin-dependent diabetes mellitus, classes B through R. Number at top of column indicates total number of cases in each time period. Reproduced with permission from Gabbe SG: Management of diabetes in pregnancy: Six decades of experience, in Pitkin RM, Zlatnik FJ (eds): 1980 *Year Book of Obstetrics and Gynecology*. Copyright © March, 1980, by Year Book Medical Publishers, Inc., Chicago.

infants of diabetic mothers (IDMs) are the important concepts in the management of diabetic pregnancies today. This chapter reviews these new concepts and their impact on fetal outcome in diabetic pregnancies.

Diabetes as a Cause of Abnormal Fetal Growth and Development

At the present time, congenital malformation has emerged as one of the major causes of perinatal mortality in diabetic pregnancy, accounting for 30 to 40% of all perinatal losses [3]. Table 8.1 lists the major developmental abnormalities in multiple systems in infants of diabetic mothers described in one current obstetric textbook [4]. These birth defects, which involve the central nervous system, the cardiovascular system, the gastrointestinal system, the genitourinary system, and the skeletal system, are described elsewhere [4–9]. Davis and Campbell [10] have reported that a specific GI abnormality, small left-side colon, was seen in up to 40% of IDMs in their study series. Mills et al [11] have reported that poor diabetic control

TABLE 8.1. Congenital malformations in infants of diabetic mothers.

Cardiovascular
    Transposition of great vessels
    Ventricular septal defect
    Atrial septal defect
    Hypoplastic left ventricle
    Situs inversus
    Anomalies of aorta
Central nervous system
    Anencephaly
    Encephalocele
    Meningomyelocele
    Microcephaly
Skeletal
    Caudal regression syndrome
    Spina bifida
Genitourinary
    Absent kidneys (Potter syndrome)
    Polycystic kidneys
    Double ureter
Gastrointestinal
    Tracheoesophageal fistula
    Bowel atresia
    Imperforate anus

Source: Samuels and Landon [4]. Used by permission from Churchill Livingstone.

during the critical period of embryonic organogenesis, prior to the eighth week of gestation, is associated with a risk of congenital malformations two to six times higher than normal for most defects. A 252:1 increase in the incidence of caudal regression in diabetes compared with the incidence in the control group was seen in this study.

Early fetal growth delay has been considered the major mechanism of fetal malformation in diabetes in animal experiments [12–16]. Severe hyperglycemia [12,13] and hypoglycemia [16] are associated with the occurrence of yolk sac damage, neural tube defects, and hypoplastic development or growth retardation of the embryo. The use of insulin [12] or arachidonic acid therapy [15] in the prevention of these embryopathies has met with some success in these animal models. In human pregnancies, early fetal growth delay has been demonstrated by ultrasound at 7 to 14 weeks of gestation in severely diabetic women [17]. Major congenital malformations were found in 27% of these pregnancies. Furthermore, women with poor diabetic control at conception have twice the normal incidence of spontaneous abortion during the first trimester [18]. These data again suggest that abnormal embryonic development may be the cause of early spontaneous abortion in insulin-dependent diabetes.

FETAL HYPERINSULINISM AND FETAL MACROSOMIA

The problem of excessive fetal growth in utero may reflect the excessive glucose and amino acids received from the mother. In the 1950s and 1960s, evidence of both hyperplastic/hypertrophic changes in the pancreatic beta-cells of IDMs and overproduction of insulin was documented [19–21]. Pedersen et al [22] then proposed the hypothesis that maternal hypergly-cemia stimulates fetal hyperinsulinism and fetal macrosomia in diabetic pregnancies. Freinkel and Metzger [23] suggested that, in addition to ex-cessive fetal insulin production, other growth factors may also play roles in fetal anabolism and increased fetal growth.

More recently, several investigators [24–26] have claimed that amniotic fluid (AF) insulin is a reliable indicator for fetal prognosis in diabetic preg-nancies, and that a high level of AF insulin may alert the obstetrician and pediatrician to the potential risks of intrauterine fetal death, fetal macro-somia, or severe hypoglycemia in the newborn infant during the immediate neonatal period. Weiss and associates [26] reported that, in poorly con-trolled diabetic pregnancies, the levels of insulin in cord serum and in urine were 20 times higher than normal values. We have studied amniotic fluid C-peptide (AFCP), insulin, and glucose levels in 33 diabetic and 126 nondiabetic pregnant women at 36 weeks or more of gestation and found that the AFCP level is the most reliable indicator of fetal outcome [27]. Levels of AFCP late in diabetic pregnancy are positively correlated with maternal diabetic control as well as with an increased risk of fetal ma-crosomia. The mean level of AFCP of the well-controlled diabetic group was not distinguishable from that of nondiabetic women, but was signif-icantly lower than that of the poorly controlled group (Fig. 8.2). Fur-thermore, the incidence of fetal macrosomia was 44% in the high AFCP level group ($\geq$1.0 pmol/ml), compared with a 12% incidence in the low

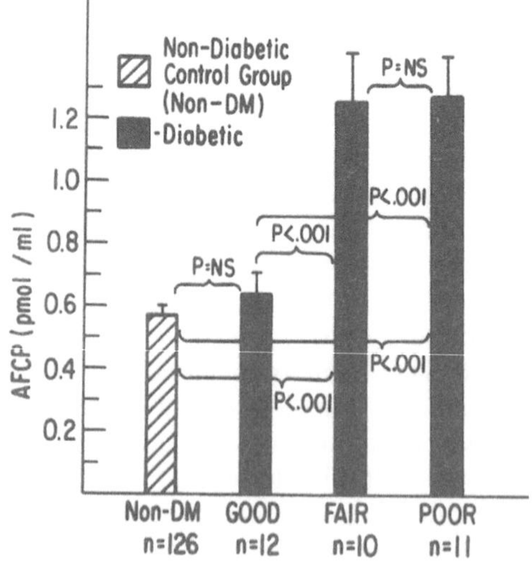

FIGURE 8.2. Statistical comparison of am-niotic fluid C-peptide (AFCP) levels (mean $\pm$ SEM) in groups with different degrees of diabetic control (good, fair, poor) and a nondiabetic control group. From Lin et al [27], used with permission from CV Mosby.

AFCP level group (p <0.05). A similar study by Tchobroutsky et al [28] indicated that levels of AFCP, but not of AF insulin, correlated well with infant birth weight or with birth weight adjusted for gestational age. This study suggested that AFCP rather than AF insulin should be used to investigate fetal hyperinsulinism in insulin-treated diabetic women.

Figure 8.3 illustrates the maternal-placental-fetal relationship in appropriate- (AGA), large- (LGA), and small-for-gestational age (SGA) infants based upon our hypothesis that insulin is an important factor in the regulation of intrauterine fetal growth [29]. Appropriate amounts of insulin secreted by the AGA infant leads to normal somatic growth, glycogen storage, and deposition of fat tissue. The maternal hyperglycemia that causes fetal hyperglycemia and hyperinsulinism is probably the main mechanism of diabetogenic fetal macrosomia and excessive storage of glycogen and fat. In contrast, the low secretion of fetal insulin secondary to chronic fetal hypoglycemia in the SGA fetus may lead to retardation of somatic growth, deficient storage of glycogen in the liver and heart, and lack of subcutaneous fat deposition. Thus, the data from our study of AFCP suggest that persistently low endogenous production of insulin in the SGA fetus and high production in the LGA fetus may lead to the different fetal growth rates observed in these two abnormal fetal growth patterns [29].

The placenta plays a central role in the delivery and regulation of maternal nutrients to the fetus. Glucose is transported across the placenta by facilitated diffusion in direct proportion to maternal blood glucose levels, up to a saturable maximum. Fetal blood glucose levels remain approximately two-thirds of the maternal glucose level, or 20 to 30 mg/dl lower than those of the maternal blood. However, Meschia and associates [30] have reported that the fetal lamb receives only one third of the glucose that the uterus takes up from the maternal circulation. Their data suggest that the uterus and placenta are important sites of glucose utilization.

In contrast, amino acids are actively transported to the fetus [31]. Neutral and basic amino acids represent the bulk of the amino acids transported across the placenta, while acidic amino acids are not transported to the fetus. In general, the level of most amino acids in fetal circulation is approximately twice that in the maternal circulation. Like glucose, some amino acids may stimulate insulin synthesis [32].

Free fatty acids cross the placenta in small amounts by gradient-dependent diffusion and are esterified to triglyceride by fetal adipocytes. Ketoacids also can diffuse across the placenta and are readily utilized by the fetus during periods of maternal starvation [33]. The placenta also serves as a modulator of maternal metabolic fuels by synthesizing hormones that are lipolytic and antagonistic to insulin, such as human chorionic somatomammotropin (hCS), estrogen, and progesterone. However, hCS stimulates lipolysis and the secretion of maternal insulin, which in turn assures the availability and adequate transfer of glucose and amino acids, particularly during the period of accelerated fetal growth in the

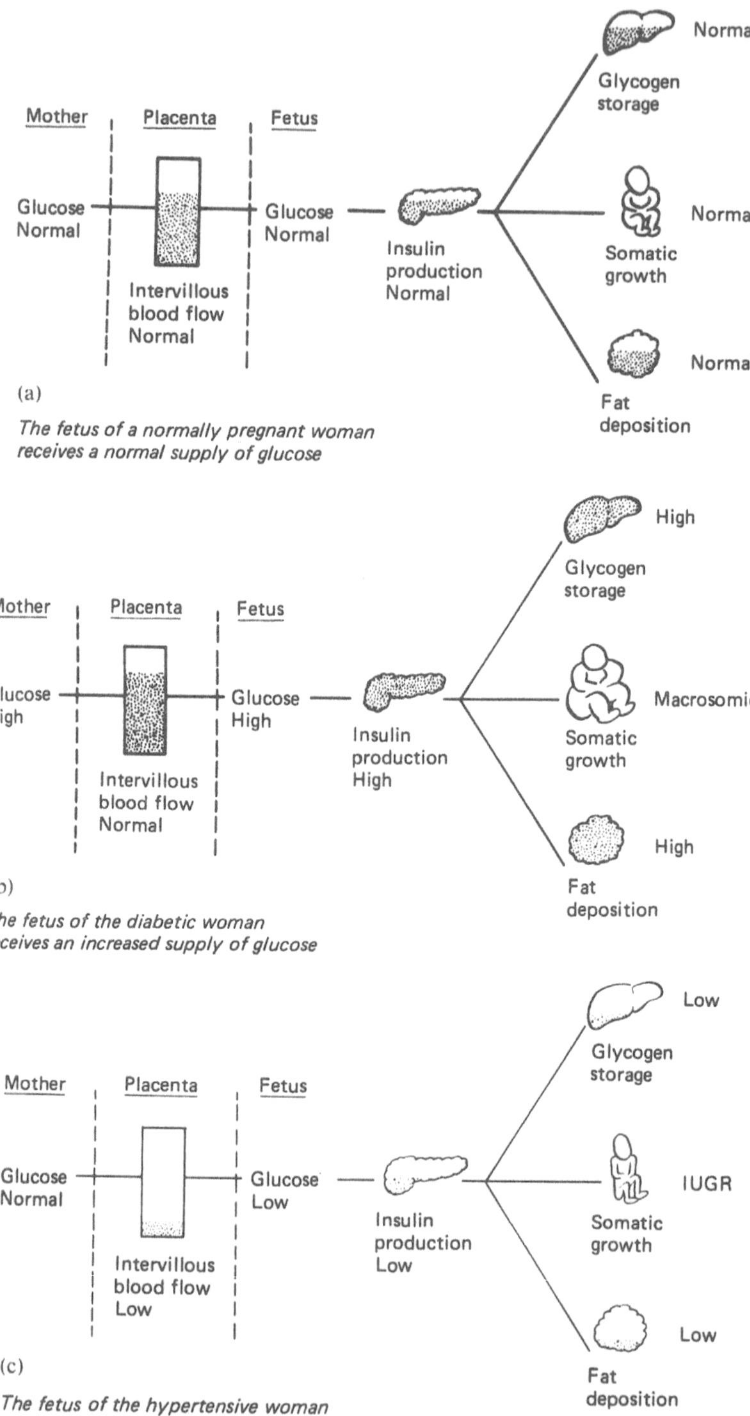

(a)

The fetus of a normally pregnant woman receives a normal supply of glucose

(b)

The fetus of the diabetic woman receives an increased supply of glucose

(c)

The fetus of the hypertensive woman receives a decreased supply of glucose

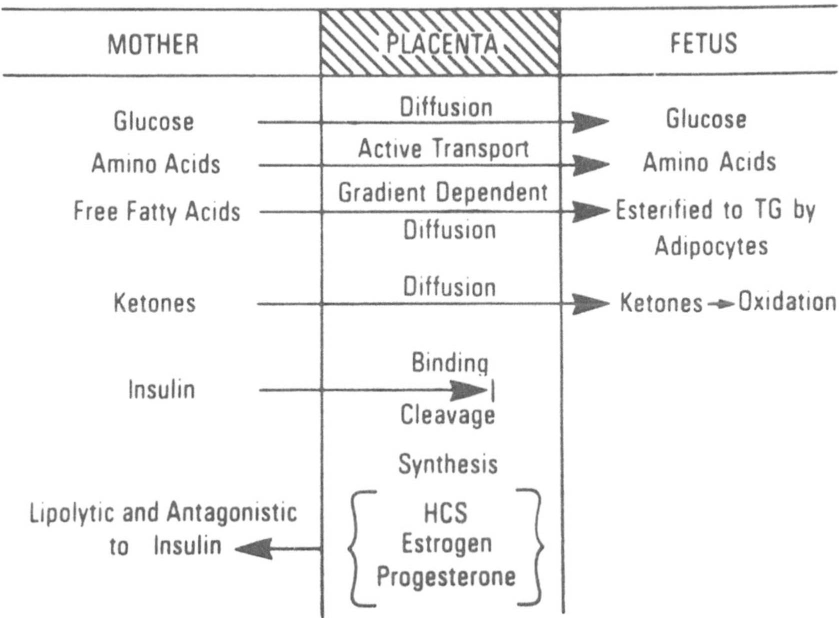

FIGURE 8.4. Maternal-placental-fetal integration of fuels for the promotion of fetal growth. HCS, human chorionic somatomammotropin; TG, triglyceride. From Hollingsworth and Cousins [9], used with permission from WB Saunders.

second half of gestation. The maternal nutrients that are transported across the placenta to the fetus are summarized in Figure 8.4.

Although macrosomic infants delivered by class A, B, or C diabetic mothers are frequently found to have a large placenta [34], the converse is not necessarily true; many growth-retarded infants of diabetic mothers with vascular complications may have placental vascular changes rather than a smaller placenta [35–37].

INTRAUTERINE FETAL DEATH

Through improved understanding of the pathophysiology of diabetes in pregnancy, as well as through development of techniques to prevent maternal and fetal complications, perinatal mortality in diabetic pregnancies has been reduced from 30% in the 1940s to 2 to 5% in the 1980s. Many

FIGURE 8.3. Insulin regulation of intrauterine growth. (a) Appropriate-for-gestational-age fetuses. (b) Large-for-gestational-age fetuses of diabetic mothers. (c) Small-for-gestational-age (intrauterine growth retardation, IUGR) fetuses of hypertensive mothers with compromised placental function. From Lin et al [29], used with permission from CV Mosby.

investigators have reported that if optimal care is delivered to diabetic pregnant women, the perinatal mortality rate, excluding infants with major congenital malformations, is equivalent to that observed in normal pregnancies [38–45]. Nevertheless, the exact mechanism that leads to sudden intrauterine fetal death in diabetic pregnancy is still not fully understood. Fetal sheep studies have demonstrated decreased fetal oxygenation in association with hyperinsulinemia and hyperglycemia [46,47]. Hyperglycemia and hypoxemia may also result in lactic acidosis and fetal death in rhesus monkeys [48]. This phenomenon of maternal hyperglycemia-induced fetal hyperlactatemia and fetal acidosis can also be observed in human pregnancies [49]. Fetal hypoxemia and acidosis may be due to a high-demand, insulin-induced anabolic state [50]; to a low-supply, diminished uteroplacental blood flow state [51]; or to both. The extreme example of fetal jeopardy, however, is encountered in the state of maternal diabetic ketoacidosis, which may result in either severe fetal distress or sudden fetal death [52–55].

In an effort to avoid sudden intrauterine fetal death, obstetricians have routinely terminated pregnancies complicated by diabetes several weeks before term. These attempts to avoid fetal death have often led to neonatal mortality from iatrogenic prematurity [1]. On the other hand, birth trauma still accounts for considerable neonatal morbidity and occasionally mortality in IDM. Shoulder dystocia secondary to vaginal delivery of a macrosomic fetus is the primary reason for perinatal mortality in this category [56,57]. Iatrogenic prematurity and birth trauma are both avoidable causes of perinatal mortality in the pregnancy complicated by diabetes mellitus.

Neonatal Morbidity

The immediate neonatal complications of IDM include hypoglycemia, hypocalcemia, hyperbilirubinemia, macrosomia with or without birth trauma, respiratory distress syndrome (RDS), and major congenital malformations. Overall neonatal morbidity correlates inversely with low gestational age, from 80% at 34 weeks of gestation to 40% at 40 weeks of gestation [58]. Table 8.2 shows the combined incidence of each category of neonatal morbidity recalculated from 12 reports in the literature dating from the late 1960s to the early 1980s. Because of a higher incidence of preterm deliveries among insulin-treated patients compared with patients with gestational diabetes, it is not surprising that the incidence of hyperbilirubinemia, hypoglycemia, hypocalcemia, and RDS are higher among infants from the former than from the latter group. It is interesting to observe that gestational diabetes is associated with a lower incidence of fetal macrosomia and major congenital malformations than is maternal insulin-dependent diabetes. Nevertheless, the incidence of these two fetal complications in gestational diabetes is still high enough to warrant concern, and the effort to reduce their incidence applies equally to the management of gestational diabetes and insulin-treated diabetes in pregnancy.

TABLE 8.2. Frequency of neonatal morbidity.*

Neonatal morbidity	Gestational diabetes mellitus (DM), class A ($N = 482$)	Insulin-treated DM, classes B–R ($N = 1,468$)	Statistical comparison (X^2-test)
Hypoglycemia (< 30 mg/dl)	32/282 (11.3%)	214/913 (23.4%)	$p < 0.001$
Hypocalcemia (< 7 mg/dl)	6/201 (3.0%)	74/617 (12.0%)	$p < 0.001$
Hyperbilirubinemia (> 12 mg/dl)	24/201 (12.0%)	252/881 (28.6%)	$p < 0.001$
Respiratory distress syndrome	2/201 (1.0%)	104/1141 (9.1%)	$p < 0.001$
Macrosomia ($\geq$ 90th percentile)	77/482 (16.0%)	249/1205 (20.7%)	$p < 0.05$
Major congential malformations	13/482 (2.7%)	75/1468 (5.1%)	$p < 0.05$

*Recalculation from 12 reports in the literature [38–45,58–61].

Management to Reduce the Incidence of Fetal Macrosomia and Congenital Malformations

Preconceptional diabetic control, diabetic screening early in pregnancy, early detection of poorly controlled cases, and tight diabetic control throughout pregnancy are the four major tasks for improving the outcome for IDMs. In addition, antepartum fetal surveillance, treatment of major complications, appropriate intrapartum management, and intensive care of the newborn IDM, particularly those infants with neonatal morbidity, will further improve perinatal outcome for these high-risk infants. Each of the above concepts and their practice will be discussed separately in subsequent sections of this chapter.

SCREENING FOR GESTATIONAL DIABETES

Early diagnosis of gestational onset diabetes is crucial, since glucose intolerance is a potential hazard to both the mother and the fetus. Traditionally, obstetricians have used a 3-hour glucose tolerance test (GTT) for pregnant women to obtain the definitive diagnosis of gestational onset diabetes. Since the GTT is a relatively difficult and time-consuming test, only patients with certain historical risk factors are screened. These risk factors include a family history of diabetes, previous stillbirth, previous macrosomic baby, previous baby with congenital anomalies, maternal age over 30, and obesity.

This method of selective screening has been shown to be inadequate. First, it is obvious that the majority of primigravida patients with gestational diabetes would not be detected because most of the high-risk factors are based on the patient's obstetric history. Second, the use of historical risk factors in diagnosis has been shown to have a sensitivity of only 63% and a specificity of only 56% [62].

Conclusions from recent investigations have led to the recommendation that a routine prenatal diabetes screening procedure be used for all pregnant women [63–68]. The screening method involves determination of the maternal plasma glucose level 1 hour after ingestion of a 50-g oral glucose challenge, known as the "50-g glucola screen." Table 8.3 demonstrates the incidence of a positive glucola test according to different plasma glucose levels in 96 pregnant women studied by Carpenter and Coustan [63]. Using a threshold of 145 mg/dl would require that further diagnostic testing (GTT) be done on 17% of the screened population, while a threshold of 135 mg/dl would require diagnostic testing on 25% of the screened population. Because of occasional cases of gestational onset diabetes with a glucola test value between 130 and 135 mg/dl, Carpenter and Coustan recommended a cutoff point of 130 mg/dl. However, a cutoff value of ≥140 mg/dl was recommended by the Second International Workshop Conference on Gestational Diabetes Mellitus [66,67]. The 50-g, 1-hour

TABLE 8.3. Incidence of positive glucose tolerance test among 96 gravidas with 50-g, 1-hour screening test values >134 mg/dl (plasma, glucose oxidase).

Screening test result (mg/dl)	Incidence of gestational diabetes (%)
135–144	14.6
145–154	17.4
155–164	28.6
165–174	20.0
175–184	50.0
>185	100.0

Source: Carpenter and Coustan [63]. Used with permission from CV Mosby.

screening protocol does not stipulate that the patient be fasting or post-prandial for the test. Thus, the test is convenient to administer at any time during pregnancy. Although one screening test at 24 to 28 weeks is widely recommended, some investigators have suggested two screening tests: one at the first prenatal visit and another during the second trimester of pregnancy [68]. Furthermore, since good health for pregnancy begins before conception, it has been suggested that all women in the reproductive age group should have regular health checkups, and that appropriate evaluation of glucose intolerance should be included as part of prospective health screenings [66].

The first well-documented criteria for the diagnosis of gestational onset diabetes are those proposed by O'Sullivan and Mahan [62], based upon a 100-g, 3-hour oral glucose tolerance test. Since then, many modified GTT criteria have been proposed, as shown in Table 8.4 [62,63,69–71]. Modern laboratories have replaced the Somogyi-Nelson method of whole blood glucose analysis with the more specific glucose oxidase method using plasma instead of whole blood. The 100-g, 3-hour oral GTT should be administered after an overnight fast and after a period of preparation

TABLE 8.4. Criteria for 100-g, 3-hour glucose tolerance test in pregnancy.

Sample	Values* (mg/dl)				
	Whole blood [62†]	Plasma [63]	Plasma [69]	Plasma [70]	Plasma [71]
Fasting	90	95	90	110	105
1-hour	165	180	205	200	190
2-hour	145	155	195	150	165
3-hour	125	140	160	130	145

*If any two values are met or exceeded, gestational diabetes is diagnosed.
†Data from studies numbered in the reference list.

consisting of at least 2 days of a diet containing at least 150 g of carbohydrates per day. This dietary priming is necessary to avoid the possibility of falsely high values on the GTT due to previous carbohydrate depletion. In addition, the patient should refrain from smoking, eating, drinking, or excessive activity during the test period.

Although a 50-g, 1-hour blood glucose screening test followed by a 100-g, 3-hour glucose tolerance test has been a widely accepted and effective way of identifying diabetic patients, there are occasional patients who cannot tolerate oral glucose loading. With such a patient it may be necessary to perform the rapid intravenous GTT with a standard 25-g dose, as proposed by Solomons et al [72]. Glucose polymer (Polycose), a tasteless mixture containing 3% glucose, 7% maltose, 5% maltotriose, and 85% polysaccharides, has also been used in oral carbohydrate tolerance testing with high efficacy and few gastrointestinal symptoms [73,74]. Recently, capillary blood glucose screening with a glucose reflectance meter has been reported to be useful [75]. However, this simpler screening method cannot be recommended until further data based on a large study population become available.

It has been reported that 22% of patients with gestational onset diabetes eventually become permanent diabetics when followed for between 2 and 8 years. Follow-up of these patients over a 16-year period showed a 60% incidence of permanent diabetes [76]. Therefore, close follow-up of gestational onset diabetes patients is highly recommended.

In a private practice setting, Dietrich et al [77] prospectively compared the efficacy of routine screening versus selective screening for gestational onset diabetes on the basis of the presence of high-risk factors. One thousand patients were tested in a routine screening group and 453 of 1,000 in a selective screening group. The incidence of gestational onset diabetes in the selectively screened group (4.2%) was twice that of the routinely screened group (2.1%). Evidence of glucose intolerance without a risk factor was found in only one case (1/1000, 0.1%) in the routinely screened group. Therefore, the authors argued that selective diabetic screening reduces office time and patient inconvenience and is very cost effective. However, we do not recommend the use of their protocol proposal for the reasons mentioned earlier in this section.

PRECONCEPTION AND EARLY POSTCONCEPTION DIABETIC CONTROL

The common goal of modern obstetrics is to maximize the quality of fetal, newborn, and infant life in such a manner as to provide every baby with the greatest potential for physical, mental, and emotional development. Thus, the concept of preventive measures in obstetrics was introduced by Aubrey and Pennington [78] and by Nesbitt [79] more than a decade ago, with an emphasis on identifying high-risk factors, on reproductive counseling and prenatal screening, and on the timing of desired pregnancies in relation to the overall medical and emotional health status of the prospective mother. During the past 10 years, efforts have been made by perinatal obstetricians and neonatologists to identify prenatally those fetuses at risk for abnormal development before and after birth. Preconception and early postconception counseling has become an important issue for obstetricians in the 1980s [80]. However, a major problem facing the obstetrician is the large number of women with poorly controlled diabetes who first request care at a gestational age many weeks beyond the critical period of fetal organogenesis.

Recent studies by Fuhrmann and associates [81,82] have demonstrated that strict metabolic control of insulin-dependent diabetes in women before conception significantly reduces the incidence of congenital malformations to a level comparable to that of the nondiabetic population. The incidence of congenital anomalies in the group with preconceptional diabetic control is less than one-tenth that of the group without preconceptional control [81]. Among 200 patients enrolled in an intensive prepregnancy metabolic treatment program, only 1 of 57 newborn infants had a congenital anomaly. In contrast, 9 of 145 newborns had major congenital anomalies in the group of 144 pregnant diabetic women who were hospitalized for evaluation and diabetic control after 8 weeks of gestation without preconceptional control [82]. Goldman et al [43] reported that among 75 pregnant women with juvenile-onset insulin-dependent diabetes, the incidence of congenital malformations was 9.6% among offspring of 31 patients who did not attend a preconceptional clinic and was zero among those of 44 women with preconceptional diabetic control. Other investigators, however, reported less dramatic results in preventing fetal anomalies by good diabetic control of insulin-dependent mothers prior to fetal organogenesis. In a study by Mills [83], the incidence of major congenital malformations was 2.1% among 389 nondiabetic controls, 4.9% among 347 insulin-dependent diabetic women with early euglycemic control prior to 21 days of conception, and 9% among 279 diabetic women with late diabetic control. Given these results, one may speculate that preconception and early postconception diabetic control could reduce by 50% the major congenital malformations caused by a diabetogenic effect, but probably not to the level of the nondiabetic population. This question will not be resolved until data from a much larger study are available.

Goldman et al [43] compared hemoglobin A_{1C} levels, blood glucose levels, and daily insulin doses between two groups: women with preconception diabetic control and those without diabetic control until late in the first trimester. All three parameters were found to be significantly higher in the latter than in the former group during the first and second trimester. By the third trimester, there were no differences between the two groups in any of the three parameters studied. Nevertheless, three congenitally malformed infants were born to the group of 31 noncontrol mothers while there were no congenital anomalies among the infants of the 44 mothers with preconceptional diabetic control. Key et al [84] reported that women with insulin-dependent diabetes had a steadily increased risk of spontaneous abortion or fetal congenital malformations once their hemoglobin A_{1C} level exceeded 9.5%. When the hemoglobin A_{1C} level reached 15.5%, virtually 100% of the conceptuses were either malformed or were spontaneously aborted (Fig. 8.5). The critical cutoff point of 9.5% or greater hemoglobin A_{1C} level effectively discriminated between the group with adverse pregnancy outcome and those with normal outcome. The sensitivity of this threshold was 97% in this particular study.

Other investigators have reported similar results using hemoglobin A_{1C} level to assign the degree of risk of giving birth to an infant with congenital malformations in diabetic pregnancies [6,85]. These data strongly support the need to assess the quality of diabetic control in all diabetic women before conception and during the early postconception weeks. Measurement of hemoglobin A_{1C} has been shown to provide an integrated, retrospective index of glucose control that reflects the mean blood glucose concentration during the 4 to 8 weeks prior to its measurement. Although measurement of hemoglobin A_{1C} is useful in identifying diabetic individuals who are poorly controlled and for counseling patients in early pregnancy

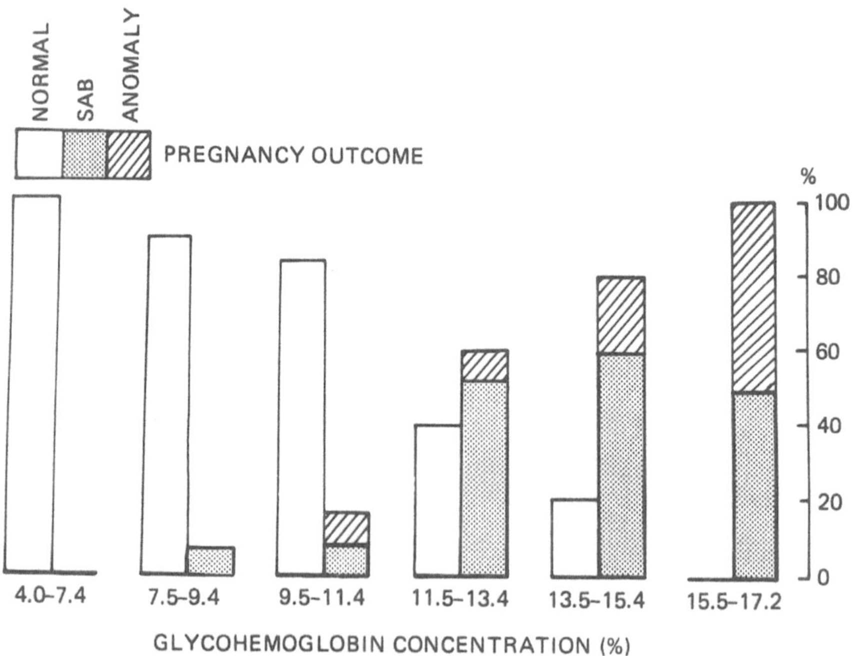

FIGURE 8.5. Incidence of adverse pregnancy outcomes, congenital anomalies, and spontaneous abortions (SAB) by glycohemoglobin (HbA$_{1C}$) concentration. From Key et al [84], used with permission from CV Mosby.

regarding their risk for fetal malformations, a recommendation for termination of pregnancy on the basis of the results of this test alone is inappropriate.

TIGHT BLOOD GLUCOSE CONTROL THROUGHOUT PREGNANCY

It is important to achieve and maintain tight glycemic control throughout the entire gestational period. It has been demonstrated that tight glycemic control of diabetes in pregnant women can result in a perinatal mortality rate similar to that seen with nondiabetic pregnancies [39,86]. In addition, it has been shown that good control early in pregnancy can decrease the incidence of fetal macrosomia and the neonatal complications [45,87].

The normal pregnant woman undergoes metabolic changes in the early part of pregnancy that result in blood glucose levels lower than those in nonpregnant women. Increased estrogen and progesterone production cause stimulation of the pancreatic β-cells, leading to an increase in insulin production. Hepatic glycogen storage is increased, while glucose production decreases. There is also increased sensitivity to insulin, with increased glucose utilization peripherally. These changes result in what Phelps et al have called "accelerated starvation," and are manifest in lower serum glucose levels [88]. In the latter half of pregnancy, production of human placental lactogen, cortisol, and prolactin rises significantly. These hormones have a contrainsulin effect and act to mobilize glycogen stores and increase glucose production.

The nondiabetic pregnant woman is able to maintain glucose values within a fairly narrow range. Hollingsworth [89] found the mean 24-hour plasma glucose level to be 84 ± 10 mg/dl, Phelps et al [88] reported a value of 96 ± 3 mg/dl, and Cousins et al [90] reported a value of 87 ± 2 mg/dl. The range of blood glucose values across the three studies was 75 to 130 mg/dl. The goal of most diabetic control programs is to achieve glucose levels within this range. Thus, "tight" diabetic control is considered a fasting glucose of less than 100 mg/dl with postprandial levels of less than 120 mg/dl.

In the pregestational insulin-dependent diabetic, an intensive program for diabetic control must be instituted. This is best accomplished by a team approach that includes a perinatologist, an internist, a dietitian, and a social worker. It is imperative for the patient who comes for prepregnancy counseling to achieve good glycemic control prior to conception. Many diabetics, however, first seek obstetric care when they are already well into the first trimester.

If poor glycemic control is noted, hospitalization is mandatory to achieve the goals mentioned above, to educate the patient, and to institute home glucose monitoring. For a poorly controlled diabetic this will usually require several days to a week. Hospitalization is followed by home monitoring with weekly visits to the clinic, rehospitalization being reserved for those patients who again develop poor control or who show signs of ketoacidosis. Home monitoring of glucose levels has been shown to have results equivalent to those achieved by hospitalizing patients [91–93]. No difference was found in duration of pregnancy, mean glucose levels, pregnancy complications, or infant morbidity when comparing hospitalized diabetics with those on a home-glucose monitoring regimen.

Diet

As in the nonpregnant diabetic, diet is one of the cornerstones of management [94]. The pregnant diabetic requires the same caloric intake as her nondiabetic counterpart: an additional 300 kcal/day to meet the energy needs of fetus, placenta, and maternal tissues [95]. A weight gain of 24 to 25 pounds (10–12 kg), similar to that for the nondiabetic pregnant woman, is recommended [95,96]. This includes a weight gain of 2 to 4 pounds (1–2 kg) in the first trimester, followed by 0.5 to 1.0 pounds (0.25–0.50 kg) per week during the last two trimesters [89,97]. To achieve this weight gain, 30 kcal/kg of the ideal body weight (IBW) is recommended in the first trimester, with an increase to 36 to 38 kcal/kg in the second and third trimesters [95,96]. In the underweight or malnourished woman this may be increased as high as 50 kcal/kg of IBW, while in the obese woman 24 to 33 kcal/kg IBW may be sufficient [97–99]. A high-protein diet (1.3–2.0 g/kg of body weight) comprising about 20% of the total daily intake is recommended for adequate growth of fetal and maternal tissues [68,96–99]. In addition, Coustan and Carpenter [68] believe that high protein intake dampens the glycemic swings induced by carbohydrates. Carbohydrates should comprise about 40 to 45% of the diet. Jovanovic and Peterson [99] suggested that a low carbohydrate intake at breakfast will help prevent the late morning hyperglycemia that is a result of the morning cortisol peak. The remainder of the diet, 35 to 40%, is composed of fat.

The caloric intake is divided among three meals and one to three snacks daily. A late evening snack, comprising about 15% of the total daily caloric intake, is essential to protect against early morning hypoglycemia [96,98,99]. Diet must be highly individualized, taking into consideration the timing and characteristics of the prescribed insulin regimen as well as the life-style, ethnic preferences, and exercise habits of the patient.

Insulin Therapy

In the long-standing diabetic, the first trimester insulin needs are usually less than prepregnancy requirements, and insulin doses need to be adjusted downward. This results from increased tissue sensitivity to insulin and, in some cases, from decreased caloric intake secondary to mild nausea or emesis [89]. Weiss and Hofmann [100] found this decrease in insulin requirement, 7.2% from weeks 10 to 17, to be so small that it might not be detected. In general, in early pregnancy the daily insulin requirement is 0.7 to 1.0 units/kg/day [101,102]. As the pregnancy progresses beyond 17 weeks, insulin requirements rise to a peak at 36 weeks, when 1.0 to 1.6 units/kg/day are needed [100–102]. Insulin levels approximately 30% higher than in the nonpregnant state are needed during this time [89]. Frequent monitoring of glucose levels, with appropriate insulin adjustments, is necessary.

Insulin therapy must be individualized for each patient. In general, good control can be achieved using a split-dose or multiple-dose regimen of intermediate and short-acting insulins. In the split-dose regimen, the morning dose, administered just before breakfast, comprises roughly two-thirds of the total daily insulin requirement, while the evening dose, given just before dinner, contains the remainder [103]. The morning dose contains NPH and regular insulin in a ratio of 2:1, while the evening dose is in a ratio of 1:1. NPH and regular insulins can be mixed in the same syringe and still retain their separate effects [104].

Jovanovic and Peterson [86,101] advocated multiple injections to more closely cover the periods of hyperglycemia after eating. The regimen includes NPH and regular insulin prior to breakfast, regular insulin prior to dinner, and NPH at bedtime. Others [96,100] have advocated multiple injections of insulin, including regular before every meal and longer acting insulin in the morning and again at dinner or at bedtime. Again, these regimens are highly individualized.

The portable open-loop continuous insulin pump has been used to treat pregnant diabetics. This system delivers a continuous subcutaneous basal level of regular insulin. Boluses of insulin are given with meals and snacks [88,103,105]. Mean serum glucose and glycosylated hemoglobin levels decrease significantly with pump therapy. Potential problems with pump therapy include episodes of hypoglycemia, or, if the pump should fail or the subcutaneous needle become dislodged, ketoacidosis. Newer models with alarm systems make the latter less likely to occur. A recent randomized clinical trial of the pump versus a multiple injection regimen in pregnant diabetics showed that there was no difference between the two groups with respect to glucose levels, symptomatic hypoglycemia, or glycosylated hemoglobin levels [102]. With either method, the patient must be highly motivated for good results to be achieved.

Human insulin, which is biosynthesized by bacteria, is now widely available. This type of insulin is less antigenic than the bovine and porcine insulins. Theoretically, it should also be less antigenic than the highly purified insulins [106]. Patients with insulin antibodies have problems with insulin resistance. Insulin antibodies in pregnant women have also been associated with higher neonatal morbidity [107]. A significant decrease in antibody titers has been noted in both pregnant and nonpregnant patients with high insulin antibody levels when the patients changed to less immunogenic insulin [107,108]. Thus, human insulin is used in many centers for newly diagnosed as well as for long-standing diabetics. In gestational diabetics requiring insulin, only those preparations that have low antigenicity are recommended [67]. These women usually will not need insulin after delivery, but a significant percentage, years later, will become insulin-requiring diabetics. Because of this, it is preferable that they do not develop insulin antibodies. As in our pregestational diabetics, we recommend human insulin for use in gestational diabetics because of its theoretical advantage over the highly purified monocomponent insulins.

Home Glucose Monitoring

Whatever insulin regimen is chosen, it is essential that the patient learn home glucose monitoring. Several studies have shown that careful self-monitoring in an ambulatory setting is equal to long-term hospitalization in achieving glycemic control [91–93,109]. Several home-monitoring methods are available using glucose oxidase-impregnated reagent strips [98,103]. A color change, the intensity of which is proportional to the glucose level, occurs when capillary whole blood obtained by finger prick is applied to the strip. The strip can be read visually by comparing the color with colors on a chart. A more accurate reading can be obtained by use of a reflectance glucose meter [110]. These meters are small battery-operated devices with a digital readout of the glucose level. Most are available for under $300. The glucose levels in capillary whole blood correlate well with plasma glucose levels [110], although it should be remembered that plasma or serum glucose levels are approximately 15% higher than in whole blood [96]. Granodos [98] reviewed in detail the various test strips, meters, and finger-pricking devices available to patients. Whatever system is chosen for monitoring, the patient must be highly motivated. All patients check their glucose level prior to each meal and at bedtime. Postprandial values may also be obtained. A daily diary of glucose values is kept by each patient.

Insulin-requiring diabetics make weekly clinic visits at which time a fasting and a 2-hour postbreakfast glucose level is obtained. The home glucose values are reviewed and insulin adjustments are made as necessary. As mentioned previously, the goal of therapy is to keep the fasting glucose level below 100 mg/dl (60–80 mg/dl is ideal) and postprandial levels below 120 mg/dl. A dietitian/educator should be available for consultation and teaching on a weekly basis.

Special Situations

Gestational Onset Diabetes

The gestational onset diabetic has an intolerance for carbohydrates. Insulin is produced by the pancreas, but there is a delay in its release; possibly there is inadequate production capacity late in pregnancy when the contrainsulin hormones are rising [89]. The vast majority of gestational onset diabetics can be managed by diet alone, but 10 to 20% will require insulin therapy. The same dietary principles discussed above hold true for the gestational onset diabetic. Caloric intake and weight gain recommendations are the same as those for nondiabetic women [67]. Calories are divided among three meals and a bedtime snack. Weight reduction is not permitted. Recent research in Europe in small patient populations suggests that caloric restriction in the obese gestational onset diabetic may improve glycemic control with no adverse effects on the outcome of the pregnancy [111,112]. Further studies with larger patient populations arc needed before diet restriction is adapted to the treatment of the obese gestational diabetic.

Gestational diabetics are also seen weekly in the clinic, at which time a fasting blood sugar is obtained. Levels greater than 105 mg/dl in a patient on diet therapy indicate the need to institute insulin therapy. Coustan and Carpenter [68] recommended a weekly glucose profile including a fasting, a 2-hour postprandial, and a late afternoon glucose level. Insulin therapy is begun if the fasting glucose level is greater than 100 mg/dl or if either of the other two levels exceeds 120 mg/dl. These levels were chosen empirically in an effort to mimic the normoglycemia of nondiabetic pregnancies [88–90]. If insulin therapy becomes necessary, the patient is managed in a manner similar to the pregestational insulin-dependent diabetic described above.

The issue of using insulin prophylactically in gestational diabetics has recently been the subject of debate. Such therapy is advocated in an effort to decrease the incidence of fetal macrosomia. In a combined prospective-retrospective study, Coustan et al have shown that prophylactic use of insulin decreases macrosomia [57,113]. Thus, in an attempt to achieve euglycemia and decrease fetal and neonatal morbidity, Coustan advocated the use of prophylactic insulin for all gestational diabetics [57,68,114].

Persson et al [115], however, found no advantage to prophylactic insulin use in a prospective randomized trial. Leikin et al [116] showed that prophylactic insulin was effective in preventing macrosomia in lean gestational diabetics but not in those who were obese. They speculated that all obese gestational diabetics may require insulin treatment rather than just prophylaxis. Because insulin therapy is not without complications (hypoglycemia, insulin antibodies, etc.), is expensive, and requires intense patient education, monitoring, and resources, we do not advocate the use of prophylactic insulin until more evidence proves it to be beneficial.

Type I Versus Type II Diabetes

Because their hormonal-metabolic adjustments are not the same, it is important to recognize the differences between type I (insulin-dependent, juvenile onset) and type II (non-insulin-dependent, mostly adult onset) diabetic women in pregnancy. Women with type I diabetes have a marked decrease in pancreatic beta cell function with a significant decrease in, or even an absence of, circulating serum insulin levels. Although type I diabetes usually develops in children, adolescents, or young adults, occasional cases may develop in middle-aged or older adults. Type II diabetes may develop anytime from childhood to the fifth decade, but in general individuals tend to be older and more obese. In type II diabetes, circulating levels of insulin may be normal or even higher than normal; rather, the physiologic release of insulin in response to the ingestion of food is delayed. This is due to either increased insulin resistance in the target tissues at the receptor level or, in some type II patients, a postreceptor defect in insulin action [8]. Women in the reproductive age group who have type II diabetes are hyperglycemic, but frequently do not require insulin to control plasma glucose level when they are not pregnant.

Hollingsworth and associates [9,117] have studied levels of C-peptide, glucagon, cortisol, and prolactin hourly around the clock during the third trimester and at 3 months postpartum in patients with type I and type II diabetes. Type I patients had barely detectable C-peptide values and very small meal-related oscillations. In contrast, women with type II diabetes had higher than normal fasting and mean 24-hour values, but decreased C-peptide release following meals. Furthermore, type I patients had a significantly lower glucagon level, a lower prolactin level, and a higher cortisol level compared with levels in type II patients.

Several variables must be considered in dietary therapy for type I diabetic gravidas. These include the state of pregnancy, life-style and food preferences, timing of meals, level of physical activity, and caloric requirements for pregnancy. Because nocturnal hypoglycemia is often a severe and common problem in type I pregnant women, emphasis is placed on the bedtime snack. A consistent dietary program of three meals plus snacks at midmorning, midafternoon, and bedtime provides ideal intervals between periods of food intake. The distribution of carbohydrate throughout the day should be balanced with the insulin regimen. The insulin dose before the evening meal must be carefully adjusted to avoid the often unrecognized hypoglycemia that can occur after midnight. Hypoglycemia due to an overdose of insulin is the most common and serious complication of type I diabetic pregnancy.

On the other hand, many obese type II diabetics with insulin resistance are unaware of impaired glucose tolerance before pregnancy. Therefore they often seek medical care late in pregnancy, resulting in the development of fetal macrosomia, polyhydramnios, and other maternal complications. These patients, because of exaggerated insulin resistance during pregnancy, may also become quite difficult to control. Although many investigators [118–120] believe that caloric restriction in obese pregnant women is contraindicated, excessive weight gain is also discouraged for the type II obese diabetic patient [117]. Ketonuria is rarely observed in such patients even if they lose weight or fail to gain a normal amount of weight. As a dietary recommendation, Ney et al [121] found that a high-carbohydrate, high-fiber, low-fat diet significantly decreases insulin requirements in both type I and type II diabetics during pregnancy.

Diabetic Ketoacidosis

Ketoacidosis occurs in approximately 9% of all pregnant diabetics. This condition is partly responsible for the tenfold increase in maternal mortality found in pregnant diabetics [122]. The pregnant diabetic is much more prone to ketoacidosis than her nonpregnant counterpart because of the state of "accelerated starvation" and insulin resistance discussed previously. Initiating events in pregnancy are similar to those in nonpregnant diabetics [53,54,123]. Insulin deficiency, whether it is associated with a relative or absolute excess of glucagon, will initiate ketotic metabolism. In addition, stress (especially secondary to infection), fasting, and dehydration all contribute to the initiation of ketoacidosis. There is decreased peripheral utilization of glucose along with increased glycogenolysis in the liver. The resulting hyperglycemia initiates a net osmotic movement of sodium and water into the extracellular space as well as causing hyperosmotic diuresis; dehydration can be severe. Free fatty acids are mobilized from the fat stores and are oxidized, increasing the number of ketone bodies in the blood circulation. Hypovolemia and hypotension cause decreased uterine blood flow and decreased placental perfusion, resulting in fetal hypoxia [54]. Fetal mortality in ketoacidosis is reported to be as high as 50 to 90% [53,54]. Maternal ketonuria has also been correlated with intellectual deficits in children [124]. Thus it behooves the obstetrician to first make the diagnosis and then to promptly begin treatment.

The pregnant patient with ketoacidosis presents with the same symptoms as a nonpregnant patient with this condition. Polydipsia, polyuria, and weight loss are early symptoms. Later the patient complains of nausea and vomiting, abdominal pain, malaise, drowsiness, and weakness. On examination one can find dry mucous membranes, poor tissue turgor, sunken eyeballs, hypotension, tachycardia, hyperventilation, oliguria, fruity odor of the breath, and, in severe cases, coma.

The urine will reveal a 4+ glucose reading and a high level of ketones. The serum glucose level is usually greater than 300 mg/dl but can be lower in the pregnant patient. The serum ketone level will be increased. Arterial blood gases will reveal metabolic acidosis, with a pH of less than 7.30; the blood bicarbonate level will be less than 15 mEq/L. Potassium level is usually elevated or normal, despite urinary losses, because potassium is being driven into the extracellular space.

In the treatment regimen that follows, immediate hydration with 0.9% NaCl must be the first step, with 1 to 2 L administered in the first hour. The solution is then changed to 0.45% NaCl, and the rate is decreased to 150 to 200 ml/hr. The total body fluid deficit can be 3 to 10 L. An intravenous bolus of regular insulin should be given, 0.4 unit/kg, followed by continuous insulin intravenous infusion at a rate of 5 to 10 units/hour. Intravenous boluses at a rate of 10 to 50 units/1 to 2 hours or subcutaneous injections of 10 to 20 units/hour may also be used. The low-dose infusion of 5 to 10 units/hour is now favored in many centers because it is thought to decrease the incidence of hypoglycemia and hypokalemia that can be seen with the other regimens. As the acidosis resolves, the infusion dosage can be adjusted downward. It is important to remember that the glucose level normalizes before the acidosis resolves and that IV insulin therapy should be continued until resolution of the acidosis occurs. Once treatment has begun, the K + level will decrease as K + is driven intracellularly. If the K + value is initially high, one can add 20 mEq KCl to the second or third liter of IV solution and monitor K + levels every hour with further potassium replacement as needed. If the K + level is normal or low, replacement is begun immediately, not to exceed a maximum of 20 mEq/hour. If KCl of this magnitude is required, a cardiac monitor should be used.

Bicarbonate is administered only if the pH is less than 7.0. As the ketones are oxidized, bicarbonate is produced, and the pH will usually normalize without bicarbonate administration. If bicarbonate is administered, 88 mEq in a liter of 0.45% NaCl solution is slowly infused over a period of 1 hour [54,123]. Blood glucose levels, arterial blood gases, pH, and K + levels should be checked every hour until the hyperglycemia and acidosis are clearly resolving. When the glucose level has reached approximately 250 mg/dl, the IV solution should be changed to D5W in 0.45% normal saline to prevent cerebral edema, a rare event that can occur because the brain continues to be hyperosmolar after the serum osmolarity has declined [54,123].

Continuous fetal heart rate monitoring is mandatory during an episode of maternal ketoacidosis. As discussed above, the fetus can suffer from hypoxia, which will be manifested as fetal tachycardia, late decelerations, or episodes of bradycardia [52,55]. Prompt, aggressive therapy of the ketoacidosis can reverse the fetal distress [52,55,125] and the pregnancy can continue. If the fetal distress does not resolve in a reasonable period of time, delivery by C-section may become necessary.

Influence of Diabetic Control on Fetal Outcome

"Degree of diabetic control" is a poorly defined phrase that varies with the opinion and experience of different investigators. However, the general consensus is that both the mean glucose level [38–45,58,59,61] and the range of fluctuation of glucose levels [60] are closely related to fetal outcome. Tables 8.5 and 8.6 illustrate the correlation between low maternal blood glucose level and low incidence of perinatal morbidity seen in a study in Sweden during the 1960s [40] and in another study in the United

TABLE 8.5. Perinatal outcome in relation to maternal blood glucose control.

Perinatal outcome	Mean maternal blood glucose values (mg/dl)		
	<100	100–150	>150
Death	2/52 (3.8%)	12/77 (16%)	9/38 (24%)
Hypoglycemia*	6/52 (12%)	8/77 (10%)	4/38 (11%)
Jaundice[†]	0/52 (0%)	6/77 (8%)	3/38 (8%)
Respiratory distress[‡]	9/52 (17%)	24/77 (31%)	9/38 (24%)
Malformation[§]	2/52 (3.8%)	12/77 (16%)	5/38 (13%)

*Includes infants with recorded blood glucose values at or below 20 mg/
dl. Only three infants had obvious clinical signs of hypoglycemia.
[†]Includes severe jaundice that required exchange transfusion.
[‡]Includes both idiopathic respiratory distress (hyaline membrane disease)
and severe aspiration.
[§]Includes both perinatally dead infants and those surviving the neonatal
period.
Source: Modified from Karlsson and Kjellmer [40], used with permission
from CV Mosby.

States during the 1980s [44]. Similarly, patients with greater glucose variability tend to have more neonatal complications [60]; Table 8.7 demonstrates this association. In other studies, tight blood glucose control during the third trimester failed to demonstrate a reduction in perinatal morbidity, as shown in Table 8.8 [61]. We used a mean fasting blood glucose level of less than 90 mg/dl with a standard deviation (SD) of less than 25 mg/dl, and a mean nonfasting blood glucose level of less than 120 mg/dl with a SD of less than 30 mg/dl as our criteria for good diabetic control in a study of 74 diabetic pregnant women in our own institution [45]. We found that good blood glucose control in pregnant diabetic patients

TABLE 8.6. Neonatal morbidity in relation to maternal glucose control.

	Mean capillary blood glucose values (mg/dl)		Significance
	< 110 ($n = 43$)	≥ 110 ($n = 32$)	
Gestational age (wk)	38.42 ± 1.4	38.15 ± 2.2	NS
Nursery days	4.72 ± 1.4	6.56 ± 2.0	$p < 0.001$
Birth weight (g)	3,199 ± 546	3,240 ± 943	NS
Large for gestational age (> 90th percentile)	4 (9.3%)	11 (34.3%)	$p < 0.05$
Hypoglycemia (< 30 mg/dl)	8 (18.6%)	13 (40.6%)	$p < 0.05$
Respiratory distress syndrome	1 (2.3%)	7 (21.8%)	$p < 0.01$
Hyperbilirubinemia (> 12 mg/dl)	10 (23.2%)	13 (40.6%)	NS
Polycythemia (> 65%)	1 (2.3%)	3 (9.3%)	—
Hypocalcemia (< 7 mg/dl)	0	2 (6.2%)	—

Source: Modified from Landon et al [44], used with permission from CV Mosby.

TABLE 8.7. Comparison of various parameters of maternal glucose control in two groups of infants, those with and those without neonatal complications.

Maternal blood glucose control	Maternal values	No. of infants without neonatal complications	Maternal values	No. of infants with neonatal complications	p*
Glucose coefficient of variation (%)	15.56 ± 1.91	49	22.08 ± 2.07	93	.023
Fasting plasma glucose level (mg/dl)	105.57 ± 3.68	54	114.57 ± 3.11	102	NS
4 PM plasma glucose level (mg/dl)	117.11 ± 3.87	54	129.26 ± 3.62	102	.024
Birth weight (g)	3,746 ± 93	54	3,615 ± 65	102	NS

*Based on two-sample tests.
Source: Modified from Atral et al [60], with permission from CV Mosby.

TABLE 8.8. Neonatal outcome in relation to maternal glucose control.

	Mean preprandial glucose (mg/dl)		
	Group I, < 115	Group II, 115–172	Group III, > 172
Morbidity*·†			
Hypoglycemia	7/18 (40%)	20/77 (26%)	5/21 (24%)
Hypocalcemia	3/18 (17%)	8/77 (10%)	5/21 (24%)
Hyperbilirubinemia	2/18 (11%)	15/77 (19%)	4/21 (19%)
Respiratory distress	0/18 (—)	6/77 (8%)	3/21 (14%)
Macrosomia*·†	5/18 (28%)	31/77 (40%)	7/21 (33%)
Malformations†	0/18 (—)	7/79 (9%)	4/24 (17%)

*Stillbirths and neonates with trisomy 18 excluded.
†No statistical differences between groups I, II, and III.
Source: Levano et al [61]. Used with permission from CV Mosby.

between 20 and 31 weeks of gestation significantly reduced the incidence of fetal macrosomia, compared with fair to poor control; the incidence of fetal macrosomia was not reduced among patients in whom good diabetic control was not achieved until after the 32nd week of gestation (Table 8.9). We concluded that the influence of maternal diabetic control on fetal growth and the development of fetal macrosomia at birth is more important in early than in late gestation. Our opinion is strongly supported by a recent study of serum fructosamine levels in the mother and ultrasound measurements of the fetus early in pregnancy [87].

The perinatal mortality rate of diabetic pregnancies in the 1980s is equivalent to that observed in normal pregnancies if infants with major congenital malformations are excluded [4]. This favorable fetal outcome can be attributed to the optimal care of pregnant diabetic women with good blood glucose control.

TABLE 8.9. Incidence of large-for-gestational-age (LGA) neonates and of high amniotic fluid C-peptide (AFCP) according to maternal blood glucose control pattern.

Maternal blood glucose control pattern			LGA		High AFCP	
Week 20–31	Week 32 to delivery	No. of patients	No.	%	No.	%
Good →	good	14	2	14.3	2	14.3
Good →	fair/poor	4	0	0	2	50.0
Fair/poor →	good	27	12	44.4*	15	55.6*
Fair/poor →	fair/poor	21	9	42.9	8	38.1*

*$p < .005$ by X^2 test compared with incidence of LGA or high AFCP in "good—good" control group.
Reprinted with permission from the American College of Obstetrics and Gynecology (*Obstetrics and Gynecology* 1986; 67:51–56.)

Antepartum Evaluation of the Mother and the Fetus

Maternal Assessment

Diabetic pregnant women with such high-risk factors as poor diabetic control, type I diabetes, White's class DFR diabetes, or poor obstetric history tend to develop complications more often than low-risk well-controlled women. These complications include pregnancy-induced hypertension, pyelonephritis, diabetic ketoacidosis, polyhydramnios, fetal macrosomia, IUGR, preterm labor, and intrauterine fetal death [2–4,126–128]. To avoid poor perinatal outcome and to assure maternal health without deterioration during the course of pregnancy [129,130], periodic maternal assessments are necessary.

Home, outpatient clinic, or in-hospital monitoring of blood glucose levels and the prevention of diabetic ketoacidosis have been discussed previously. Renal function is assessed at the first prenatal visit and every 2 months thereafter, along with creatinine clearance, blood urea nitrogen level, and uric acid level. A urine culture is obtained at least once each trimester. An ophthalmologic examination is also performed each trimester to detect vascular changes or proliferative retinopathy. Blood pressure is monitored closely because hypertension appears with increased frequency in diabetic patients. Hypertension is the most dangerous complication of diabetic pregnancy, since it frequently causes poor fetal outcome.

Antepartum Fetal Surveillance

Both biochemical and biophysical monitoring are used to ascertain normal fetal growth and development throughout pregnancy.

Hemoglobin A_{1C}, Fructosamine, and Amniotic Fluid C-Peptide Levels

During the first trimester, glycosylated hemoglobin (HbA_{1C}) level has been used to determine the degree of risk for diabetic women of giving birth to an infant with congenital malformations [6,59,84,85]. Recently it has been found that the HbA_{1C} concentration correlates well with the mean maternal glucose level [131–135], with birth weight, and with birth weight corrected for gestational age [135]. Therefore, in addition to maternal glucose level monitoring, the HbA_{1C} level should be assayed at least once a month during the second and third trimesters of pregnancy.

More recently, the concentration of fructosamine, an indicator for serum glycosylated protein levels, was found to be higher in the serum of mothers of diabetic macrosomic infants. Fructosamine levels were highest in women with established diabetes, intermediate in women with gestational onset diabetes, and lowest in nondiabetic women [136]. The same investigators found that serum fructosamine concentrations were significantly elevated in mothers of macrosomic infants during the first trimester;

ultrasonic measurements revealed that sustained elevation of the fructosamine level correlated well with the development of a macrosomic fetus during the first and second trimesters [87].

The relationship between amniotic fluid C-peptide and fetal growth has been described in previous sections of this chapter [27–29]. Increased cord blood C-peptide levels were seen in infants of diabetic mothers, particularly infants with macrosomia and neonatal hypoglycemia [137]. In addition, amniotic fluid C-peptide has been shown to respond positively to an arginine challenge in insulin-treated diabetic women in late pregnancy [138]. These investigators also found that C-peptide concentration was correlated with both insulin concentration and birth weight. Both the insulin and C-peptide levels were significantly higher in diabetic pregnancies associated with fetal morbidity than in those without fetal morbidity. Thus, amniotic fluid C-peptide level is useful in detecting fetal hyperinsulinism in late pregnancy, and a diagnosis of fetal macrosomia can be made with its use in conjunction with the ultrasonic measurements to be discussed in the following section.

Ultrasound Evaluation

Ultrasonography is an extremely valuable tool in evaluating fetal size and fetal growth pattern and in detecting polyhydramnios and congenital malformations. In the first trimester it is used to detect early fetal growth delay [17], a missed abortion, or a blighted ovum [139,140]. For detection of fetal congenital malformations, initial ultrasonography may be performed at 16 to 18 weeks of gestation. Determination of maternal serum alpha-fetoprotein (AFP) should be employed at this time in association with ultrasonography in an attempt to detect neural tube defects [141,142]. In general, CNS anomalies account for approximately 40% of all fetal anomalies, while fetal cardiac anomalies account for another 20 to 30% [143]. In a large series of ultrasound studies for the detection of major fetal malformations, Manning et al [144] reported a detection rate of 70% in 2,175 referred high-risk patients. Campbell and Pearce [145] correctly diagnosed 95% of 425 fetuses with malformations, based on 2,372 patients screened. During the second and third trimester, ultrasound studies may be repeated at 4- to 6-week intervals to assess fetal growth and amniotic fluid volume.

Macrosomia is the leading risk factor for shoulder dystocia. Several studies have employed ultrasound measurements to predict fetal size [146–148]. In most infants weighing more than 4,000 g, the chest diameter will be at least 1.4 cm greater than the biparietal diameter [146]. In a study by Bracero and associates [148], mean values of both the abdominal diameter/femur length ratio and the abdominal diameter/biparietal diameter ratio were highest in the LGA diabetic group. When both ratios were used together, the accuracy of diagnosis of LGA reached 92%.

Diabetic halo, a double-ring outline of the fetal head on ultrasonography, has been described in association with poorly controlled diabetic pregnancies [149]. In a study of 42 diabetic patients, diabetic halo, with a space of 4 mm or more between the fetal scalp and parietal bone, was present in 12 cases. Nine of the 12 pregnancies with halo resulted in the birth of LGA infants.

While the various methods of diagnosing fetal macrosomia described above have a relatively high sensitivity, false-positive predictions cannot be totally eliminated. Therefore, decisions regarding the best route of delivery for an infant suspected to be macrosomic should be based on both ultrasound data and clinical assessment.

Plasma Unconjugated Estriol and Urinary Estriol Assays

Estriol assays were once a widely used antepartum test to evaluate fetal well-being in diabetic pregnancies. Because estriol levels in maternal serum or maternal urine are a reflection of the status of the fetoplacental unit, pregnant diabetic patients tend to have high estriol values until a sudden deterioration of placental function occurs, prior to fetal death. Goebelsmann et al [150] advocated daily measurements of urinary estriol in diabetic pregnancies in order to closely monitor placental function and detect a compromised fetus. Subsequently, unconjugated plasma estriol was reported to be more useful [151]. However, many clinicians avoid this test because the complicated assay procedure leads to delays in reporting results to the doctor. It is also not as effective as fetal heart rate monitoring or biophysical profile scoring in determining the fetal status. Dooley et al [152] reviewed 138 pregnancies in which more than 3,000 urinary estriol assays were performed. Twenty-one assays revealed a significant drop in the estriol/creatinine ratio, but only two cases were actually associated with fetal distress. These data confirm the observations of others that there is limited clinical value for the urinary estriol assay in pregnancies complicated by diabetes [152].

Biophysical Methods

Maternal monitoring of fetal movement is an easy and practical method that has proven useful in assessing the fetal condition in a variety of high-risk pregnancies [153,154]. Either the total number of fetal movements throughout the day or many recordings of the number of fetal movements during 30- to 60-minute periods within 1 day may be used. A marked decrease in fetal movements to fewer than 10 in a 12-hour period may indicate fetal jeopardy, and fetal heart rate testing should be performed immediately. Today, fetal heart rate (FHR) testing, both the nonstress test (NST) and the contraction stress test (CST), remain in the front line among various methods of evaluating fetal well-being in diabetic pregnancies. In view of the subsequent sharp decline in the incidence of intrauterine fetal deaths, the application of the CST to the management of diabetic pregnancy a decade ago marked an important milestone in perinatal care [69].

Positive CSTs have been observed in the fetuses of approximately 10% of insulin-dependent diabetic patients and are associated with an increased incidence of perinatal mortality, late decelerations in labor, low Apgar scores, RDS, and reduced birth weight [69]. In our experience, both non-reactive NSTs and positive CSTs in diabetic pregnancies were less than 10%, while the incidence of abnormal tests in IUGR was approximately 30% [153–155]. Nevertheless, testing should begin at 30 weeks in diabetic pregnancies and should be performed twice weekly [156]. In patients with vascular disease, hypertension, poor diabetic control, or a history of previous stillbirth, for whom the incidence of abnormal tests and intrauterine deaths is greater, testing is often performed daily. At the present time, most medical centers in the United States use the NST as a screening test, backed up by either the CST or the biophysical profile score [157] to evaluate fetal health in various high-risk pregnancies.

The variables constituting the biophysical profile proposed by Manning [158] are the nonstress test, fetal breathing movements, fetal movements, fetal tone, and amniotic fluid volume. Baskett [159] tested 1,996 high-risk fetuses with the biophysical profile and found that an abnormal biophysical profile score had a positive predictive value of perinatal complications of 79%. A normal profile score obtained within a week before delivery, with the amniotic membranes intact at the time of testing, was associated with a perinatal mortality rate of 0.5/1,000 total births, compared with an overall rate of 4.4/1,000 births when lethal anomalies are excluded. In insulin-requiring diabetic pregnancies, a fetal biophysical profile score of 8 was at least as reliable as a reactive NST or a negative CST [156].

Recently, umbilical velocity waveforms and calculated systolic/diastolic (S/D) ratios appear to offer promise for the clinical assessment of placental-umbilical circulation function in high-risk pregnancies [160–163]. In diabetic pregnancies, many patients demonstrate an S/D ratio of 3 or more [164], in contrast to an S/D ratio of 2.5 in normal pregnancies between 31 and 39 weeks of gestation [160]. A significant positive correlation between S/D ratios and serum glucose level has been shown to exist in diabetic pregnancies [164]. Furthermore, those diabetic pregnancies with an S/D ratio of 3 or more were associated with an increased number of stillbirths and neonatal morbidity.

Fetal Maturity Studies

The amniotic fluid lecithin/sphingomyelin ratio (L/S ratio) has proven to be an invaluable index of fetal pulmonary maturity. Although the reliability of the L/S ratio in diabetic pregnancies has been questioned, most diabetic study series report a low incidence of RDS with a mature L/S ratio of 2.0 or greater. In one study of 93 insulin-dependent diabetic patients, an L/S ratio of 2.0 or greater was associated with a 3% risk of RDS [69]; this result was no higher than that observed in a nondiabetic population. The presence of phosphatidylglycerol (PG) is a final marker of fetal pulmonary maturation. Fetal hyperinsulinism in diabetic pregnancies is believed to be associated with a delayed appearance of PG and an increased incidence of RDS [165]. Infants of diabetic mothers have been reported to develop RDS after an L/S ratio between 2.0 and 3.0 and a negative PG were obtained [165]. Therefore, caution must be used in planning the delivery of a diabetic patient with a mature L/S ratio but absent PG. If the antepartum assessment of fetal well-being remains reassuring, delivery may be delayed for 1 to 2 weeks.

Brazy et al [166] studied amniotic fluid cortisol in normal and diabetic patients and found that the incidence of RDS was 26% when the amniotic fluid cortisol level was less than 4.3 ng/dl and only 2 to 9% RDS if the cortisol level was above the 4.3 ng/dl cutoff point. In normal pregnancies the cortisol level was low until 35 weeks' gestation; it rose sharply at 36 weeks and continued in an upward trend to 39 weeks. In many diabetic pregnancies, the rise in cortisol level after 35 weeks was delayed or absent. This observation may help to explain the phenomenon of delayed fetal lung maturity in diabetic pregnancies.

Timing of Delivery

Management protocols developed during the 1970s advocated routine hospitalization 4 to 5 weeks before delivery for patients with insulin-dependent diabetes mellitus. Gabbe et al [58] employed daily estriol monitoring and weekly CSTs for fetal surveillance for their series of 260 patients. Pregnancy was rarely terminated for fetal indications before 38 weeks in the absence of documented pulmonary maturity. Using such a protocol, perinatal mortality was less than 5% and fetal death rates were no higher than those in the nondiabetic population.

With the availability of daily home glucose testing to maintain normoglycemic control, as well as outpatient FHR testing twice per week, obstetricians are now better able to manage well-controlled diabetic pregnant women as outpatients until the decision is made for delivery [156]. Expectant management has permitted more patients to enter spontaneous labor. Inpatient care is reserved for those patients who require daily fetal surveillance as well as intensive diabetic control. Women with severe vascular disease, hypertension, fetal compromise, fetal growth retardation, or poor diabetic control belong in this category. These complications may dictate delivery prior to 38 weeks' gestation. Although documentation of a mature L/S ratio before premature delivery is the general rule, such documentation may not be necessary in the management of diabetic pregnancies with any of these complications. Today, fewer elective cesarean sections are being performed, and the criteria for induction of labor have been loosened somewhat for the management of the diabetic pregnant women at term.

Intrapartum Management

Since the focus of prenatal care has changed to maintaining euglycemia throughout pregnancy, there has been a remarkable decrease in intrauterine deaths and neonatal mortality in insulin-dependent diabetics. Much less attention has been focused on the intrapartum control of glucose levels and neonatal morbidity. Euglycemia during the intrapartum period is also desirable. In studies of chronic sheep preparations, hyperinsulinemia and hyperglycemia produced fetal hypoxia [46,47]. Glucose-induced hypoxemia may contribute to the fetal distress and demise seen in poorly controlled diabetic pregnancies. Neonatal hypoglycemia, which can lead to seizures, has been shown to result from transient or sustained maternal hyperglycemia. Soler and Malin [167] have demonstrated a direct relationship between maternal intrapartum glucose level and neonatal hypoglycemia. In their study series, when maternal blood glucose was greater than 130 mg/dl, the incidence of neonatal hypoglycemia was 41.1%, whereas when the glucose level was less than 90 mg/dl, the incidence was only 7.4%. Midovnik et al [168] showed that when the maternal glucose level was greater than 90 mg/dl, neonatal hypoglycemia occurred in 47.0% of the neonates, compared with 14.0% when the glucose level was less than 90 mg/dl. Euglycemia in labor, however, does not totally eradicate neonatal hypoglycemia [167–169]; another mechanism must also contribute to this condition. Jovanovic and Peterson [170] postulated that tight long-term as well as intrapartum diabetic control is the key to the eradication of neonatal morbidity. Euglycemia in labor is also thought to decrease other neonatal complications including hypocalcemia, polycythemia, and hyperbilirubinemia.

Jovanovic and Peterson [170] have shown that in tightly controlled euglycemic diabetic parturients, insulin requirements decrease to zero during active labor while glucose requirements remain relatively constant at 2.55 mg/kg/min. The work of Golde et al [169] supports these findings. It is postulated that contractions may decrease the supply of placental antiinsulin hormones to the maternal circulation. In the second stage of labor, however, insulin requirements return. Insulin requirements decrease rapidly with delivery of the placenta; there is a sudden decrease in placental lactogen and a decrease in growth hormone release, with a concomitant increase in sensitivity to insulin. Oxytocin is frequently used to induce or enhance labor in diabetic pregnancies. However, oxytocin has been shown to have no influence on patients' insulin requirements.

The key points in the intrapartum management of diabetics include (1) frequent blood glucose determinations, most easily done with a bedside reflectance meter, (2) D5W intravenously to assure a constant supply of glucose to the fetus, (3) insulin administration as needed, and (4) a decrease in insulin administration at the time the placenta delivers.

Bearing these points in mind, one must evaluate intrapartum subcutaneous insulin regimens compared with intravenous regimens. The advantage of the subcutaneous regimens is that they are fairly simple, no IV pumps are required, and they are controlled mainly by varying the rate of the IV glucose infusion. However, less constant insulin levels are achieved compared with an IV insulin regimen, and if the delivery is more rapid than expected the patient may have a large amount of circulating insulin at delivery, resulting in maternal hypoglycemia. Management of the intrapartum patient with a constant intravenous infusion of insulin and glucose provides a more consistent insulin level that can be rapidly decreased after delivery.

White [2] proposed only an IV infusion of D5W with no insulin for those undergoing short labor or C-section, and administration of the prepregnancy insulin dose after delivery. Long inductions are managed with 50% of the prepregnancy dose of insulin as NPH and the other half administered after delivery. Soler and Malen [167] suggested a uniform 24 units of NPH subcutaneously in the morning of an induction or elective C-section. This is repeated 14 to 16 hours later if the patient still has not delivered. Haigh et al [171] suggested giving one-third of the usual dose as NPH if delivery is expected in 4 to 6 hours, two-thirds of the usual dose as NPH if delivery is expected in 6 to 10 hours, and the full dose as NPH if delivery is more than 10 hours away. Additional coverage is given with regular insulin as needed. At the first meal after delivery, one-third of the pregnancy dose or two-thirds of the prepregnancy dose is given.

Nathass et al [172] described a closed-loop computerized system that reads a glucose level constantly and administers IV solutions of normal saline, saline with insulin, or normal saline with D5W. Insulin rates vary from 0.2 to 9.8 units/hour with an immediate decrease in the rate at the time of delivery. This system, however, is not practical except in a research setting. Cohen and Gabbe [173] described an open-loop system using a continuous subcutaneous insulin infusion pump along with the usual D5W IV infusion. The pump delivers 0.1 unit of regular insulin every 8 minutes, and the rate is adjusted as needed.

The easiest regimen suggested is one in which 10 units of regular insulin are added to 1 L of D5W and run at 100 to 125 cc/hour, thus administering 1.0 to 1.25 units of insulin per hour [127,174]. The insulin concentration is increased as needed by the addition of regular insulin to the IV solution, keeping the IV rate constant. Bowen et al [175] suggested a similar regimen but used D10W with twice the concentration of insulin. An alternative is that the insulin can be "piggy-backed" into the D5W IV solution via a pump as needed [169,176,177]. Jovanovic and Peterson [86] suggested having three IV solutions at the bedside with a three-way stopcock. The patient is begun on 0.9 NS and a blood sugar level is determined. If the glucose level is less than 70 mg/dl, D10W is administered; if the glucose level is from 70 to 110 mg/dl, D5W is given; and for a glucose level greater than 110 mg/dl, 0.9 NS with 2 units of regular insulin IV is given. Midovnik et al [168] used a similar regimen but substituted D5W with lactated Ringer's or lactated Ringer's with 2 units of regular insulin, respectively. In all regimens, blood glucose levels are checked every 1 to 2 hours and adjustments in the rates of the infusions are made accordingly.

Continuous intrapartum fetal heart rate monitoring is essential in all diabetic pregnancies. In those patients undergoing induction of labor, an intrauterine pressure catheter is helpful in assuring adequate labor. An ongoing assessment of the progress of labor is also important. Fetal scalp blood sampling should be used if appropriate. One should be watchful for shoulder dystocia in macrosomic infants. If the second stage of labor is prolonged, the incidence of shoulder distocia approaches 25% [178,179]. Macrosomia is associated with traumatic delivery in 15% of these pregnancies and the obstetrician should be prepared to perform various maneuvers to deliver such an infant [180]. If signs of cephalopelvic disproportion occur, a C-section should be performed without delay.

Management of immediate neonatal complications such as perinatal asphyxia, hypoglycemia, hypocalcemia, polycythemia, hyperbilirubinemia, RDS, congenital malformations, and birth trauma are largely the responsibility of the neonatologist and the pediatric nurses in the intensive care nursery. A detailed discussion of pediatric management will not be offered in this chapter.

Table 8.10 summarizes antepartum maternal management as well as fetal surveillance in insulin-dependent diabetic pregnancies. Each category of these management procedures has been discussed in detail in this chap-

TABLE 8.10. Protocols for antepartum maternal management and fetal surveillance in insulin-dependent diabetic pregnancies.

Maternal management	Fetal surveillance
Preconception and early postconception control	Hemoglobin A_{1C} measurement at initial visit, then once per month
Tight antepartum glycemic control	Ultrasonography, initially at 16–18 weeks,
Individualized diet adjustment	then at 4–6-week intervals (fetal
Home glucose monitoring four times	growth, major malformations,
daily	macrosomia, polyhydramnios)
Clinic visits weekly for fasting/	Plasma/urinary estriol levels not
postprandial glucose	necessary in the 1980s
Readjustment of insulin doses	Nonstress test (NST) twice weekly after
Hospitalization for:	30 weeks, daily in severely ill cases
Poor diabetic control	Contraction stress test (CST) or
Diabetic ketoacidosis	biophysical profile score (BPS) only if
Severe complications	NST is nonreactive
Fetal compromise	Amniocentesis for L/S ratio and PG*
Planned delivery	levels at 37–38 weeks
Fetal maturity	
Fetal jeopardy	

*L/S ratio, lecithin/sphingomyelin ratio; PG, phosphatidylglycerol.

ter. To achieve the best maternal and fetal outcome, a continuous, meticulous effort by a team that includes the obstetrician, the pediatrician, ultrasonographers, nurse educators, laboratory technicians, and dietitians must be employed throughout the antepartum, intrapartum, and neonatal periods. Of course, the cooperation of the patients themselves is the most important factor leading to a successful perinatal outcome in diabetic pregnancies.

REFERENCES

1. Gabbe SG: Management of diabetes in pregnancy: Six-decades of experience. In Pitkin RM, Zlatnik FJ (Eds): *The Year Book of Obstetrics and Gynecology.* Chicago: Year Book, 1980, pp. 37–49.
2. White P: Pregnancy complicating diabetes. *Am J Med* 7:609, 1949.
3. Pedersen J, Pedersen LM, Andersen B: Assessors of fetal perinatal mortality in diabetic pregnancy. *Diabetes* 23:302–305, 1974.
4. Samuels P, Landon MD: Medical complication. In Gabbe SG, Niebyl JR, Simpson JL (Eds): *Obstetrics: Normal and Problem Pregnancies.* New York: Churchill Livingstone, 1986, pp. 865–977.
5. Molsted-Pedersen L: Pregnancy and diabetes: A survey. *Acta Endocrinol* **94** (suppl 238):13–19, 1980.
6. Miller E, Hare JW, Cloherty JP, et al: Elevated maternal HbA_{1c} in early pregnancy and major congenital anomalie in infants of diabetic mothers. *N Engl J Med* **304:**1331–1334, 1981.
7. Grix A Jr, Curry C, Hall BD: Patterns of multiple malformations in infants of diabetic mothers. In March of Dimes Birth Defects Foundation: *Prenatal Diagnosis and Mechanisms of Teratogenesis.* Vol. 18. New York: Alan R. Liss, 1982, pp. 55–77.
8. Hollingsworth DR: *Pregnancy, Diabetes and Birth: A Management Guide.* Baltimore: Williams & Wilkins, 1984.
9. Hollingsworth DR, Cousins L: Disorder of carbohydrate metabolism. In Creasy RK, Resnik R (Eds): *Maternal-Fetal Medicine: Principles and Practice.* Philadelphia: WB Saunders, 1984, pp. 833–896.
10. Davis WS, Campbell JB: Neonatal small left colon syndrome. *Am J Dis Child* **129:**1024–1027, 1975.
11. Mills JL, Baker L, Goldman AS: Malformations in infants of diabetic mothers occur before the seventh gestational week. *Diabetes* **28:**292–293, 1979.
12. Eriksson V, Dahlstrom E, Larsson KS, et al: Increased incidence of congenital malformations in the offspring of diabetic rats and their prevention by maternal insulin therapy. *Diabetes* **31:**1–6, 1982.
13. Pinter E, Reece EA, Leranth CS, et al: Yolk sac failure in embryopathy due to hyperglycemia: Ultrastructural analysis of yolk sac differentiation associated with embryopathy in rat conceptuses under hyperglycemic conditions. *Teratology* **33:**73–84, 1986.
14. Reece EA, Pinter E, Leranth CS, et al: Ultrastructural analysis of malformations of the embryonic neural axis induced by hyperglycemic conceptus culture. *Teratology* **32:**363–373, 1985.
15. Pinter E, Reece EA, Leranth CZ, et al: Arachidonic acid prevents hyper-

glycemia associated yolk sac damage and embryopathy. *Am J Obstet Gynecol* **155**:691–702, 1986.

16. Sadler TW, Hunter III ES: Hypoglycemia: How little is too much for the embryo? *Am J Obstet Gynecol* **157**:190–193, 1987.
17. Pedersen JF, Molsted-Pedersen L: Early fetal growth delay detected by ultrasound marks increased risk by congenital malformation in diabetic pregnancy. *Br Med J* **1**:18–19, 1979.
18. Sutherland HW, Pritchard CW: Increased incidence of spontaneous abortion in pregnancies complicated by maternal diabetes mellitus. *Am J Obstet Gynecol* **155**:135–138, 1986.
19. Cardell BS: Hypertrophy and hyperplasia of pancreatic islets in newborn infants. *J Pathol Bacteriol* **66**:335–346, 1953.
20. Driscoll SG, Benirschke K, Curtis GW: Neonatal deaths among infants of diabetic mothers. *Am J Dis Child* **100**:818–835, 1960.
21. Steinke J, Driscoll SG: The extractable insulin content of pancreas from fetuses and infants of diabetic and control mothers. *Diabetes* **14**:573–578, 1965.
22. Pedersen J, Bojsen-Moller B, Poulsen H: Blood sugar in newborn infants of diabetic mothers. *Acta Endocrinol.* (Copenh.) **15**:33–52, 1954.
23. Freinkel N, Metzger BE: Pregnancy as a tissue culture experience: The critical implications of maternal metabolism for fetal development. In *CIBA Foundation Symposium 63: Pregnancy, Metabolism, Diabetes, and the Fetus*. Amsterdam: Excerpta Medica, 1979, pp. 3–28.
24. Spellacy WN, Buhi WC, Bradley B, et al: Maternal, fetal, and amniotic fluid levels of glucose, insulin, and growth hormone. *Obstet Gynecol* **41**:323–331, 1973.
25. Newman RI, Tutera G: The glucose-insulin ratio in amniotic fluid. *Obstet Gynecol* **47**:599–601, 1976.
26. Weiss PAM, Lichtenegger W, Winter R, et al: Insulin levels in amniotic fluid: Management of diabetes in pregnancy. *Obstet Gynecol* **51**:393–398, 1978.
27. Lin CC, River P, Moawad AH: Prenatal assessment of fetal outcome by amniotic fluid C-peptide levels in pregnant diabetic women. *Am J Obstet Gynecol* **141**:671–676, 1981.
28. Tchobroutsky G, Heard I, Tchobroutsky C, et al: Amniotic fluid C-peptide in normal and insulin-dependent diabetic pregnancies. *Diabetologia* **18**:289–292, 1980.
29. Lin CC, Moawad AH, River P, et al: Amniotic fluid C-peptide as an index for intrauterine fetal growth. *Am J Obstet Gynecol* **139**:390–396, 1981.
30. Meschia G, Battaglia FC, Hay WW, et al: Utilization of substrates by the ovine placenta in vivo. *Fed Proc* **39**:245–249, 1980.
31. Battaglia FC: Principal substrates of fetal metabolism: Fuel and growth requirements of the ovine fetus. In *CIBA Foundation Symposium 63: Pregnancy, Metabolism, Diabetes, and the Fetus*. Amsterdam: Excerpta Medica, 1979.
32. Milner RGG: Amino acids and beta cell growth in structure and function. In Merkatz IR, Adam PAJ (Eds): *The Diabetic Pregnancy: A Perinatal Perspective*. New York: Grune & Stratton, 1979.
33. Felig P: Maternal and fetal fuel homeostasis in human pregnancy. *Am J Clin Nutr* **26**:998–1005, 1973.
34. Fox H: Pathology of the placenta in maternal diabetes mellitus. *Obstet Gynecol* **34**:792–798, 1979.

35. Robertson WB, Brosens I, Landells WN: Abnormal placentation. In Wynn RM (Ed): *Obstetrics and Gynecology Annual.* Vol. 14. Norwalk, CT: Appleton-Century-Crofts, 1985, pp. 411–426.

36. Fox H: Placental pathology: A contemporary approach. In Wynn RM (Ed): *Obstetrics and Gynecology Annual.* Vol. 14. Norwalk, CT: Appleton-Century-Crofts, 1985, pp. 427–440.

37. Driscoll SC: The pathology of pregnancy complicated by diabetes mellitus. *Med Clin North Am* **49**:1053–1067, 1965.

38. Lavin JP, Lovelace DR, Miodovnik M, et al: Clinical experience with one hundred seven diabetic pregnancies. *Am J Obstet Gynecol* **147**:742–752, 1983.

39. Lemons JA, Vargas P, Delaney JJ: Infant of the diabetic mother: Review of 225 cases. *Obstet Gynecol* **57**:157–192, 1981.

40. Karlsson K, Kjellmer I: The outcome of diabetic pregnancies in relation to the mother's blood sugar level. *Am J Obstet Gynecol* **112**:213–220, 1972.

41. Adashi EY, Pinto H, Tyson JE: Impact of maternal euglycemia on fetal outcome in diabetic pregnancy. *Am J Obstet Gynecol* **133**:268–274, 1979.

42. Ylinen K, Raivio K, Teramo K: Hemoglobin A_{1C} predicts the perinatal outcome in insulin dependent diabetic pregnancies. *Br J Obstet Gynecol* **88**:961–967, 1981.

43. Goldman JA, Dicker D, Feldberg D, et al: Pregnancy outcome in patients with insulin-dependent diabetes mellitus with preconceptional diabetic control: A comparative study. *Am J Obstet Gynecol* **155**:293–297, 1986.

44. Landon MB, Gabbe SG, Piana R, et al: Neonatal morbidity in pregnancy complicated by diabetes mellitus: Predictive value of maternal glycemic profiles. *Am J Obstet Gynecol* **156**:1089–1095, 1987.

45. Lin CC, River J, River P, et al: Good diabetic control early in pregnancy and favorable fetal outcome. *Obstet Gynecol* **67**:51–56, 1986.

46. Carson BS, Philips AF, Simmons MA, et al: Effects of a sustained insulin infusion upon glucose uptake and oxygenation of the ovine fetus. *Pediatr Res* **14**:147–152, 1980.

47. Philips AF, Dubin JW, Matty PJ, et al: Arterial hypoxemia and hyperinsulinemia in the chronically hyperglycemic fetal lamb. *Pediatr Res* **16**:653–658, 1982.

48. Kitzmiller JL, Phillipe M, VonOeyen P, et al: Hyperglycemia, hypoxia, and fetal acidosis in Rhesus monkey. Paper presented at the 28th Annual Meeting of the Society of Gynecologic Investigation, St. Louis, 1981.

49. Lawrence GR, Brown VA, Parsons RJ, et al: Feto-maternal consequences of high-dose glucose infusion during labor. *Br J Obstet Gynaecol* **89**:27–32, 1982.

50. Philips AF, Dubin JW, Raye JR: Fetal metabolic responses to endogenous insulin release. *Am J Obstet Gynecol* **139**:441–445, 1981.

51. Nylund L, Lunell NO, Lewander R, et al: Utero-placental blood flow in diabetic pregnancy. *Am J Obstet Gynecol* **144**:298–302, 1982.

52. LoBue C, Goodlin RC: Treatment of fetal distress during diabetic ketoacidosis. *J Reprod Med* **20**:101–104, 1978.

53. Kitzmiller JL: Diabetic ketoacidosis and pregnancy. *Contemp OB/GYN* **20**:141–168, 1982.

54. Coustan DR: Diabetic ketoacidosis. In Berkowitz RL (Ed): *Critical Care of the Obstetric Patient.* New York: Churchill Livingstone, 1983, pp. 411–429.

55. Hughes AB: Fetal heart rate changes during diabetic ketosis. *Acta Obstet Gynecol Scand* **66**:71–73, 1987.
56. Gross TL, Sokol RJ, Williams T, et al: Shoulder dystocia: A fetal-physician risk. *Am J Obstet Gynecol* **156**:1408–1418, 1987.
57. Coustant DR, Imarah J: Prophylactic insulin treatment of gestational diabetics reduces the incidence of macrosomia, operative delivery, and birth trauma. *Am J Obstet Gynecol* **150**:836–842, 1984.
58. Gabbe SG, Mestman JH, Freeman RK, et al: Management and outcome of diabetes, classes B to R. *Am J Obstet Gynecol* **129**:723–732, 1977.
59. Roversi GD, Garbiulo M, Nicolini V, et al: A new approach to the treatment of diabetic pregnant women: Report of 479 cases seen from 1963 to 1975. *Am J Obstet Gynecol* **135**:567–576, 1979.
60. Atral R, Golde SH, Dorey F, et al: The effect of plasma glucose variability on neonatal outcome in the pregnant diabetic patient. *Am J Obstet Gynecol* **147**:537–541, 1983.
61. Levano KJ, Hauth JC, Gilstrap LC, et al: Appraisal of "rigid" blood glucose control during pregnancy in the overtly diabetic woman. *Am J Obstet Gynecol* **135**:853–862, 1979.
62. O'Sullivan JB, Mahan CM: Criteria for the oral glucose tolerance test in pregnancy. *Diabetes* **13**:278–285, 1964.
63. Carpenter MW, Coustan DR: Criteria for screening tests for gestational diabetes. *Am J Obstet Gynecol* **144**:768–773, 1982.
64. Lavin JP, Barden TP, Miodovnik M: Clinical experience with a screening program for gestational diabetes. *Am J Obstet Gynecol* **141**:491–494, 1981.
65. Merkatz IR, Duchon MA, Yamashita TS, et al: A pilot community-based screening program for gestational diabetes. *Diabet Care* **3**:453–457, 1980.
66. Gabbe SG: Definition, detection and management of gestational diabetes. *Obstet Gynecol* **67**:121–125, 1986.
67. Summary and Recommendations of the Second International Workshop-Conference on Gestational Diabetes Mellitus. *Diabetes* **34** (suppl 2):123–126, 1985.
68. Coustan DR, Carpenter MW: Detection and treatment of gestational diabetes. *Clin Obstet Gynecol* **28**:507–515, 1985.
69. Forest J-C, Garrido-Russo M, Lemay A, et al: Reference values for the oral glucose tolerance test at each trimester of pregnancy. *Am J Clin Pathol* **80**:828–831, 1983.
70. Mestman J: Medical management of the pregnant diabetic. *Contemp OB/GYN* **1**:61–64, 1973.
71. National Diabetes Data Group: Classification and diagnosis of diabetes mellitus and other categories of glucose intolerance. *Diabetes* **28**:1039–1057, 1979.
72. Solomons E, Silverstone FA, Posner NA: Obstetric factors suggesting diabetes evaluated by the rapid intravenous glucose tolerance test. *Obstet Gynecol* **22**:50–55, 1963.
73. Court DJ, Stone PR, Killip M: Comparison of glucose and a glucose polymer for testing oral carbohydrate tolerance in pregnancy. *Obstet Gynecol* **64**:251–255, 1984.
74. Reece EA, Holford T, Tuck S, et al: Screening for gestational diabetes: One-hour carbohydrate tolerance test performed by a virtually tasteless polymer of glucose. *Am J Obstet Gynecol* **156**:132–134, 1987.

75. Landon MB, Cembrowski GS, Gabbe SG: Capillary blood glucose screening for gestational diabetes: A preliminary investigation. *Am J Obstet Gynecol* **155**:717–721, 1986.

76. O'Sullivan JB: Establishing criteria for gestational diabetes. *Diabet Care* **3**:437–439, 1980.

77. Dietrich ML, Dolnicek TF, Rayburn WF: Gestational diabetes screening in a private, midwestern American population. *Am J Obstet Gynecol* **156**:1403–1408, 1987.

78. Aubrey RH, Pennington JC: Identification and evaluation of high risk pregnancy: The perinatal concept. *Clin Obstet Gynecol* **16**:3–27, 1973.

79. Nesbitt REL Jr: Perinatal identification of the fetus at risk. *Clin Perinatol* **1**:213–228, 1974.

80. Hollingsworth DR, Jones OW, Resnik R: Expanded care in obstetrics for the 1980's: Preconception and early postconception counseling. *Am J Obstet Gynecol* **149**:811–814, 1984.

81. Fuhrmann K, Reiher H, Semmler K, et al: Prevention of congenital malformations in infants of insulin-dependent diabetic mothers. *Diabet Care* **6**:219–223, 1983.

82. Fuhrmann K, Reiher H, Semmler K, et al: The effect of intensified conventional insulin therapy before and during pregnancy on the malformation rate in offspring of diabetic mothers. *Exp Clin Endocrinol* **83**:173–177, 1984.

83. Mills JL: Euglycemic control during early pregnancy does not guarantee prevention of malformations in infants of insulin-dependent diabetic mothers. Paper presented at American Diabetes Association Meeting, Indianapolis, 1987 (*abstract in OB/GYN New* **22** (13):1, 1987).

84. Key TC, Giuffrida R, Moore TR: Predictive value of early pregnancy glycohemoglobin in the insulin-treated diabetic patient. *Am J Obstet Gynecol* **156**:1096–1100, 1987.

85. Ylinen K, Aula P, Steman UH, et al: Risk of minor and major fetal malformations in diabetes with high hemoglobin A_{1C} values in early pregnancy. *Br Med J* **289**:345–346, 1984.

86. Jovanovic L, Peterson CM: Management of the pregnant, insulin-dependent diabetic woman. *Diabet Care* **3**:63–68, 1980.

87. Roberts AB, Baker JR: Relationship between fetal growth and maternal fructosamine in diabetic pregnancy. *Obstet Gynecol* **70**:242–246, 1987.

88. Phelps RL, Metzger BE, Freinkel N: Carbohydrate metabolism in pregnancy. *Am J Obstet Gynecol* **140**:730–736, 1981.

89. Hollingsworth DR: Maternal metabolism in normal pregnancy and pregnancy complicated by diabetes mellitus. *Clin Obstet Gynecol* **28**:457–472, 1985.

90. Cousins L, Rigg L, Hollingsworth D, et al: The 24-hour excursion and diurnal rhythm of glucose, insulin, and C-peptide in normal pregnancy. *Am J Obstet Gynecol* **136**:483–488, 1980.

91. Peacock I, Hunter JC, Walford S, et al: Self-monitoring of blood glucose in diabetic pregnancy. *Br Med J* **2**:1333–1336, 1979.

92. Hanson U, Persson B, Lennerhagen P, et al: Self-monitoring of blood glucose by diabetic women during the third trimester of pregnancy. *Am J Obstet Gynecol* **150**:817–821, 1984.

93. Tyden O, Berne C: Obstetric care in diabetic pregnancy. *Acta Pediatr Scand* (suppl. 320):94–99, 1985.

94. American Diabetes Association's Committee on Food and Nutrition: Principles of nutrition and dietary recommendations for individuals with diabetes mellitus, 1979. *Diabetes* **28**:1027–1030, 1979.
95. Committee on Dietary Allowances Food and Nutrition Board National Research Council: Recommended dietary allowances. Washington, D.C.: *National Academy of Sciences,* 1980.
96. Freinkel N, Dooley SL, Metzger BE: Care of the pregnant woman with insulin-dependent diabetes mellitus. *N Engl J Med* **313**:96–101, 1985.
97. Schulman PK, Gyves MT, Merkatz IR: Role of nutrition in the management of the pregnant diabetic patient. *Sem. Perinatol* **2**:353–360, 1978.
98. Granodos JL: Recent developments in the outpatient management of insulin-dependent diabetes mellitus during pregnancy. *Obstet Gynecol Ann* **13**:83–98, 1984.
99. Jovanovic L, Peterson CM: Intensified treatment of pregnant insulin-dependent diabetic women. *Acta Endocrin Scand* (suppl 227):77–80, 1986.
100. Weiss PAM, Hofmann H: Intensified conventional insulin therapy for the pregnant diabetic patient. *Obstet Gynecol* **64**:629–637, 1984.
101. Jovanovic L, Peterson CM: Optimal insulin delivery for the pregnant diabetic patient. *Diabet Care* **5** (suppl 1):24–37, 1982.
102. Coustan DR, Reece EA, Sherwin RS, et al: A randomized clinical trial of the insulin pump vs. intensive conventional therapy in diabetic pregnancies. *JAMA* **255**:631–636, 1986.
103. Landon MB, Gabbe SG: Glucose monitoring and insulin administration in the pregnant diabetic patient. *Clin Obstet Gynecol* **28**:496–506, 1985.
104. Galloway JA, Spradlin CT, Nelson RL, et al: Factors influencing the absorption, serum insulin concentration, and blood glucose responses after injections of regular insulin and various insulin mixtures. *Diabet Care* **4**:366–376, 1981.
105. Mancuso S, Caruso A, Langone A, et al: Continuous subcutaneous insulin infusion (CSII) in pregnant diabetic women. *Acta Endocrin* **277** (suppl):112–116, 1986.
106. Skyler JS, Pferffer EF, Raptis S, et al: Biosynthetic human insulin: Progress and prospects. *Diabet Care* **4**:140–143, 1981.
107. Mylvaganam R, Stowers JM, Steel JM, et al: Insulin immunogenicity in pregnancy: Maternal and fetal studies. *Diabetologia* **24**:19–25, 1983.
108. Heding LG, Larssen Y, Ludvigssen J: The immunogenicity of insulin preparation: Antibody levels before and after transfer to highly purified porcine insulin. *Diabetologia* **19**:511–515, 1980.
109. Stubbs SM, Brudenell JM, Puke DA, et al: Management of the pregnant diabetic: Home or hospital, with or without glucose meters? *Lancet* **1**:22–24, 1980.
110. Reeves ML, Forham SE, Skyler JS, et al: Comparison of methods for blood glucose monitoring. *Diabet Care* **4**:404–406, 1981.
111. Bompiani GD, Botta RM: Treatment of noninsulin-dependent diabetic women during pregnancy. *Acta Endocrin* **277** (suppl):56–59, 1986.
112. Gillmer MDG, Maresh M, Beard RW, et al: Low energy diets in the treatment of gestational diabetes. *Acta Endocrin* **277** (suppl):44–49, 1986.
113. Coustan DR, Lewis SB: Insulin therapy for gestational diabetes. *Obstet Gynecol* **51**:306–310, 1978.

114. Coustan DR: Is insulin necessary for gestational diabetes? *Contemp Obstet Gynecol* **30**:35–51, 1987.
115. Persson B, Stangenberg M, Hannsson U, et al: Gestational diabetes mellitus: Comparative evaluation of two treatment regimens, diet versus insulin and diet. *Diabetes* **34** (suppl 2):101–105, 1985.
116. Leikin E, Jenkins JH, Graves WL: Prophylactic insulin in gestational diabetes. *Obstet Gynecol* **70**:587–592, 1987.
117. Hollingsworth DR, Krans P, Cousins L, et al: Heterogeneity of serum C-peptide responses in pregnant diabetics. Paper presented at Endocrine Society Meeting, 1981. (Cited in Hollingsworth and Cousins [9]).
118. Pitkin RM: Nutritional influences during pregnancy. *Med Clin N Am* **61**:3–15, 1977.
119. Mintz DH, Skyler JS, Chez RA: Diabetes mellitus and pregnancy. *Diabet Care* **1**:49–63, 1978.
120. Schulman PK, Gyves MT, Merkatz IR: Role of nutrition in the management of the pregnant diabetic patient. In Merkatz IR, Adam PAJ (eds): *The Diabetic Pregnancy: A Perinatal Perspective*. New York: Grune & Stratton, 1979.
121. Ney D, Hollingsworth DR, Cousins L: Decreased insulin requirement and improved control of diabetes in pregnant women given a high-carbohydrate, high-fiber, low fat diet. *Diabet Care* **5**:529–533, 1982.
122. Cousins L: Pregnancy complications among diabetic women: Review 1965–1985. *Obstet Gynecol Surv* **42**:140–149, 1987.
123. Brumfield CG, Huddleston JF: The management of diabetic ketoacidosis in pregnancy. *Clin Obstet Gynecol* **27**:50–59, 1984.
124. Stehbens JA, Baker GL, Kitchell M: Outcome at ages 3 and 5 years of children born to diabetic women. *Am J Obstet Gynecol* **127**:408–413, 1977.
125. Rhodes RW, Ogburn PL: Treatment of severe diabetic ketoacidosis in the early third trimester in a patient with fetal distress (a case report). *J Reprod Med* **29**:621–624, 1984.
126. Cousins L: Pregnancy complications among diabetic women: Review 1965–1985. *Obstet Gynecol Surv* **42**:140–149, 1987.
127. Coustan DR: Recent advances in the management of diabetic pregnant women. *Clin Perinatol* **7**:299–311, 1980.
128. Gabbe SG: Application of scientific rational to the management of the pregnant diabetic. *Semin Perinatol* **2**:361–371, 1978.
129. Dibble CM, Kochenour NK, Worley RJ, et al: Effect of pregnancy on diabetic retinopathy. *Obstet Gynecol* **59**:699–704, 1982.
130. Kitzmiller JL, Brown ER, Phillipe M, et al: Diabetic nephropathy and perinatal outcome. *Am J Obstet Gynecol* **141**:741–751, 1981.
131. Schwartz HC, Kig KC, Schwartz AL, et al: Effects of pregnancy on hemoglobin A_{1c} in normal, gestational diabetes, and diabetic women. *Diabetes* **25**:1118–1122, 1976.
132. Kjaergaard JJ, Ditzel J: Hemoglobin A_{1c} as an index of long-term blood glucose regulation in diabetic pregnancy. *Diabetes* **28**:694–696, 1979.
133. O'Shaughnessy R, Russ J, Zuspan FP: Glycosylated hemoglobin and diabetes mellitus in pregnancy. *Am J Obstet Gynecol* **135**:783–790, 1979.
134. Leslie RDG, Pyke DA, John PN, et al: Hemoglobin A_{1c} in diabetic pregnancy. *Lancet* **2**:958, 1978.
135. Widness JA, Schwartz HC, Thompson D, et al: Hemoglobin A_{1c} (glyco-

hemoglobin) in diabetic pregnancy: Indicator of glucose control and fetal size. *Br J Obstet Gynaecol* **85**:812–817, 1978.

136. Roberts AB, Court DJ, Henley JR, et al: Fructosamine in diabetic pregnancy. *Lancet* **2**:998–1000, 1983.

137. Sosenko IR, Kitzmiller JL, Loo SW, et al: Infant of diabetic mother: Correlation of increased cord C-peptide levels with macrosomia and hypoglycemia. *N Engl J Med* **301**:859–862, 1979.

138. Falluca F, Gargiulo P, Troili F: Amniotic fluid insulin, C-peptide concentrations, and fetal morbidity in infants of diabetic mothers. *Am J Obstet Gynecol* **153**:534–540, 1985.

139. Robinson HP: The diagnosis of early pregnancy failure by sonar. *Br J Obstet Gynaecol* **82**:849–857, 1975.

140. Sanders RC: Ultrasound and the diagnosis of fetal death. In Sanders RC, Jame AE Jr (Eds): *Ultrasonography in Obstetrics and Gynecology* 2nd ed. New York: Appleton-Century-Crofts, 1980, p. 291.

141. Milunsky A, Alpert E, Kizmiller JL, et al: Prenatal diagnosis of neural tube defects. VIII. The importance of serum alpha-fetoprotein screening in diabetic pregnant women. *Am J Obstet Gynecol* **142**:1030–1032, 1982.

142. Hobbins J, Grannum P, Berkowitz R, et al: Ultrasound in the diagnosis of congenital anomalies. *Am J Obstet Gynecol* **134**:331–345, 1979.

143. Gabbe SG: Antepartum fetal evaluation. In Gabbe SG, Neibyl JR, Simpson JL (Eds): *Obstetrics: Normal and Problem Pregnancies*. New York: Churchill Livingstone, 1986, pp. 269–323.

144. Manning F, Morrison I, Lange I: Antepartum detection of congenital anomalies: A prospective study in 2175 referred pregnancies. Paper presented at the Society of Obstetrics and Gynecology of Canada, Quebec City, 1979. (Cited by Gabbe et al [143])

145. Campbell S, Pearce J: The prenatal diagnosis of fetal structural anomalies by ultrasound. *Clin Obstet Gynaecol* **10**:475–490, 1983.

146. Elliot JP, Garite TJ, Freeman RK, et al: Ultrasonic prediction of fetal macrosomia in diabetic patients. *Obstet Gynecol* **60**:159–162, 1982.

147. Ogata ES, Sabbagha R, Metzer BE, et al: Serial ultrasonography to assess evolving fetal macrosomia: Studies in 23 pregnant diabetic women. *JAMA* **243**:2405–2408, 1980.

148. Bracero LA, Baxi LV, Rey HR, et al: Use of ultrasound in antenatal diagnosis of large-for-gestational-age infants in diabetic gravid patients. *Am J Obstet Gynecol* **152**:43–47, 1985.

149. Miller JM, Horger EO III: Diabetic halo. *South Med J* **76**:1484–1486, 1983.

150. Goebelsmann U, Freeman RK, Mestman JH, et al: Estriol in pregnancy. II. Daily urinary estriol assays in the management of the pregnant diabetic woman. *Am J Obstet Gynecol* **115**:795–802, 1973.

151. Whittle MJ, Anderson D, Lowensohn RI, et al: Estriol in pregnancy. VI. Experience with unconjugated plasma estriol assays and antepartum fetal heart rate testing in diabetic pregnancies. *Am J Obstet Gynecol* **135**:764–772, 1979.

152. Dooley SL, Depp R, Socol ML, et al: Urinary estriols in diabetic pregnancy: A reappraisal. *Obstet Gynecol* **64**:469–475, 1984.

153. Shulman H, Lin CC, Saldana L, et al: Quantitative analysis in the oxytocin challenge test. *Am J Obstet Gynecol* **129**:239–244, 1977.

154. Lin CC, Moawad AH, River P, et al: An OCT-reactivity classification to predict fetal outcome. *Obstet Gynecol* **56**:17–23, 1980.

155. Lin CC, Devoe LD, River P, et al: Oxytocin challenge test and intrauterine growth retardation. *Am J Obstet Gynecol* **140**:282–288, 1981.

156. Golde SH, Montoro M, Good-Anderson B, et al: Role of nonstress tests, fetal biophysical profile, and contraction stress tests in outpatient management of insulin-requiring diabetic pregnancies. *Am J Obstet Gynecol* **148**:269–273, 1984.

157. Manning FA, Baskett TF, Morrison I, et al: Fetal biophysical profile scoring: A prospective study in 1,184 high-risk patients. *Am J Obstet Gynecol* **140**:289–294, 1981.

158. Manning FA, Platt LD, Sipas L: Antepartum fetal evaluation: Development of a fetal biophysical profile. *Am J Obstet Gynecol* **136**:787–795, 1980.

159. Baskett TF, Gray SJ, Prewett LM, et al: Antepartum fetal assessment using a fetal biophysical profile score. *Am J Obstet Gynecol* **148**:630–633, 1984.

160. Schulman H, Fleischer A, Stern W, et al: Umbilical velocity wave ratios in human pregnancy. *Am J Obstet Gynecol* **148**:985–990, 1984.

161. Erskine RLA, Ritchie JWK: Umbilical artery blood flow characteristics in normal and growth retarded fetuses. *Br J Obstet Gynaecol* **92**:605–610, 1985.

162. Trudinger BJ, Giles WB, Cook CM: Flow velocity waveforms in the maternal uteroplacental and fetal placental circulations. *Am J Obstet Gynecol* **152**:155–163, 1985.

163. Fleischer A, Schulman H, Farmakides G, et al: Umbilical artery velocity waveforms and intrauterine growth retardation. *Am J Obstet Gynecol* **151**:502–505, 1985.

164. Bracero L, Schulman H, Fleischer A, et al: Umbilical artery velocimetry in diabetes and pregnancy. *Obstet Gynecol* **68**:654–658, 1986.

165. Hallman H, Teramo K: Amniotic fluid phospholipid profile as a prediction of fetal maturity in diabetic pregnancies. *Obstet Gynecol* **54**:703–707, 1979.

166. Brazy JE, Crenshaw C, Brumley GW: Amniotic fluid cortisol in normal and diabetic pregnant women and its relation to respiratory distress in the neonate. *Am J Obstet Gynecol* **132**:567–570, 1978.

167. Soler NG, Malins JM: Diabetic pregnancy: Management of diabetes on the day of delivery. *Diabetologia* **15**:441–446, 1978.

168. Miodovnik M, Mimouni F, Tsang R, et al: Management of the insulin-dependent diabetic during labor and delivery. *Am J Perinatol* **4**:106–114, 1987.

169. Gold SH, Good-Anderson BG, Montaro M, et al: Insulin requirements during labor: A reappraisal. *Am J Obstet Gynecol* **144**:556–612, 1982.

170. Jovanovic L, Peterson CM: Insulin and glucose requirements during the first stage of labor in insulin dependent diabetic women. *Am J Med* **75**:607–612, 1983.

171. Haigh SE, Tevaarwerk GJM, Harding PEG, et al: A method for maintaining normoglycemia during labor and delivery in insulin-dependent diabetic women. *Can Med J* **126**:487–490, 1982.

172. Nattrass M, Alberti KGMM, Dennis KJ, et al: A glucose controlled insulin infusion system for diabetic women during labor. *Br Med J* **2**:599–601, 1978.

173. Cohen AW, Gabbe SG: Intrapartum management of the diabetic patient. *Clin Perinatol* **8**:165–172, 1981.

174. Yeast JD, Porreco RP, Ginsberg HN: The use of continuous insulin infusion

for the peripartum management of pregnant diabetic women. *Am J Obstet Gynecol* **131**:861–864, 1978.
175. Bowen DJ, Daykin AP, Nancekievill ML, et al: Insulin-dependent diabetic patients during surgery and labour. *Anaesthesia* **39**:407–411, 1984.
176. West TET, Lowy D: Control of blood glucose during labor in diabetic women with combined glucose and low-dose insulin infusion. *Br Med J* **1**:1252–1254, 1977.
177. Caplan RH, Pagliara AS, Begium EA, et al: Constant intravenous insulin infusion during labor and delivery in diabetes mellitus. *Diabet Care* **5**:6–10, 1982.
178. Benedetti TJ, Gabbe SG: Shoulder dystocia: A complication of fetal macrosomia and prolonged second stage of labor with midpelvic delivery. *Obstet Gynecol* **52**:526–529, 1978.
179. Sack RA: The large infant: A study of maternal, obstetrical, fetal, and newborn characteristics, including a long-term pediatric follow-up. *Am J Obstet Gynecol* **104**:195–204, 1969.
180. Horger EO III, Miller MC III, Counner ED: Relation of large birthweight to maternal diabetes mellitus. *Obstet Gynecol* **45**:150–154, 1975.

9
The Immune Immature Newborn

Leigh G. Donowitz

The fetus and neonate are immune-compromised patients with increased susceptibility to infection when compared with older children or adults. Deficiencies have been documented in each of the main components of the immune system in the neonate.

Mechanical Barrier to Infection

The skin and mucous membranes of newborns have been shown to be more permeable to exogenous antigen then those in older patients. The stratum corneum is poorly developed before 26 weeks of gestation. This usual barrier to exogenous antigen is only a few cells thick and is poorly keratinized. Harpin and Rutter [1] studied 70 infants born between 25 to 41 weeks of gestation and showed that skin application of phenylephrine, a powerful alpha-agonist, caused no skin blanching and no water loss in babies with gestational ages greater than 37 weeks. In contrast, there was marked skin blanching and water loss at the site of phenylephrine application in neonates born before 32 weeks of gestation. Regardless of gestational age, at 2 weeks of age the neonate develops skin maturity. Before this, this immature barrier to infection is a very real source of bacterial entry, especially for the premature newborn.

Phagocyte Function

Migration of polymorphonuclear leukocytes (PMNs) toward a site of exogenous antigen, ingestion of the foreign substance, and successful completion of bactericidal mechanisms make up a complex biologic phenomenon. Current information shows that the neonatal granulocyte demonstrates abnormalities in migration and ingestion but has fairly reliable intracellular bacterial killing ability.

Miller [2] showed that neonatal PMNs were significantly less effective than adult PMNs in migrating toward any of the usual chemotactic stimuli. Similarly, Pahwa et al [3] demonstrated that cord blood PMNs were significantly less effective in movement than adult PMNs. Klein et al [4] looked at PMN and monocyte migration with agarose gel technique and showed that PMNs in newborns migrated at levels less than 50% those of normal adult chemotaxis, and monocytes migrated at approximately 25% of adult values. Other studies have documented the decreased phagocytic cell movement, decreased deformability of the cell membranes, decreased lectin-induced aggregation [5], and decreased capping of PMNs when exposed to conconavolin A [6]. The significance of the latter finding is that PMN receptors do not orient normally or cap as they would in the adult or older child, suggestive of a functional and developmental membrane defect in the neonatal PMN.

Data on ingestion reliably show that neonatal PMNs in the presence of adult sera have normal phagocytic properties [7–9]. At adult serum concentrations of less than 3%, neonatal PMNs did not phagocytize as well as adult PMNs [10]. Thus there appears to be a serum factor in neonates responsible for defective phagocytosis.

Bacterial intracellular killing of ingested microorganisms by PMNs obtained from normal term and preterm infants has been shown to be normal in many studies [8,11,12]. Mills et al[13] showed decreased chemoluminescence of PMNs in the newborn and concluded that neonates have decreased oxidative metabolic responsiveness and lowered bactericidal activity. Other authors have found variations in premature bactericidal activity of PMNs and abnormalities in PMN bactericidal activity in sick infants. These data suggest that intracellular PMN killing ability is at normal adult levels against most microorganisms in the well newborn.

Immunoglobulins

IgM is the first immunoglobulin synthesized by the fetus at 30 or more weeks of age, but normal IgM production occurs as a result of stimulation from gastrointestinal colonization. IgM is the major antibody that is synthesized during the first few months of extrauterine life, and levels are at approximately 80% of adult values by 1 year of age. Identification of a newborn with elevated IgM levels suggests that there has been increased fetal antigenic stimulation and is suggestive of intrauterine infection [14].

Maternal IgG is transferred to the fetus in only negligible quantities until the second trimester of pregnancy. By term, the levels of IgG measured in the fetus generally exceed the maternal levels because an active transport of IgG takes place during the third trimester [15]. Significant synthesis of IgG commences at 6 months of extrauterine life and reaches 60% of adult levels by 1 year. With rapid disappearance of maternal IgG, the newborn is essentially hypogammaglobulinemic from 3 to 6 months of age.

The infant born to a mother with high circulating levels of antibody against a specific antigen such as measles or rubella is protected. If the immune mother's antibody levels are low and her own immunity is based on a brisk anamnestic response such as prior immunization against tetanus or diphtheria, the infant will have only partial or poor immunity. Mothers who have had diseases that primarily result in the production of IgM antibodies for protection (e.g., Salmonella, infection, *Escherichia coli* infection) confer no immunity to their newborns because IgM is not transplacentally transferred.

Complement

Complement studies have shown a decrease in classic pathway activity in the neonate, but the most pronounced deficiencies are those of the alternate pathway. Activation of the classic and alternate complement systems appears to be normal. The most important deficiency in the complement system is markedly decreased opsonic activity compared with adult values [16]. Fibronectin, a large opsonic glycoprotein that promotes reticuloendothelial clearance of bacteria, has been studied by Gerdes et al [17] and has been shown to be present at approximately 50% of normal adult values in the term infant. The fibronectin serum level reaches adult values at 2 months of age.

Reticuloendothelial System

The reticuloendothelial system and specifically the spleen in newborns has been shown to be deficient in removal of exogenous antigen from the circulating blood. Holyrode and colleagues [18] looked at red blood cell (RBC) pocking as a measure of asplenia or functional asplenia. They demonstrated that 2.6% of RBCs are pocked in the normal adult, 24% are pocked in the term infant, and 47.2% are pocked in the preterm infant. The last value compares with the prevalence of pocked RBCs seen in traumatically splenectomized or autosplenectomized adult patients.

Multiple factors affect the infection risk of the developing fetus and newborn. The sterile fetal environment is rapidly replaced by microorganisms from the inanimate environment, the mother, hospital personnel and visitors. Organisms that normally colonize are potentially invasive in the newborn because of the immature immune system. For these reasons, careful surveillance for infection, rapid evaluation, and initiation of empiric therapies are required for optimal care of this immune-compromised host.

REFERENCES

1. Harpin VA, Rutter N: Barrier properties of the newborn infant's skin. *J Pediatr* **102**(3):419–425, 1983.
2. Miller ME: Chemotactic function in the human neonate: Humoral and cellular aspects. *Pediatr Res* **5**:487–492, 1971.
3. Pahwa S, Pahwa R, Grines E, et al: Cellular and humoral components of monocyte and neutrophil chemotaxis in cord blood. *Pediatr Res* **11**:677–680, 1977.
4. Klein RB, Fischer TJ, Gard SE, et al: Decreased mononuclear and polymorphonuclear chemotaxis in human newborns, infants, and young children. *Pediatrics* **60**(4):467–472, 1977.
5. Mease AD, Fischer GW, Hunter KW, et al: Decreased phytohemagglutinin-induced aggregation and C5a-induced chemotaxis of human neutrophils. *Pediatr Res* **14**:142–146, 1980.
6. Kimura GM, Miller ME, Leake RD, Raghunathan R, Cheung ATW: Reduced cancanavolin A capping of neonatal polymorphonuclear leucocytes. *Pediatr Res* **15**:1271–1273, 1981.
7. McCracken GH, Eichenwald HF: Leucocyte function and the development of opsonic and complement activity in the neonate. *Am J Dis Child* **121**:120–126, 1971.
8. Coen R, Grush O, Kauder E: Studies of bactericidal activity and metabolism of the leukocyte in full term neonates. *J Pediatr* **75**(3):400–406, 1969.
9. Dassett JH, Williams RC Jr, Quie PG: Studies on interaction of bacteria, serum factors and polymorphonuclear leucocytes in mothers and newborns. *Pediatrics* **44**:49–57, 1969.
10. Miller ME: Phagocytosis in the newborn infant: Humoral and cellular factors. *J Pediatr* **74**:255–259, 1969.
11. Park BH, Holmes B, Good RA: Metabolic activities in leucocytes in newborn infants. *J Pediatr* **76**:237–241, 1970.
12. Cocchi P, Marianelli L: Phagocytosis and intracellular killing of *Pseudomonas aeruginosa* in premature infants. *Helv Paediatr Acta* **22**:110–118, 1967.
13. Mills EL, Thompson T, Bjorksten B, et al: The chemoluminescence response and bactericidal activity of neutrophils from newborns and their mothers. *Pediatrics* **63**:429–434, 1979.
14. Stiehm ER, Ammann AJ, Cherry JD: Elevated cord macroglobulins in the diagnosis of intrauterine infections. *N Engl J Med* **275**:971–977, 1966.
15. Kohler PF, Farr RS: Elevation of cord over maternal IgG immunoglobulin: Evidence for an active placental IgG transport. *Nature* **210**:1070–1071, 1966.
16. Farman ML, Stiehm ER: Impaired opsonic activity but normal phagocytosis in low birth weight infants. *N Engl J Med* **281**:926–931, 1969.
17. Gerdes JS, Yoder MC, Douglas SD, et al: Decreased plasma fibronectin in neonatal sepsis. *Pediatrics* **72**(6):877–881, 1983.
18. Holroyde CP, Oski FA, Gardner FH: The "pocked" erythrocyte: Red-cell surface alterations in reticuloendothelial immaturity of the neonate. *N Engl J Med* **281**(10):516–520, 1969.

10
Diagnosis of Neonatal Infection: Utilization of the Absolute Neutrophil Count

CHARLES R. ROSENFELD

Sepsis and pneumonia occur in one to two neonates per 1,000 live births in most nurseries in Western nations. Diagnosis of the newborn with suspected bacterial infection, however, continues to be a dilemma of significant concern, impacting not only the duration of antimicrobial therapy but also the duration and cost of hospitalization. Although numerous laboratory tests have been suggested as diagnostically useful, no single test in particular has been shown to be "the best test." Therefore, it is important to delineate a reasonable approach to the diagnosis and evaluation of the infant at risk for bacterial infection, whether of intrauterine or extrauterine etiology. This chapter provides such an approach, with particular emphasis on the utilization of peripheral neutrophil values in establishing the diagnosis of neonatal infection.

Risk Factors

In approaching this diagnostic dilemma, the age of the infant is an important consideration, since age in days impacts on the source and type of infection that occurs. Neonates should be divided into groups younger than and older than 1 week of age. In the neonate less than 3 days of age one must be concerned with the maternal antepartum and intrapartum course as well as the outcome of prior pregnancies. For example, it is imperative that the physician know whether there was intrapartum maternal fever, prolonged rupture of the membranes (i.e., >24 hours), evidence of chorioamnionitis (e.g., maternal fever and uterine tenderness), foul-smelling or purulent amniotic fluid, or administration of antibiotics to the mother. Although each of these is considered an important factor in the occurrence of neonatal infection, the predictive value of each remains unclear. For example, it is unclear what foul-smelling amniotic fluid or infant really means and how this actually correlates with the incidence of neonatal sepsis and/or pneumonia. In the case of intrapartum administration of antibiotics to the mother, it is important to determine if such administration was to treat suspected disease or to prevent subsequent postpartum infection. If the latter is the case, it is extremely unlikely that the infant requires any evaluation other than routine physical examination and close observation [1].

Consideration also should be given to whether delivery was term or preterm, since the risk for infection in the preterm infant exposed to prolonged ruptured membranes, with evidence of chorioamnionitis, might be somewhat higher than the risk in the term infant. Also, it has been suggested that preterm delivery might be reflective of the effects of bacterial invasion of the fetal membranes, which would expose this particular group of infants to a somewhat greater risk for infection [2]. This, however, remains speculative at best.

Finally, if a woman has had a prior pregnancy complicated by neonatal group B streptococcal infection, there may be increased risk for neonatal infection in subsequent pregnancies, especially if the woman remains a carrier of this particular pathogen. In this instance cervical and/or rectal cultures at 28 to 30 weeks of gestation should be considered, as should intravenous administration of ampicillin to the mother during labor [3,4]. In other instances screening cultures for group B streptococcus are not cost effective and thus have little or no role in the assessment of neonatal risk for infection in large unspecified populations, because of the low incidence of neonatal disease [5–7].

Clinical Signs of Neonatal Infection

Clinical manifestations of neonatal bacterial disease may be nonspecific, and as noted in Table 10.1, are quite variable in their association with infection. Furthermore, they are commonly seen in the presence of other problems. For example, if the incubator heating mechanism is malfunctioning, the preterm infant may develop hypothermia or hyperthermia due to changes in the environmental temperature. It also must be remembered that if an infant is on servo-control for temperature regulation, the development of relative hypothermia may be masked by the automated rise in incubator temperature. The opposite may be the case with hyperthermia. Thus, it is important to routinely examine temperature changes in both the incubator and the infant, looking for an increase in incubator or environmental temperature to offset hypothermia and a decrease in environmental temperature associated with hyperthermia.

Hypoglycemia also occurs frequently in association with neonatal sepsis. Like the other manifestations, it is not specific and may be seen in circumstances unrelated to infection, for example, in the unidentified small-for-gestational-age infant. However, when sepsis is present, hypoglycemia may be preceded by the development of glycosuria and sometimes hyperglycemia due to impaired glucose utilization, especially in the small

TABLE 10.1. Clinical manifestations associated with neonatal sepsis.

Clinical sign	Percent of neonates affected
Temperature instability	50–60
Respiratory distress	>33
Neurologic abnormality	15–25
Hyperbilirubinemia	35
Gastrointestinal disturbances	10–30

infant [8]. In the case of neurologic abnormalities, it is of course necessary to first determine whether an intracranial hemorrhage has occurred, especially in the preterm infant weighing less than 1,500 g at birth.

Although the clinical signs associated with neonatal sepsis may be relatively nonspecific, when taken into context with other clinical signs or manifestations and the maternal history, they generally provide a very strong index of suspicion that must *not* be ignored. For example, because of the relatively rare occurrence of respiratory distress in infants weighing more than 1,500 g at birth in our hospital, a diagnosis of pneumonia is entertained in any infant with respiratory distress until proven otherwise. In the past, we have seen group B streptococcus as a major cause of respiratory dysfunction in these infants [9].

Diagnosis of Neonatal Infection

CULTURES

The most definitive method for determining whether bacterial infection has occurred is to obtain a positive culture of a bacterial pathogen. This, however, is not always possible; in many instances negative blood cultures are found in cases where the clinical evidence of disease is overwhelming. It should be noted that urine cultures, that is, suprapubic bladder aspirations, are *not* indicated in the first week after birth because of their very low yield [10]; however, they should be considered in the evaluation for neonatal infection thereafter.

Use of the spinal tap to obtain cerebrospinal fluid for culture and other studies in the first 1 to 3 days after birth is less clear. At Parkland Memorial Hospital we documented only five cases of neonatal meningitis in the first week after birth over a 5-year period, 1978 to 1982, among some 60,000 live births. This incidence of approximately 1 in 10,000 live births raises the question of the utility, cost effectiveness, and necessity of performing routine lumbar punctures in all infants being evaluated for suspected infection in the first 3 days of life, especially the term infant with questionable indications. Furthermore, one also could question the advisability of lumbar puncture and assessment of spinal fluid in the infant with substantial respiratory distress, regardless of gestational age, since there is evidence that the procedure itself may lead to worsening of the disease and the yield is so low. This question is presently under study in our institution.

LABORATORY TESTS

Turning our attention to the laboratory, it is obvious that numerous diagnostic tests for establishing a diagnosis of neonatal infection are presently available to the clinician (Table 10.2). In order to use these tests optimally, knowledge of their *sensitivity* (i.e., the probability that a result will be positive in the presence of a specific disease) and *specificity* (i.e., the probability that a result will be negative in the absence of a specific disease) must be obtained. These data, however, are not available for many if not most of the available tests.

In our experience, the gastric aspirate has been associated with an extremely high incidence of false-positive cultures and/or smears (i.e., positive cultures in infants not considered at risk for infection; unpublished observations); this is similar to the experience of others [11,12]. Moreover, it has been shown that the white cells seen on smears of the gastric aspirate, and probably of the external ear fluid, are more likely to represent maternal than fetal cells [13]. The chest radiograph also can be misleading. For example, it has been our experience and that of others that group B streptococcal sepsis and pneumonia frequently present with chest x-ray findings not different from those seen in the preterm infant with hyaline membrane disease or the term infant with transient tachypnea [9,14–16]. We and others also have seen this nonspecific radiographic pattern with early-onset infection with *Escherichia coli* and other pathogens in the preterm infant. However, we have recently observed that the urine latex fixation test for group B streptoccocus is extremely useful in the diagnosis of this particular type of neonatal infection, especially when the cultures are positive. Nevertheless, this too requires documentation of sensitivity and specificity.

TABLE 10.2. Suggested laboratory tests for the evaluation of suspected neonatal sepsis or pneumonia.

Examination of the buffy coat
Limulus assay for endotoxin
Counterimmunoelectrophoresis
Latex agglutination test
Measurement of C-reactive protein
Erythrocyte sedimentation rage
Umbilical cord or placental histology
Culture/smears of gastric aspirate or fluid from the external ear
Amniocentesis
Chest radiograph
Peripheral neutrophil count

The final laboratory test noted in Table 10.2 is the peripheral neutrophil count, a test that is available in every hospital and easily done. In early studies it was demonstrated that the total white blood cell count was non-specific and of little use in the diagnosis of neonatal infection [17,18]. However, it was suggested that absolute peripheral neutrophilic values might be of some utility in diagnosing neonatal infection [19–23]. For accurate use of this or any other test in the neonatal period, it is of paramount importance to first determine what perinatal factors might affect the distribution of peripheral neutrophilic values and to establish reference ranges (the range of values considered normal) that take these factors into account, thereby increasing the usefulness of this or any other laboratory test used in the neonate. Such a study was performed at our institution on infants in the first 28 days after birth. The study included 434 infants who were considered either normal or without significant complications; 905 blood counts were obtained from these neonates [24]. Using these counts we established normal reference ranges (Fig. 10.1 and 10.2) for the total absolute neutrophil values (i.e., the sum of mature plus immature neutrophilic forms), the total absolute immature neutrophil values (the sum of all immature forms), and the "ratio" or proportion of the total immature forms to total neutrophil values (I/T ratio). To obtain the absolute

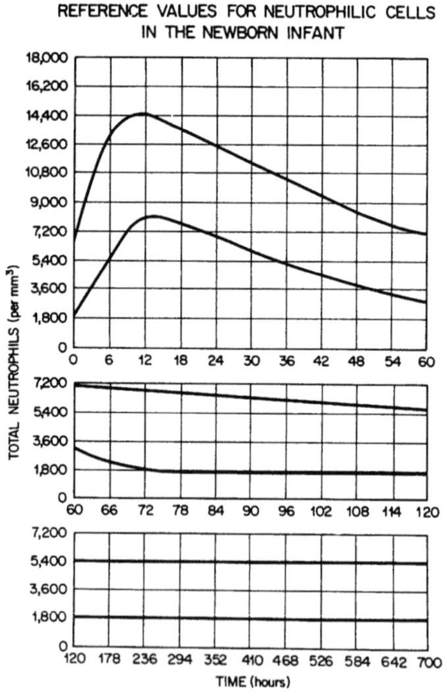

FIGURE 10.1. Reference ranges for total absolute neutrophil values from birth to 28 days of life. Data modified from Monroe et al [24].

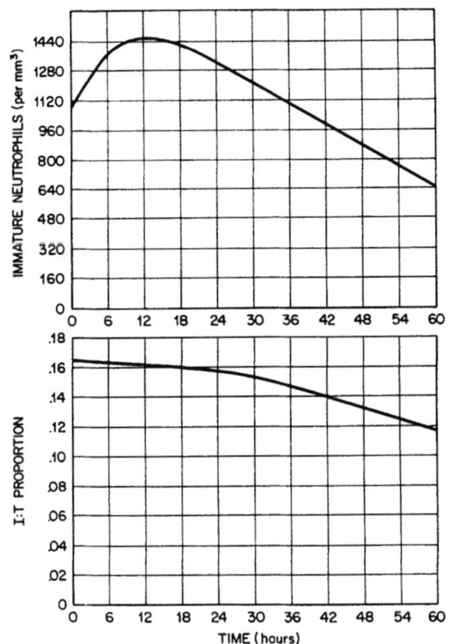

FIGURE 10.2. Reference ranges for total absolute immature neutrophil values and the ratio of total immature to total absolute neutrophil values from birth to 60 hours of age. Data modified from Monroe et al [24].

neutrophil values, a corrected white blood cell count must be used. This can be obtained from the Coulter Counter white blood cell count (WBC_{cc}) value using the following equation, which removes the effects of nucleated red blood cells (NRBC):

$$WBC = WBC_{cc} \times \frac{100}{NRBC + 100}$$

In our studies we found that a number of common perinatal events had no effect on the absolute neutrophil values [24] (Table 10.3). However, numerous other perinatal events had, in some instances, rather striking effects on these values (Table 10.4). Most impressive was the development of significant neutropenia in two groups—infants of hypertensive mothers and infants who had experienced perinatal asphyxia, that is, who had Apgar scores below 6 at 1 and 5 minutes. In nearly all other instances the effect on neutrophil dynamics was to cause neutrophilia. In the majority of cases this was associated with a proportionate increase in the immature neutrophil values, resulting therefore in no change in the I/T ratio, for example, pneumothorax, surgery, seizures, and meconium aspiration

TABLE 10.3. Perinatal factors with no significant effect on peripheral neutrophil values.

Duration of ruptured membranes without maternal fever
Birth weight
Gestational age
Route of delivery
Duration of ruptured membranes without maternal fever
Uncomplicated hyaline membrane disease
Uncomplicated transient tachypnea
Phototherapy
Prophylactic use of antibiotics
Meconium staining without lung disease

Source: Monroe et al [24].

syndrome. From these observations and the development of the normal reference ranges, two things became obvious: (1) that the absolute peripheral neutrophilic values cannot be adequately evaluated in the absence of complete knowledge of the intrapartum and neonatal course, and (2) that the age after birth at which the count is obtained *must* be known for the first 72 hours to correctly interpret the values reported by the laboratory.

Using our reference ranges and knowledge of the perinatal factors listed in Table 10.4, we examined the predictive value of the absolute neutrophil counts for neonatal infection. In our study, 156 infants had a diagnosis of infection and all were screened by the neutrophil counts as abnormal; thus, the sensitivity was extremely good. When the neutrophil counts obtained from these infants and noninfected infants were further examined, we found that of 459 counts with *no* abnormality in any of the three neutrophilic parameters, only 4 occurred in infants with confirmed or sus-

TABLE 10.4. Perinatal events affecting peripheral neutrophil values.

Event	Total neutrophil counts		Immature neutrophil counts
	↓	↑	↑
Maternal hypertension	76	0	6
Periventricular hemorrhage	62	23	31
Asphyxia	14	28	28
Hemolytic disease	0	47	53
Asymptomatic hypoglycemia	0	44	63
Maternal fever	0	46	65
Surgery	0	100	90
Stressful labor	0	67	81
Meconium aspiration syndrome	0	78	56
Seizures	0	71	71
Pneumothorax	0	80	80
Oxytocin induction ≥ 6 hours	0	27	50

Source: Monroe et al [24]. Values represent the percent of counts increased or decreased.

pected bacterial disease. That is, fewer than 1% of normal counts were seen in infected infants, whereas 99% of these normal counts occurred in infants without evidence of infection or with noninfectious complications. When counts were examined for the types of abnormalities that occurred, for example, neutrophilia or neutropenia, and for the distribution between infected and noninfected neonates, the specificity was observed to be relatively low—34% of the abnormal counts had occurred among infants without evidence of infection. Neutropenia, however, was substantially more frequent in neutrophil counts from infected infants, 77% versus 23%. The relatively poor specificity occurs because of the substantial number of common perinatal events that tend to alter neutrophil dynamics and mimic the effects of bacterial disease. However, since sepsis is a life-threatening yet treatable disease and false-positive results do little harm, the greater sensitivity of this test is preferred. Furthermore, the reduced specificity can be balanced by a greater awareness of those factors that result in false-positive values (Table 10.4).

When these reference ranges were applied to infants with group B streptococcal infection in the first 24 hours after birth [9], 39 of 45 infants (87%) had abnormal total absolute neutrophil values, 19 (42%) had elevated immature neutrophil counts, and 41 (91%) had an abnormal I/T ratio. All infants (100%) were correctly identified when both the total absolute neutrophil count and the I/T ratio were used. Among infants under 37 weeks of gestation with group B streptococcal infection, neutropenia was observed in 70%, whereas in term infants the findings were variable, that is, neutrophilia occurred as commonly as neutropenia. The I/T ratio, however, was abnormal in 83% and 88% of the preterm and term infants, respectively. The usefulness of these reference ranges for the absolute neutrophil values in screening infants at risk for infection has since been confirmed by others [25].

Since neutropenia has been considered a frequent finding in newborn infants with neonatal sepsis, especially preterm infants, and we had shown it to occur commonly within the context of other settings [24], we studied the pattern of peripheral neutrophil values in three groups of infants with a high likelihood of developing neutropenia [26], that is, those with perinatal asphyxia, sepsis, or a maternal history of hypertension. In these studies the mean total absolute neutrophil value was below the lower limits of the normal reference range in infants with perinatal asphyxia ($n = 13$) and maternal hypertension ($n = 20$). Moreover, mean values remained in the neutropenic range throughout the first 60 to 70 hours of life. In contrast, the mean value for septic infants ($n = 13$), most of whom were term, was within the reference range from birth to 12 hours, and significant neutrophilia was observed thereafter.

When the infants within these groups were examined individually, neutropenia was observed in 8 of 13 asphyxiated neonates (62%) and 10 of 20 infants delivered of hypertensive mothers (50%) (all of whom had pregnancy-induced hypertension); within these two groups of infants, more than 80% remained neutropenic at 60 hours. However, when the immature neutrophil counts and I/T ratio were examined in infants of hypertensive mothers, values were abnormal in only 2 of 47 counts (4%) and 6 of 47 counts (13%), respectively. Thus, the presence of neutropenia alone among these infants should not be considered suggestive or reflective of infection. In contrast, the immature neutrophil count and I/T ratio were more likely to be abnormal in septic infants, 46% and 61%, respectively. Unfortunately, the neutrophilic values from the asphyxiated infants were somewhat intermediate; that is, 4 of 35 counts (11%) and 8 of 35 counts (23%) had either an abnormal immature neutrophil value or I/T proportion, respectively. The former values, however, were not significantly different from the normal range ($p > .05$), but the latter were ($p < .05$). Thus, an asphyxiated infant may present with significant neutropenia and an elevated I/T ratio, making the initial cell count difficult to interpret and the clinical information of utmost importance. If all three neutrophilic values are abnormal, however, a diagnosis of bacterial infection should be strongly considered.

Guidelines for Using Peripheral Absolute Neutrophil Values

In view of the above discussion, the following guidelines can be suggested for use of the peripheral absolute neutrophil values in the diagnosis and evaluation of neonatal infection. First, a thorough maternal intrapartum history and neonatal physical exam must be obtained. If these are strongly supportive of a diagnosis of or risk for bacterial disease, antibiotics should be administered after obtaining a blood culture and a complete white blood cell count with differential count, repeating the differential count at 8 to 12 hours. If the absolute neutrophil values are abnormal on both counts, especially the I/T ratio, and factors affecting the counts are not present, then 5 to 7 days of antibiotic therapy should be considered with a follow-up cell count at 24 and 72 hours. If the intrapartum history is only suggestive, for example, prolonged rupture of membranes without maternal fever or foul-smelling infant; Apgar scores are good; and the infant is term, one should obtain a differential white blood cell count and maybe a blood culture and closely observe the infant while monitoring peripheral neutrophil values at 12 and 24 hours of age. The presence of normal neutrophil values would result in no antibiotic therapy. If, in this situation, the infant is preterm, antibiotics might be started shortly after birth but discontinued at 48 to 72 hours if (1) the absolute neutrophil values are normal, (2) the clinical course does not suggest infection, and (3) blood cultures are negative. This approach has been used in our institution over the past 4 to 5 years and has shortened the course of antibiotic therapy by 3 to 5 days.

This also has proven especially useful as an approach to the term infant, resulting in earlier discharge and a decreased cost for hospitalization in our institution.

REFERENCES

1. Cunningham FG, Leveno KJ, DePalma RT, et al: Perioperative antimicrobials for cesarean delivery: Before or after cord clamping? *Obstet Gynecol* **62:**151–154, 1983.
2. Regan JA, Chao S, James LS: Premature rupture of membranes, preterm delivery, and group B streptococcal colonization of mothers. *Am J Obstet Gynecol* **141:**184–186, 1981.
3. Yow MD, Mason ED, Leeds LJ, et al: Ampicillin prevents intrapartum transmission of group B streptococcus. *JAMA* **24:**1245–1247, 1979.
4. Boyer KM, Gadzala CA, Kelly PD, et al: Selective intrapartum chemoprophylaxis of neonatal group B streptococcal early-onset disease. III. Interruption of mother-to-infant transmission. *J Infect Dis* **148:**810–816, 1983.
5. Hall RT, Barnes W, Krishnan L, et al: Antibiotic treatment of parturient women colonized with group B streptococcus. *Am J Obstet Gynecol* **124:**630–634, 1976.
6. Baker CJ, Barrett FF: Transmission of group B streptococci among parturient women and their neonates. *J Pediatr* **83:**919–925, 1973.
7. Eickhoff TC, Flein JP, Mortimer EA, et al: The issue of prophylaxis of neonatal group B streptococcal infections. *J Pediatr* **83:**1097–1098, 1973.
8. Popow C, Pollak A, Schilling R, et al: Glucose disposal in very low birth weight infants. *Wien Klin Wochenschr* **94:**285–288, 1982.
9. Manroe BL, Rosenfeld CR, Weinberg AG, et al: The differential leukocyte count in the assessment and outcome of early-onset neonatal group B streptococcal disease. *J Pediatr* **91:**632–637, 1977.
10. Visser VE, Hall RT: Urine culture in the evaluation of suspected neonatal sepsis. *J Pediatr* **94:**635–638, 1979.
11. Pole JRG, McAllister TA: Gastric aspirate analysis in the newborn. *Acta Pediatr Scand* **64:**109–112, 1975.
12. Hosmer ME, Sprunt K: Screening method for identification of infected infant following premature rupture of maternal membranes. *Pediatrics* **49:**283–285, 1972.
13. Vasan U, Lim DM, Greenstein RM, et al: Origin of gastric aspirate polymorphonuclear leukocytes in infants born after prolonged rupture of membranes. *J Pediatr* **91:**69–72, 1977.
14. Ablow RC, Driscoll SG, Effman EL, et al: A comparison of early-onset group B streptococcal neonatal infection and the respiratory distress syndrome of the newborn. *N Engl J Med* **292:**65–70, 1976.
15. Hemming VG, McCloskey DW, Hill HR: Pneumonia in the neonate associated with group B streptococcal septicemia. *Am J Dis Child* **130:**1231–1233, 1976.
16. Lillien LD, Harris VJ, Pildes RS: Significance of radiographic findings in early-onset group B streptococcal infection. *Pediatrics* **60:**360–363, 1977.
17. Weitzman M: Diagnostic utility of white blood cell counts and differential cell counts. *Am J Dis Child* **129:**1183–1189, 1975.
18. Franciosi RA, Knostman JD, Zimmerman RA: Group B streptococcal neonatal infant infections. *J Pediatr* **82:**707–718, 1973.

19. Xanthou M: Leukocyte blood picture in healthy full-time and premature babies during neonatal period. *Arch Dis Child* **45**:242–249, 1970.
20. Xanthou M: Leukocyte blood picture in ill newborn babies. *Arch Dis Child* **47**:741–746, 1972.
21. Gregory J, Hey E: Blood neutrophil response to bacterial infection in the first month of life. *Arch Dis Child* **47**:747–753, 1972.
22. Akenzua GI, Hui YT, Milner R, et al: Neutrophil and band counts in the diagnosis of neonatal infection. *Pediatrics* **54**:38–42, 1974.
23. Zipursky A, Palko J, Milner R, et al: The hematology of bacterial infections in premature infants. *Pediatrics* **57**:839–853, 1976.
24. Monroe BL, Weinberg AG, Rosenfeld CR, et al: The neonatal blood count in health and disease. I. Reference values for neutrophilic cells. *J Pediatr* **95**:89–98, 1979.
25. Benuck J, David RJ: Sensitivity of published neutrophil indices in identifying newborn infants with sepsis. *J Pediatr* **103**:961–963, 1983.
26. Engle WD, Rosenfeld CR: Neutropenia in high-risk neonates. *J Pediatr* **105**:982–986, 1984.

11
Group B Streptococci at Parturition:
I. A Case-Control Study

V. Schauf, P. Holobaugh, K. Nelson, K. Mallin,
M. Ismail, and The Collaborative Group B
Streptococcus Research Group

Group B streptococcus (GBS) infection acquired from the mother in the perinatal period continues to contribute importantly to neonatal morbidity and mortality [1–3]. Antimicrobial treatment of GBS carrier mothers prior to onset of labor proved disappointing because the carrier state was not eradicated [4]. Other strategies for treatment during pregnancy, including simultaneous treatment of husbands or treatment until the time of delivery, failed or were impractical to prevent most cases [5,6]. Penicillin treatment of the infant immediately after delivery was not effective in reducing GBS morbidity or mortality in premature infants, who account for a large fraction of GBS disease [7]. As early as 1978, Baker [8] suggested that many GBS infections are acquired in utero and that studies of prophylaxis should be directed toward women.

Intrapartum antibiotics have been shown to interrupt transmission of GBS from mother to infant [9,10] and have been claimed to prevent early-onset disease [11,12] (Tuppurainen et al. Abstract 1455, Society for Pediatric Research, 1986). Thus, current interest in early intervention focuses on the intrapartum period. Because GBS colonization may not be routinely evaluated [13] and varies during pregnancy [14–17], the colonization status of many parturients is unknown. Because most GBS colonized pregnancies are not associated with fetal or maternal morbidity, the problem has been to identify at-risk pregnancies readily in the delivery room.

Epidemiologic methods used to identify at-risk pregnancies have included comparison of early- versus late-onset disease [18], comparison of perinatal events in colonized versus uncolonized mothers and/or infants [3,19,20], calculation of disease attack rates [10–12], and clinical observation [21,22]. However, results using the case-control method to evaluate at-risk pregnancies have not been reported.

To help plan an effective strategy to prevent this disease, we prospectively collected data on the incidence of GBS disease in five Chicago-area hospitals. To identify risk factors of importance, we performed a case-control study in four of the hospitals. On the basis of these results, the use of intrapartum antibiotics for certain high-risk pregnancies is discussed.

Methods

The prospective study was conducted from 1979 to 1981 at Christ Hospital, Cook County Hospital, Foster G. McGaw Hospital of Loyola University, the University of Chicago Hospital, and the University of Illinois Hospital. Infants with invasive GBS infection documented by blood and/or cerebrospinal fluid GBS isolates were identified prospectively by daily surveillance of nurseries, pediatric wards, and microbiology laboratories. In addition, disease rates for 1976 to 1979 were determined retrospectively by chart review in two of the study hospitals. Infants with GBS isolated from blood or CSF in the first 5 days of life were designated as having early-onset infections. Late-onset infections were those occurring after age 5 days.

The case-control study employed the methodologic standards of Horwitz and Feinstein [23]. Data collected for the case-control study described the course of the perinatal period for mothers and infants. Infants with early-onset GBS infection were identified prospectively in four of the hospitals; data for these infants were compared with data for control infants born in the same hospital and within 2 weeks of each affected infant. Where possible, four control infants were included for each infant with early-onset GBS infection.

The control infants had participated as placebo recipients in a double-blind trial of penicillin prophylaxis for GBS infection [5]. Three infants with early-onset GBS infection had likewise received placebo and 22 had not participated in the trial.

Over 200 data items concerning the maternal and neonatal hospital course were collected from hospital records, entered onto a precoded data collection form, manually edited, entered into a computer, and given further edits by computer. The statistical analysis system was used to analyze the data. Fisher's exact test, Student's T test, chi-square, or chi-square with Yates' correction was performed to determine statistical significance.

Results

During the period of prospective case identification, there were 34 babies with early-onset and 11 babies with late-onset GBS infection. Of these, 25 with early-onset disease and 8 with late-onset disease were born in the study hospitals. The remaining infants had been transferred to these hospitals after birth.

The overall incidence of early-onset GBS infection in the study hospitals was 0.9/1,000 live births (Table 11.1). The rate varied in the different hospitals (maximum 1.3/1,000 live births; minimum 0/1,000 live births). The retrospectively determined yearly rates shown in Table 11.2 ranged from a minimum of 0 to a maximum of 2.6/1,000 live births.

TABLE 11.1. Incidence of group B streptococcus (GBS) infection during period of prospective observation.

Hospital	Period	No. of live births	No. of GBS cases		No. of EOGBS* cases	
			Born in study hospital	Per 1,000 live births	Born in study hospital	Per 1,000 live births
Christ	12/79– 2/81	4,650	10	2.2	3	0.6
Cook County	1/80–12/81	12,237	23	1.9	16	1.3
Foster McGaw	2/80–11/81	2,818	1	0.4	0	0.0
University of Chicago	1/80– 3/81	4,376	6	1.4	3	0.7
University of Illinois	11/79–11/80	2,499	5	2.0	3	1.2
Total		26,580	45	1.7	25	0.9

*EOGBS, early-onset GBS.

TABLE 11.2. Group B streptococcus (GBS) infection in neonates born in two study hospitals in the years 1976 to 1979.

Hospital	Year	No. of live births	Total GBS cases/ 1,000 live births	No. of EOGBS* cases/ 1,000 live births
University of Illinois	1977	2,430	2.9	1.6
	1978	2,306	3.0	2.6
	1979	2,311	0.0	0.0
Foster McGaw	7/76–6/77	1,918	1.0	0.5
	7/77–6/78	1,649	0.6	0.6
	7/78–6/79	1,503	2.0	2.0

*EOGBS, early-onset GBS.

Table 11.3 shows the age of onset of GBS infection for infants identified during the prospective observation period. Cases occurred most frequently on the first day of life. One of the affected infants was one of a pair of twins. There were five deaths among the infants with early-onset disease, a case fatality rate of 20%.

The control infants came from the four hospitals experiencing early-onset GBS disease during the period of prospective GBS case identification. There were 97 control infants, two of them twins from separate sets.

The perinatal course of infants with early-onset GBS infection differed significantly from that of the control infants (Table 11.4). Pregnancies of mothers of infected infants were characterized significantly more frequently by short gestation, long duration of rupture of membranes, cesarean section, maternal fever, and endometritis. Pregnancies of mothers of infected infants did not differ significantly with respect to age, race, source of medical payment, gravidity, parity, abortion history, meconium staining of infant or amniotic fluid, use of anesthetic, fetal monitoring,

TABLE 11.3. Days from birth to onset of group B streptococcus (GBS) infection.

Day	No. of babies
1	21
2	6
3	2
4	1
5	2
6	2
7	1
8–15	2
16–23	3
24–31	1
32–42	1

TABLE 11.4. Perinatal risk factors for early-onset group B streptococcus (GBS) infection.

Risk factor	GBS	Control	X^2	p	Odds ratio
Premature labor (<38 weeks)	12/25	3/97	32.7	< .005	28.9
Cesarean section	6/24	7/97	4.5	< .05	4.3
Membrane rupture					
> 48 hours	5/25	1/97		.003*	24.0
> 24 hours	11/25	10/97	13.6	< .005	6.8
> 12 hours	15/25	13/97	24.7	< .005	9.7
Maternal temperature ≥ 100.4°F	13/24	20/96	10.7	< .005	4.5
Endometritis	7/23	2/97	18.0	< .005	20.8

*Fisher's exact test.

maternal urinary tract infection, unexplained maternal fever, or maternal diabetes.

Affected infants were significantly more likely to have low Apgar scores; to be premature and small for gestational age; to require resuscitation, intubation, intensive care, transfusions, and antibiotics; to experience jaundice, apnea, and shock; and to have abnormal chest x-rays and a diagnosis of hyaline membrane disease. Affected infants required significantly more days in the hospital and in neonatal intensive care units than control infants (4.4 days vs. 16.0 days, p <.0001, and 0.8 days vs. 11.2 days, p <.0001, respectively). Five affected premature infants died, but no control infants died. When twins were excluded from the analysis of both groups, the results were not significantly changed.

The case-control study was also analyzed separately for 16 cases and 59 controls from the one hospital contributing the largest number of cases and four of five deaths, Cook County Hospital. The perinatal course in a single hospital again revealed significant differences between pregnancies of mothers of infected infants and mothers of controls (Table 11.5). The pattern of differences was similar to that shown in Table 11.4. Also a

TABLE 11.5. Perinatal risk factors for early-onset group B streptococcus (GBS) infection, Cook County Hospital.

Risk factor	GBS	Control	X^2	p	Odds ratio
Abortions ≥ 2	3/16	4/58		.026*	3.1
Premature labor (<38 weeks)	9/16	0/59	33.0	< .005	75.9
Antibiotics before delivery	2/15	0/59		.039*	9.1
Cesarean section	5/15	2/59	9.5	< .005	14.2
Rupture of membranes					
> 48 hours	3/16	0/57		.008*	13.6
> 24 hours	8/16	6/59	10.6	< .005	8.8
> 12 hours	10/16	8/50	14.2	< .005	10.6
Maternal temperature ≥ 100.4°F	9/15	13/59	6.4	.025	5.3
Endometritis	5/15	2/59	9.5	< .005	14.2
Antibiotics after delivery	9/15	3/57		.039*	27.0

*Fisher's exact test.

history of abortions or antibiotic use before and/or after delivery was found significantly more often in mothers of infected infants. Affected infants experienced significant morbidity, as noted for the entire study group. Four of 16 infants died, a case fatality rate of 25%.

Discussion

The GBS disease rates reported for this study (Tables 11.1 and 11.2) are slightly lower than those reported for 1974 by us (3/1,000) [14], those reported for Cook County Hospital during 1972 to 1979 [24], and those reported recently in Chicago [17] and for other parts of the United States [2,3]. The variations in incidence noted among the hospitals (Table 11.1), over time (Table 11.2), and among various reports [3,14,17,20,24,25] may reflect the difficulty in establishing reliable incidence rates for a disease of low incidence rather than true differences in incidence [26]. In any case, the rates of GBS disease in our study hospitals were within the range of statistical variations of the rates found in previous studies in Chicago.

The mortality rate of 20% in our present series of early-onset GBS infection is similar to that in our earlier report [27] and compares favorably with the rates in several other reports [17,24,25]. We did not analyze our data on the affected infants to determine which components of their illness were attributable to GBS infection, which to prematurity, and which to the combination. Both GBS infection and prematurity may be important prognostic variables, considering the severe disease that occurs in some term infants and the high mortality in infected premature infants.

During the years of our study, there were approximately 3.5 million live births yearly in the United States (National Center for Health Statistics). Assuming a rate for early-onset GBS infection of 1 in 1,000 live births and a 20% mortality rate, an estimated 700 deaths would occur yearly. The annual years of potential life lost to this disease in the United States can be estimated at 700×65 or 45,500 years, about 10% the loss due to prematurity [28]. Additionally, GBS infection was reported to be associated with 10% of all neonatal deaths in Winnipeg, Manitoba, in the last decade [11]. GBS infection remains an important cause of perinatal morbidity and infant mortality despite extensive awareness of the disease, several proposed preventive strategies [5,6,9,10,12,17,29,30], and effective antimicrobial therapy [5,27].

Even though GBS infection is relatively common, currently culture results may not be available for all women in labor, nor is it feasible to treat all women in labor with antibiotics [13,31]. While there is hope that rapid screening tests may prove useful in selecting women for antimicrobial prophylaxis [32], at present these are not generally available. Similarly, although culture results would have been helpful in identifying at-risk women in our study, it was not feasible for us to include cultures for all subjects. Thus, we performed a case-control study to identify clinical risk factors that might help identify women whose infants could benefit from intrapartum therapy.

Premature labor, prolonged rupture of membranes, cesarean section, fever, or endometritis are many times more likely in pregnancies in which there is a GBS-affected infant than in normal pregnancies (Tables 11.4 and 11.5). Some of these risk factors have previously been identified using different approaches, including comparison of parameters of early- versus late-onset disease [18] and calculations of disease attack rates [10]. In our study, these risk factors were identified when the data from all hospitals were examined, and also when the data from Cook County Hospital were analyzed separately, which indicates that these risk factors are of importance across the socioeconomic spectrum of our study. The additional risk factors identified in the more uniform population of a single hospital included a history of abortions and use of antibiotics before and/or after delivery. Some of the factors that our study and others reported in the literature have identified as "risk factors" for early-onset neonatal GBS disease may in fact be "early markers" of the effects of GBS infection. Nevertheless, from the perspective of the clinician armed with an effective antimicrobial, knowledge of perinatal events that suggest early intervention might be helpful in devising a strategy to reduce the morbidity and mortality of early onset GBS infection.

Even when premature labor was excluded from the analysis, the other maternal risk factors remained significant, indicating that the several significant risk factors were not dependent on the presence of premature labor. In general, exclusion from analysis of patients with each of the other risk factors did not remove the significance of the remaining factors. Not enough cesarean deliveries occurred to distinguish the risk of primary versus secondary procedures. However, most of the cesarean sections analyzed were primary.

Several previously reported associations had no demonstrated significance in our study. These included maternal GBS bacteriuria [33], race [34], and persistent fetal circulation [35]. The sample size is adequate to have documented the proposed racial association; however, it may not have been large enough to detect associations with maternal bacteriuria or persistent fetal circulation.

Our findings in the case-control study (Tables 11.4 and 11.5) and the high frequency of cases on the first day of life (Table 11.3) underline the importance of maternal infection as a determinant of early-onset GBS infection. The actual costs and benefits of intrapartum antibiotics for women at risk of delivering an infant with early-onset GBS infection need further evaluation. It will be necessary to determine if placentally transferred intrapartum antibiotics such as ampicillin [36] increase neonatal morbidity by obscuring results of neonatal bacterial cultures. This might conceivably occur if antibiotics given to the mother perinatally were transferred to the infant in sufficient concentration to cause the infant's cultures to be "falsely negative," but not in sufficient amount to treat effectively or prevent a GBS infection in an infant. Intrapartum ampicillin administration has been advocated for GBS-colonized women with certain perinatal risk factors [12]. In addition, intrapartum penicillin or ampicillin may be appropriate for at-risk women who are not allergic to beta-lactam antibiotics and for whom colonization status is unknown.

Summary

To help form a basis for an effective strategy to prevent neonatal group B streptococcal (GBS) infection, we prospectively collected data on its incidence in five Chicago area hospitals from 1979 to 1981 and performed a case-control study in four of the hospitals to identify risk factors of importance. Data describing the perinatal course for infants identified prospectively with early onset GBS infection were compared to data for control infants born in the same hospital and within two weeks of each affected infant. The incidence of early onset GBS infection was 0.9/1000 live births. Cases occurred most frequently on the first day of life. The case fatality rate was 20%. Maternal risk factors included gestation <38 weeks, prolonged rupture of membranes, Cesarean section, fever, and endometritis. The selective use of intrapartum antibiotics for certain high risk pregnancies is discussed.

Acknowledgments. This work was supported by NIAID contract 92610. Members of the Collaborative Group B Streptococcus Research Group were: H. Evenhouse, M.D., M. Rathi, M.D., and D. Terry, R.N., Christ Hospital; N. Cooperman, M.D., U. Freese, M.D., N. McMahon, R.N., and W. Semenek, R.N., Cook County Hospital; S. Aladjem, M.D., C. Anderson, M.D., S. Basalik, R.N., and C. Caldwell, M.D., Foster G. McGaw Hospital of Loyola University; M. Ismail, M.D., E. Larsen, R.N., A. Moawad, M.D., and D. Woo, M.D., University of Chicago Hospital; C. Chakinis, B.S., A. Deveikis, M.D., K. Ghaey, M.D., B. Kontelas, R.N., P. Levy, D. Sc., K. Mallin, Ph.D., P. Nell, M.D., K. Nelson, M.D., L. Riff, M.D., V. Schauf, M.D., M. Tolpin, M.D., D. Vidyasagar, M.D., and B. Work, M.D., University of Illinois Hospital.

REFERENCES

1. Eickhoff TC, Klein JO, Daly KA, et al: Neonatal sepsis and other infections due to group B beta-hemolytic streptococci. *N Engl J Med* **271**:1221–1228, 1964.
2. Fischer G, Horton RE, Edelman R: Summary of the National Institutes of

Health Workshop on group B streptococcal infection. *J Infect Dis* **148**:163–166, 1983.

3. Dillon HC, Santosh K, Gray BM: Group B streptococcal carriage and disease: A 6-year prospective study. *J Pediatr* **110**:31–36, 1987.

4. Hall RT, Barnes W, Krishnan L, et al: Antibiotic treatment of parturient women colonized with group B streptococci. *Am J Obstet Gynecol* **124**:630–634, 1976.

5. Schauf V, Nelson K, Riff L: Neonatal group B streptococcal infection: An analysis of preventive and therapeutic strategies. In Rathi M (Ed): *Clinical Aspects of Perinatal Medicine.* Vol. II. New York: Macmillan, 1986, pp. 188–200.

6. Merenstein GB, Todd WA, Brown G, et al: Group B β-hemolytic streptococcus: Randomized controlled treatment study at term. *Obstet Gynecol* **55**:315–318, 1980.

7. Pyati SP, Pildes RS, Jacobs NM: Penicillin in infants weighing two kilograms or less with early-onset group B streptococcal disease. *N Engl J Med* **308**:1383–1388, 1983.

8. Baker CJ: Early onset group B streptococcal disease. *J Pediatr* **93**:124–125, 1978.

9. Yow MD, Mason ED, Leeds LJ, et al: Ampicillin prevents intrapartum transmission of group B streptococcus. *JAMA* **241**:1245–1247, 1979.

10. Boyer KM, Gadzala CA, Kelly PD, et al: Selective intrapartum chemoprophylaxis of neonatal group B streptococcal early-onset disease. *J Infect Dis* **148**:795–816, 1983.

11. Allardice JG, Baskett TF, Seshia MMK, et al: Perinatal group B streptococcal colonization and infection. *Am J Obstet Gynecol* **142**:617–620, 1982.

12. Boyer KM, Gotoff SP: Prevention of early-onset neonatal group B streptococcal disease with selective intrapartum chemoprophylaxis. *N Engl J Med* **314**:1665–1669, 1986.

13. Bobitt JR, Damato JD, Sakakini J Jr: Perinatal complications in group B streptococcal carriers: A longitudinal study of prenatal patients. *Am J Obstet Gynecol* **151**:711–717, 1985.

14. Schauf V, Hlaing V: Group B streptococcal colonization in pregnancy. *Obstet Gynecol* **47**:719–721, 1979.

15. Baker CJ, Barrett FF, Yow MD: The influence of advancing gestation on group B streptococcal colonization in pregnant women. *Am J Obstet Gynecol* **122**:820–823, 1975.

16. Anthony BF, Okada DM, Hobel CJ: Epidemiology of group B streptococcus: Longitudinal observations during pregnancy. *J Infect Dis* **137**:524–530, 1978.

17. Boyer KM, Gotoff SP: Strategies for chemoprophylaxis of GBS early-onset infections. *Antibiot Chemother* **35**:267–280, 1985.

18. Baker CJ, Barrett FF, Gordon RC, et al: Suppurative meningitis due to streptococci of Lancefield group B: A study of 33 infants. *J Pediatr* **82**:724–729, 1973.

19. Regan JA, Solan C, James LS: Premature rupture of membranes, preterm delivery, and group B streptococcal colonization of mothers. *Am J Obstet Gynecol* **141**:184–186, 1981.

20. Pass MA, Gray BM, Khare S, et al: Prospective studies of group B streptococcal infections in infants. *J Pediatr* **95**:437–443, 1979.

21. Pass MA, Gray BM, Dillon HC: Puerperal and perinatal infections with group B streptococci. *Am J Obstet Gynecol* **143**:147–152, 1982.
22. Pasnick M, Mead PB, Philip AGS: Selective maternal culturing to identify group B streptococcal infection. *Am J Obstet Gynecol* **138**:480–484, 1980.
23. Horwitz RI, Feinstein AR: Methodologic standards and contradictory results in case-control research. *Am J Med* **66**:556–564, 1979.
24. Pyati SP, Pildes RS, Ramamurthy RS, et al: Decreasing mortality in neonates with early-onset group B streptococcal infection: Reality or artifact? *J Pediatr* **98**:625–627, 1981.
25. Baker CJ, Barrett FF: Transmission of group B streptococci among parturient women and their neonates. *J Pediatr* **83**:919–925, 1973.
26. Mayon-White RT: The incidence of GBS disease in neonates in different countries. *Antibiot Chemother* **35**:17–27, 1985.
27. Schauf V, Manroe B, Gupta M, et al: Therapy of GBS infection. *Perinatol-Neonatol* **3**:67–70, 1979.
28. Centers for Disease Control: Estimated years of potential life lost before age 65 and cause-specific mortality, by cause of death—United States, 1984. *MMWR* **35**:27, 1986.
29. Siegel JJ: Prevention and treatment of group B streptococcal infections. *Pediatr Infect Dis* **4**:S33–S36, 1985.
30. Minkoff H, Mead P: An obstetric approach to the prevention of early onset group B β-hemolytic streptococcal sepsis. *Am J Obstet Gynecol* **154**:973–977, 1986.
31. Easmon CSF, Hastings MJG, Neill J, et al: Is group B streptococcal screening during pregnancy justified? *Br J Obstet Gynaecol* **92**:197–201, 1985.
32. Morales WJ, Lim DV, Walsh AF: Prevention of neonatal group B streptococcal sepsis by the use of a rapid screening test and selective intrapartum chemoprophylaxis. *Am J Obstet Gynecol* **155**:979–983, 1986.
33. Moller M, Thomsen AC, Borch K, et al: Rupture of fetal membranes and premature delivery associated with group B streptococci in urine of pregnant women. *Lancet* **2**:69–70, 1984.
34. Anthony BF, Okada DM: The emergence of group B streptococci in infections of the newborn infant. *Annu Rev Med* **28**:355–369, 1977.
35. Shankaran S, Farooki ZQ, Desai R: β-Hemolytic streptococcal infection appearing as persistent fetal circulation. *Am J Dis Child* **136**:725–727, 1982.
36. Adamkin DH, Marshall E, Weiner LB: The placental transfer of ampicillin. *Am J Perinatol* **1**:310–311, 1984.

12
Group B Streptococci at Parturition:
II. Infant Intervention

V. Schauf, L. Riff, K. Nelson, and
The Collaborative Group B Streptococcus
Research Group

Prophylactic use of antibiotics has been proposed for prevention of group B streptococcal infection of infants, the most frequent cause of sepsis neonatorum in the United States. In the preceding chapter, strategies for intrapartum antibiotics were discussed [1,2]. The alternative strategy, prophylaxis for the neonate, was evaluated in the study reported here.

Penicillin has been used to prevent neonatal infection by penicillin-susceptible gonococci, group A streptococci, and other susceptible bacteria [3–5]. Parenteral penicillin has been claimed to be effective for prevention of neonatal colonization and early-onset infection due to group B streptococcus (GBS) [6,7], but was not effective in premature infants with intrapartum infection [8]. Parenteral penicillin appears safe for neonates, and anaphylaxis has not been reported. None of the studies of penicillin for GBS prophylaxis employed a placebo to control for subjective clinical decisions, such as the decision to evaluate an infant for sepsis neonatorum. The risks and benefits of routine use of prophylactic penicillin have not been fully determined.

To evaluate penicillin prophylaxis, the Chicago Collaborative GBS Research Group performed a randomized, double-blind trial of the effects of intramuscular penicillin given in the first minutes of life. Over 2,800 infants born in five Chicago-area hospitals participated in the study, which included safety observations for all subjects. All subjects were observed for the occurrence of GBS infection; a subgroup was evaluated for GBS colonization, a recognized risk factor for early-onset disease.

Patients and Methods

The study was conducted from 1979 to 1981 at Christ Hospital, Cook County Hospital, Foster G. McGaw Hospital of Loyola University, the University of Chicago Hospital, and the University of Illinois Hospital. Excluded at Cook County Hospital were infants weighing less than 2,000 g; they were enrolled in another research protocol [8]. Also excluded were women from whom informed consent was not obtained and women delivering when the injection could not be administered because research staff were off duty.

Nurse research assistants obtained informed consent from the parturient women before or on admission for delivery. The protocol had been approved by the institutional research review committee of each hospital in the study. Then infants were randomized to receive intramuscular penicillin or placebo as soon as possible after delivery. Syringes containing 100,000 U aqueous penicillin G or 0.9% saline placebo were prepared, coded, stored at 4°C for no longer than 2 (usually 1) weeks, and used in random order. Penicillin in syringes stored at 4°C were shown to retain full activity for at least 15 days (see below).

All infants received standard pediatric care. Because over 2,800 infants were studied, it was not feasible to include a blood culture before injection of penicillin or placebo for all subjects. Blood samples for culture were taken when an infant had signs suggestive of sepsis neonatorum or because of prolonged rupture of membranes. Infants with signs of sepsis neonatorum were not excluded from the study unless recognition, evaluation, and treatment took place immediately at delivery. Thus, cultures may have been obtained after the injection of penicillin or placebo. Additional antibiotics were administered to infants upon diagnosis of possible sepsis neonatorum. When available, serum, urine, and cerebrospinal fluid (CSF) were stored at $-70°C$; urine was concentrated 50-fold and counterimmunoelectrophoresis (CIE) was performed [9]. The code was broken and replaced on only three occasions at the request of the clinicians caring for the infants. All mothers received standard obstetric care. Bacterial cultures were obtained as clinically indicated.

Infants with GBS isolated from blood or CSF in the first 5 days of life were designated as having early-onset infection. Late-onset infection was that occurring after age 5 days. To identify subsequent infectious morbidity and/or mortality after subjects' discharge, we conducted surveillance of participating hospital microbiology records for blood and/or CSF GBS isolates and of pediatric wards for readmission of subjects. A questionnaire was mailed to parents, in English and Spanish, to determine subsequent illnesses, physician visits, and hospitalizations.

Mothers and infants enrolled in four of the study hospitals during designated culture survey periods were evaluated for GBS colonization. Included were 348 mothers during labor, 479 infants at delivery, and 400 infants at hospital discharge, 12%, 17%, and 14% of all subjects, respectively.

We obtained maternal cultures from vagina and rectum at admission for labor; from infant ear canal and umbilicus shortly after birth; and from infant rectum and throat at discharge. Samples were inoculated immediately into selective media containing Todd-Hewitt broth with nalidixic acid (15 μg/ml), polymixin (1.0 μg/ml), and 0.1 μg/ml of crystal violet [10].

Hemolytic and nonhemolytic colonies of appropriate morphology were screened by the CAMP test [11]. Final identification was by the Lancefield method [12,13].

Syringes containing 100,000 U aqueous penicillin G per 0.5 ml were stored at 4°C for 6, 7, 8, 14, 15, and 22 days and tested for penicillin activity by the agar-well diffusion technique [14]. Full penicillin activity was present at all time points except for day 22.

The efficacy of penicillin in reducing GBS colonization at discharge in babies of colonized mothers was defined as

$$\text{Efficacy} = \frac{(\text{placebo GBS positive/total placebo}) - (\text{penicillin GBS positive/total penicillin})}{\text{placebo GBS positive/total placebo}}$$

Over 200 data items concerning the maternal and neonatal hospital course were collected from hospital records, entered onto a precoded data collection form, manually edited, entered into a computer, and given further edits by computer. The statistical analysis system was used to perform standard statistical tests (e.g., Fisher's exact test, Student's T test, and the Chi-square test).

Results

PATIENT POPULATION

The subjects were of diverse racial and socioeconomic background (Table 12.1). The penicillin and placebo groups were similar in distribution by hospital, race, and source of medical payment. Mothers of the two study groups did not differ significantly in age, gravidity, parity, abortion history, blood group distribution, history of penicillin allergy, frequency of induction of labor, duration of rupture of membranes or labor, frequency of vaginal examinations, use of general anesthetic, internal fetal monitoring, or route of delivery. The infants in the two groups were similar in weight, gestational age, Apgar scores, and birth weight distribution in categories 1,500 g, 1,501 to 1,999 g, 2,000 to 2,499 g, and 2,500 g or over. By chance, mothers of penicillin recipients had more often received intrapartum and postpartum antibiotics, even though maternal infectious morbidity data did not differ between the groups.

PENICILLIN ADMINISTRATION

There were 1,441 placebo and 1,432 penicillin injections given at a mean of 12 minutes after birth in both groups. Over 85% of injections of penicillin and placebo were administered within 15 minutes of birth.

TABLE 12.1. Demography of mothers of penicillin and placebo recipients.

	Placebo	Penicillin
Hospital (no.)		
University of Illinois	171	187
University of Chicago	246	252
Christ	454	443
Loyola	157	152
Cook County	413	398
Total	1,441	1,432
Race (%)		
Caucasian	39.2	40.3
Black	47.6	47.2
Hispanic	11.9	11.1
Other	1.3	1.4
Third party medical payment (%)		
None	7.5	8.4
Public	30.0	30.5
Private insurance	41.1	40.8
Unknown	21.4	20.3

GBS COLONIZATION

GBS were present in the vagina and/or rectum of 16.1% of the 348 mothers evaluated for GBS colonization. Mothers receiving intrapartum antibiotics had a GBS recovery rate similar to the rate in those who received no antibiotics (2/15 = 13.3% vs. 54/333 = 16.2%). However, the group of antibiotic-treated women was too small and heterogeneous to allow a valid conclusion regarding an antibiotic effect on maternal GBS recovery.

The results for all infants evaluated prospectively for GBS colonization at birth and/or at discharge from hospital are shown in Table 12.2. Penicillin and placebo recipients had a similar rate of colonization at birth. At discharge, penicillin recipients had significantly reduced throat colonization compared with placebo recipients (7.1% vs. 1.6%, p <.025). Rectal colonization was also less in the penicillin recipients at discharge; however, statistical significance was not achieved.

Penicillin was effective in reducing GBS colonization in infants of colonized mothers. The infants of 31 mothers with GBS-positive cultures at delivery had selective cultures obtained for GBS at birth and at discharge (Table 12.3). These mothers had not received antibiotics in the 48 hours preceding delivery. There were 17 mother-infant pairs in the placebo group and 14 in the penicillin group. GBS was present at birth in approximately half of the infants in each group. At discharge, the colonization rate in the placebo group had not changed significantly. In contrast, only one infant in the penicillin group still harbored GBS. Penicillin was 84.9%

TABLE 12.2. Neonatal colonization with group B streptococcus (GBS).

| Infant cultures | No. of infants positive for GBS /no. of infants tested (% positive) | | X^2 | P |
	Placebo[†]	Penicillin[†]		
At birth				
Ear	17/250 (6.8)	16/229 (7.0)		
Umbilicus	12/228 (5.3)	10/251 (4.0)		
At discharge				
Throat	15/211 (7.1)	3/189 (1.6)	5.83[‡]	<.025
Rectal	12/211 (5.7)	5/189 (2.6)		

[†]Received at delivery.
[‡]Yates correction.

effective in reducing GBS colonization at discharge in babies of colonized mothers; from Table 12.3:

$$\frac{(8/17 - 1/14)}{8/17} = 84.9\%$$

GBS INFECTIONS

Three placebo recipients had early-onset GBS infection, a rate of 2.1/1,000. No penicillin recipient developed early-onset infection. Two placebo and two penicillin infants developed late-onset infection. Early-onset plus late-onset GBS infection occurred in five placebo recipients (3.5/1,000) and in two penicillin recipients (1.4/1,000).

The status of the seven infants with GBS infection and their mothers was evaluated. The four female and three male babies were of 38 weeks' gestation or more, weighed over 2,500 g, and all but one were Caucasian.

TABLE 12.3. Colonization with group B streptococcus (GBS) of infants of colonized mothers (longitudinal study).

| Infant cultures | No. of infants positive for GBS /No. of infants tested (% positive) | |
	Placebo*	Penicillin*
At birth	9/17 (52.9)	6/14 (42.9)[†]
At discharge	8/17 (47.1)[‡]	1/14 (7.1)[†]

*Received at delivery.
[†]Penicillin recipients, discharge vs. delivery, $p = .04$.
[‡]Discharge culture, penicillin vs. placebo, $p = .02$.

Six of the infants had Apgar scores equal to or greater than 6; six were born in one private hospital and developed fever, respiratory, and/or neurologic signs of infection, requiring intensive treatment. The asymptomatic infant was identified by blood culture because of prolonged rupture of membranes and did not receive any antibiotic treatment; that infant was the only one to receive triple-dye prophylactic cord care.

Fever, GBS isolate, and/or postpartum antibiotic use was present in three mothers of placebo recipients with GBS infection and in neither of the two mothers of penicillin recipients with GBS infection. One mother in each group was delivered by cesarean section.

TABLE 12.4. Bacterial isolates from neonates requiring diagnostic culture of blood, CSF, and/or urine during first hospitalization.

	No. of positive infants/total infants cultured (%)	
Organisms isolated*	Placebo[†]	Penicillin[†]
Blood cultures	16/148(10.8)	8/125(6.4)
GBS[‡]	4	0
α-streptococcus	4	0
Staphylococcus epidermidis	8	8
S. aureus	1	0
Diphtheroids	1	1
Fusobacterium nucleatum	0	1
Neisseria sicca	0	1
Escherichia coli	0	4
Pseudomonas	0	1
Total	18	16
CSF cultures	5/79(6.3)	4/69(5.8)
GBS[‡]	1	0
Group D streptococcus	1	0
S. epidermidis	2	1
E. coli	0	1
Bacillus sp.	2	1
No indentification	2	0
Total	8	3
Urine cultures	20/71(28.2)	14/58(24.1)
GBS[‡]	4	0
S. epidermidis	8	3
S. aureus	2	0
E. coli	7	8
Klebsiella pneumoniae	0	2
Other	12	4
Total	33	17

*Some cultures contained more than one organism and some patients had several positive cultures counted.
[†]Received at delivery.
[‡]GBS isolates only during first hospital admission.

INFANT OUTCOME

Penicillin prophylaxis had no deleterious effect on hospital course, duration of hospital stay, or neonatal respiratory or central nervous system status, compared with placebo. Infectious morbidity or suspicion of neonatal infection during hospitalization was similar in the penicillin and placebo groups, as judged by the percent of infants requiring antimicrobial therapy (6.6% vs. 6.5%), diagnostic lumbar puncture (4.8% vs. 5.5%), blood culture (8.7% vs. 10.4%), or urine culture (4.3% vs. 5.0%).

The frequency of positive cultures from blood, CSF, or urine was similar in penicillin and placebo recipients (Table 12.4). However, streptococcal isolates were obtained only from placebo recipients. In contrast, *Escherichia coli* was isolated from blood and/or CSF of penicillin recipients only. Serum, urine, and/or CSF was negative for GBS antigen by CIE in 10 culture-negative penicillin recipients and in 4 culture-negative placebo recipients suspected of sepsis neonatorum.

More than 95% of the subject's parents were queried after discharge about subsequent illnesses and physician visits; parents were asked to describe all illnesses. The response rate in the first 2 years was 57%. There was remarkable similarity between the penicillin and placebo recipients in the reported prevalence of infections, febrile illnesses, and allergies. Penicillin and placebo recipients' parents reported similar rates of yeast infections (16/776 vs. 12/786) and total infectious morbidity (273/776 vs. 287/786).

TOLERANCE OF INJECTION

The saline and penicillin injections were well tolerated. No hypersensitivity reactions were observed. Minor reactions, including local swelling, redness, and nonspecific rashes, occurred in 2.7% of placebo and 2.6% of penicillin recipients.

TABLE 12.5. Mortality of subjects by study group.

	Placebo	Penicillin
During nursery stay	4 (2)*	8 (2)
After nursery stay	4 (2)	2
Total deaths	8 (4)	10 (2)
Total enrolled	1,441	1,432
Total deaths/1,000 infants	6.9	5.5

*Number of infants in whom infection may have contributed to death is shown in parentheses.

MORTALITY

Neonatal and postneonatal mortality as determined from hospital records, hospital surveillance, and follow-up letters was similar in the two groups (Table 12.5). There were 8 deaths in the placebo group and 10 in the penicillin group. None was attributed to GBS infection. No evidence of GBS pneumonia was seen in any autopsy. In the penicillin group, one premature 1,020-g infant with respiratory distress syndrome and necrotizing enterocolitis died with late-onset invasive *E. coli* infection.

Discussion

Penicillin G was effective in reducing neonatal GBS colonization and was well tolerated. This randomized, double-blind trial differed in design from earlier studies [1–4,6–8,15] in that the use of a placebo made it possible to control for subjective clinical decisions, such as the decision to evaluate infants for sepsis neonatorum, and decreased the chance of attributing to penicillin an effect due to other factors.

Penicillin decreased the frequency of GBS throat carriage in the cross-sectional study of babies at the time of hospital discharge (Table 12.2). In infants of GBS-colonized mothers, penicillin significantly decreased throat and rectal GBS carriage at hospital discharge, even though both the penicillin and placebo recipient infants were equally exposed to GBS at delivery (Table 12.3). This decrease in GBS colonization was not due to intrapartum antimicrobial treatment, since mothers of infants in this group had received no intrapartum antibiotics. Reduced rectal colonization was also observed in the cross-sectional study (Table 12.2), but was not statistically significant. The efficacy of penicillin for GBS carriage demonstrated in our study expands previous observation [6] by studying the infants of GBS-colonized mothers as well as unselected infants.

Our study excluded infants born at Cook County Hospital weighing less than 2,000 g, who were in another trial [8]. In the latter trial, penicillin administered at birth was not effective in reducing GBS infection. Therefore, practices based on the present study should be limited to infants weighing more than 2,000 g.

Reduction of GBS colonization may be important in preventing GBS infection, as first suggested by Yow et al [1]. Heavily colonized infants are at risk to develop invasive early-onset GBS disease [16]. Penicillin reduction of neonatal GBS carriage has been associated with a reduction in GBS disease [6].

Penicillin was reported effective in preventing invasive early-onset GBS infection in a series of over 30,000 subjects in Dallas [6,7]. However, a change in mortality rate could not be evaluated because too few deaths occurred [6,7]. In our study, no early-onset GBS infections occurred in the penicillin group, despite the occurrence of three early-onset GBS infections in the placebo group. However, the number of GBS infections was too small to confirm statistically whether penicillin was effective in reducing GBS disease.

We observed GBS infection in term infants that produced morbidity but not mortality. Symptomatic neonatal GBS infection occurred in only one hospital, which does not use triple-dye cord care. This observation raises the question whether triple dye may have a role in preventing GBS infection from an umbilical portal of entry. Studies of triple dye for preventing GBS colonization have not revealed a consistent effect [17–19]. Signs of maternal infection were present in three mothers of infants with GBS infection who had received placebo. Since so few GBS infections occurred, this observation may be of no significance. Alternatively, by chance, infants of infected mothers may have been randomized more often to placebo than to penicillin.

The occurrence and/or demonstration of infection in penicillin recipients may have been obscured by the greater use of intrapartum antibiotics. Also, it is possible that the penicillin prophylaxis led to false-negative streptococcal cultures and underdiagnosis of streptococcal disease. Importantly, there was no increase in late-onset GBS cases in penicillin recipients and no evidence of culture-negative GBS infection in clinical specimens examined by CIE or at autopsy. In GBS-infected mice, a single dose of ampicillin often did not sterilize the blood [20]. However, infected infants treated with antibiotics before or after delivery may subsequently have negative bacterial cultures, and decisions regarding continued antimicrobial therapy would have to take this possibility into account.

Penicillin had no effect on the rate of subsequent antibiotic use or on the culture yield (Table 12.4). No streptococcal isolates were obtained from the blood, urine, or CSF of penicillin recipients. In contrast, *E. coli* were isolated from blood and/or CSF of four penicillin recipients, including a premature infant whose infection may have been secondary to necrotizing enterocolitis. No *E. coli* were isolated from blood and/or CSF of placebo recipients.

The number of patients was too small to demonstrate whether penicillin prophylaxis had an effect on bacterial infection. However, both groups of infants had similar requirements for diagnostic procedures and similar rates of positive culture and posthospital illness. These similarities suggest that GBS colonization can be reduced without increasing overall infectious morbidity. The isolation of *E. coli* in our penicillin group and the increase in infections in the first year, but not later years, of the Dallas study [6,7] are of concern. Further experience with penicillin prophylaxis is needed to see if possible improvement in morbidity due to control of susceptible organisms is offset by morbidity and/or mortality due to penicillin-resistant organisms, including *E. coli*.

No detrimental effects of penicillin were detected either by direct observation or by questionnaire survey. In earlier trials, severe reactions to penicillin were not reported in the neonate, apart from the possible occurrence of Herxheimer phenomena with congenital syphilis [21]. The prevalence of IgM penicilloyl antibodies in 5-year-old children was not influenced by neonatal penicillin administration [22]. Some infants in our trial underwent additional studies of their microbial flora and of the frequency of β-lactam hypersensitivity, and no late detrimental effects of penicillin were seen [23,24].

In this study penicillin was well tolerated and effective for reducing GBS colonization without increasing overall infectious morbidity. None of the GBS disease we observed occurred in premature infants, who have the highest incidence of GBS disease and the highest mortality from GBS infection [25]. Premature infants may already be infected at birth; penicillin at delivery was not effective in these infants [8]. Whether early-onset GBS infection in term infants occurs often enough and is severe enough to justify widespread penicillin prophylaxis at birth remains to be determined.

Intrapartum ampicillin administration to carrier mothers also rendered infants GBS culture negative, even on the first day of life [1,26]. However, attempts to identify pregnant women at high risk of delivering a GBS-infected preterm infant using cultures taken early in pregnancy have been frustrated because such cultures are not entirely predictive of culture status at delivery [13,27].

The decision to implement widespread routine chemoprophylaxis of GBS infection needs further study. The impact of penicillin prophylaxis on prevention of invasive infection was not established in our study, and was not the same in the Dallas versus the Cook County studies [6–8]. For now, where GBS disease rates are excessive, intrapartum antibiotic administration might be considered for mothers who may harbor GBS if the estimated fetal weight is less than 2,000 g. For infants weighing more than 2,000 g, 100,000 U of aqueous penicillin G could be given to the infant intramuscularly at delivery to reduce GBS colonization. Surveillance for penicillin-resistant infections is necessary if penicillin prophylaxis is to be implemented.

Summary

Infants participated in a randomized, double-blind comparison of a single dose of intramuscular penicillin G or placebo for safety and effect against group B streptococci (GBS). Over 2,800 infants were studied for safety. A subgroup of infants and mothers were evaluated for GBS colonization during periodic culture surveys. Penicillin significantly decreased infant GBS throat carriage and was 84.9% effective in reducing GBS colonization at discharge from hospital in babies of colonized mothers. Early-onset GBS infection occurred in three placebo and no penicillin recipients. Penicillin was well tolerated and total infectious morbidity was similar in the two groups. Among infants requiring diagnostic evaluation, blood or CSF contained streptococcal isolates only in placebo recipients, and *E. coli* only in penicillin recipients. In late survey of participants, no detrimental effects of penicillin were detected. Penicillin appears safe and effective for reducing GBS colonization. Where GBS disease is producing excessive morbidity in term infants, GBS colonization may be decreased with penicillin. The question of routine, widespread penicillin prophylaxis needs further study.

Acknowledgments. This project was supported by NIAID contract 92610. The work was made possible by the contributions of many physicians, nurses, administrators, parents, and infants. Drs. R. Horton, R. Edelman, I. Rosenthal, P. Quie, and P. Wehrle made many valuable contributions to design and implementation. Members of The Collaborative Group B Streptococcus Research Group were H. Evenhouse, M.D., M. Rathi, M.D., and D. Terry, R.N., Christ Hospital; N. Cooperman, M.D., U. Freese, M.D., N. McMahon, R.N., and W. Semenek, R.N., Cook County Hospital; S. Aladjem, M.D., C. Anderson, M.D., S. Basalik, R.N., and C. Caldwell, M.D., Foster G. McGaw Hospital of Loyola University; M. Ismail, M.D., E. Larsen, R.N., A. Moawad, M.D., and D. Woo, M.D., University of Chicago Hospital; C. Chakinis, B.S., A. Deveikis, M.D., K. Ghaey, M.D., B. Kontelas, R.N., P. Levy, D. Sc., K. Mallin, Ph.D., P. Nell, M.D., K. Nelson, M.D., L. Riff, M.D., V. Schauf, M.D., M. Tolpin, M.D., D. Vidyasagar, M.D., and B. Work, M.D., University of Illinois Hospital.

REFERENCES

1. Yow MD, Mason EO, Leeds LJ, et al: Ampicillin prevents intrapartum transmission of group B streptococcus. *JAMA* **241**:1245–1247, 1979.
2. Boyer KM, Gotoff SP: Prevention of early-onset neonatal group B streptococcal disease with selective intrapartum chemoprophylaxis. *N Engl J Med* **314**:1665–1669, 1986.
3. Steigman AJ, Bottone EJ, Hanna BA: Intramuscular penicillin administration at birth: Prevention of early onset group B streptococcal disease. *Pediatrics* **62**:842–843, 1978.
4. Steigman AJ, Bottone EJ, Hanna BA: Does intramuscular penicillin at delivery prevent group B beta hemolytic streptococcal disease of the newborn infant? *J Pediatr* **87**:496–497, 1975.
5. Nelson JD, Dillon HC, Howard JB: A prolonged nursery epidemic associated with a newly recognized type of group A streptococcus. *J Pediatr* **89**:792–796, 1976.
6. Siegel JD, McCracken GH, Threlkeld N, et al: Single-dose penicillin prophy-

laxis against neonatal group B streptococcal infections. *N Engl J Med* **303**:770–775, 1980.

7. Siegel JD, McCracken GH, Threlkeld N, et al: Single-dose penicillin prophylaxis of neonatal group B streptococcal disease. *Lancet* **1**:1426–1430, 1982.

8. Pyati SP, Pildes RS, Jacobs NM, et al: Penicillin in infants weighing two kilograms or less with early-onset group B streptococcal disease. *N Engl J Med* **308**:1383–1388, 1983.

9. Siber GR, Skapriwsky P: Counterimmunoelectrophoresis for detection of microbial antigens: Increased sensitivity with dextran-containing gels. *J Clin Microbiol* **7**:392–393, 1978.

10. Gray BM, Pass MA, Dillon HC Jr: Laboratory and field evaluation of selective media for isolation of group B streptococcus. *J Clin Microbiol* **9**:466–470, 1979.

11. Christie R, Atkins NE, Munch-Peterson E: A note on a lytic phenomenon shown by group B streptococci. *Aust J Exp Biol Med Sci* **22**:197–200, 1944.

12. Lancefield RC: A microprecipitin-technic for classifying hemolytic streptococci, and improved methods for producing antisera. *Proc Soc Exp Biol Med* **38**:473–478, 1938.

13. Schauf V, Hlaing V: Group B streptococcal colonization in pregnancy. *Obstet Gynecol* **47**:719–721, 1976.

14. Sabath LD, Casey JI, Ruch PA, et al: Rapid microassay for circulating nephrotoxic antibiotics. *Antimicrob Agents Chemother* **10**:83–90, 1970.

15. Lloyd DJ, Belgaumkar TK, Scott KE, et al: Prevention of group B beta haemolytic streptococcal septicaemia in low-birth weight neonates by penicillin administered within two hours of birth. *Lancet* **1**:713–715, 1979.

16. Pass MA, Gray BM, Khare S, et al: Prospective studies of group B streptococcal infections in infants. *J Pediatr* **95**:437–443, 1979.

17. Wald ER, Snyder MJ, Gutberlet RL: Group B β-hemolytic streptococcal colonization. *Am J Dis Child* **131**:178–180, 1977.

18. Wong P, Mason EO, Barrett FF: Group B streptococcal colonization in a newborn nursery: Effects of iodophor and triple dye cord care. *Southern Med J* **70**:978–979, 1977.

19. Speck WT, Driscoll JM, Polin RA, et al: Staphylococcal and streptococcal colonization of the newborn infant. *Am J Dis Child* **131**:1005–1008, 1977.

20. Deveikis A, Schauf V, Mizen M, et al: Antimicrobial therapy of experimental group B streptococcal infection in mice. *Antimicrob Agents Chemother* **11**:817–820, 1977.

21. Davidson HH, Hill JH, Eastman NJ: Penicillin in the prophylaxis of ophthalmia neonatorum. *JAMA* **145**:102–105, 1951.

22. Fellner MJ, Klaus MV, Baer RL, et al: Antibody production in normal children receiving penicillin at birth. *J Immunol* **107**:1440–1447, 1971.

23. Schauf V, Nell P, Ghaey K, et al: Hypersensitivity to β-lactam antibiotics in children given penicillin G or placebo at birth. *J Infect Dis* **152**:1074–1075, 1985.

24. Ghaey K, Tolpin M, Schauf V, et al: Penicillin prophylaxis and the neonatal microbial flora. *J Infect Dis* **152**:1070–1073, 1985.

25. Pyati SP, Pildes RS, Ramamurthy RS, et al: Decreasing mortality in neonates with early-onset group B streptococcal infection: Reality or artifact? *J Pediatr* **98**:625–627, 1981.

26. Boyer KM, Gadzala CA, Kelly PD, et al: Selective intrapartum chemoprophylaxis of neonatal group B streptococcal early-onset disease. III. Interruption of mother-to-infant transmission. *J Infect Dis* **148**:810–816, 1983.
27. Boyer KM, Gadzala CA, Kelly PD, et al: Selective intrapartum chemoprophylaxis of neonatal group B streptococcal early-onset disease. II. Predictive value of prenatal cultures. *J Infect Dis* **148**:802–809, 1983.

13
Respiratory Distress Syndrome (RDS)

Martha D. Mullett

Premature infants have been known to die from pulmonary failure for many years. In the 1950s this cause of mortality in the neonatal period was treated supportively with temperature regulation, oxygen, and antibiotics. In the early 1960s it was determined that pulmonary failure was caused by lack of a surface active substance in the lung [1]. This substance was named pulmonary surfactant, and the clinical disorder was named respiratory distress syndrome (RDS). The pathologic description of the disorder led to the name "hyaline membrane disease" [2]. Therapies encompassing more specific measures, such as continuous positive airway pressure, ventilatory support, nutrition, and medications such as sodium bicarbonate, were devised to improve survival in infants with RDS [3,4]. Even with the utilization of these measures, RDS was still the major factor contributing to death in 11,900 infants per year in the years 1969 to 1973. The average contribution of RDS to the neonatal mortality rate—20%—made it the highest single factor associated with death in neonates [5].

In 1968 Liggans and Howie [6] described the prevention of RDS in sheep by the prenatal use of steroids. Results of a controlled multicenter study completed in 1982 revealed that prenatal steroids are effective in girl singletons but that boys and twins do less well [7]. In 1982 Herron et al [8] aimed at preventing RDS by preventing prematurity.

While obstetric interventions were being tried in the late 1970s and early 1980s, research was also being directed by many different disciplines toward understanding the surface active substances in the lung and determining what properties of these substances are necessary for normal lung function. Since then many breakthroughs in understanding of surfactant composition and function have been made.

Production and Physiology of Surfactant

Microscopically the lung appears as multiple thin-walled chambers, called alveoli, that are lined with two types of cells. A thin flat epithelial cell covering most of the surface of the alveolus is the type I pneumocyte. A few rounded cells containing dark-staining laminated inclusions are also present and are called type II pneumocytes. Capillaries are numerous in the alveolar walls and the interstitial spaces are thin, giving the lung a lacy appearance microscopically.

The source of surfactant in the lung is the type II pneumocyte. Dark granules in these pneumocytes, called lamellar bodies, contain bilayers of surfactant. The surfactant is synthesized in the endoplasmic reticulum, then stored in lamellar bodies, and finally extruded at the surface of the cell into the layer of fluid lining the alveolus, called the subphase. In the subphase the initial form in which surfactant is found is thought to be tubular myelin. This form can be seen as a regular reticular pattern when specimens are carefully prepared. Tubular myelin is thought to change into the functional form of surfactant, a monolayer at the air/liquid interface (Fig. 13.1) [9,10].

Surfactant is obtained for study from animal sources by fractionating lung homogenates or by alveolar washes [11]. The composition of whole surfactant obtained is very similar in many different animal species [12]. It is composed primarily of phosphatidylcholine, but contains other lipids and a small amount of protein [13] (Table 13.1). The protein appears to

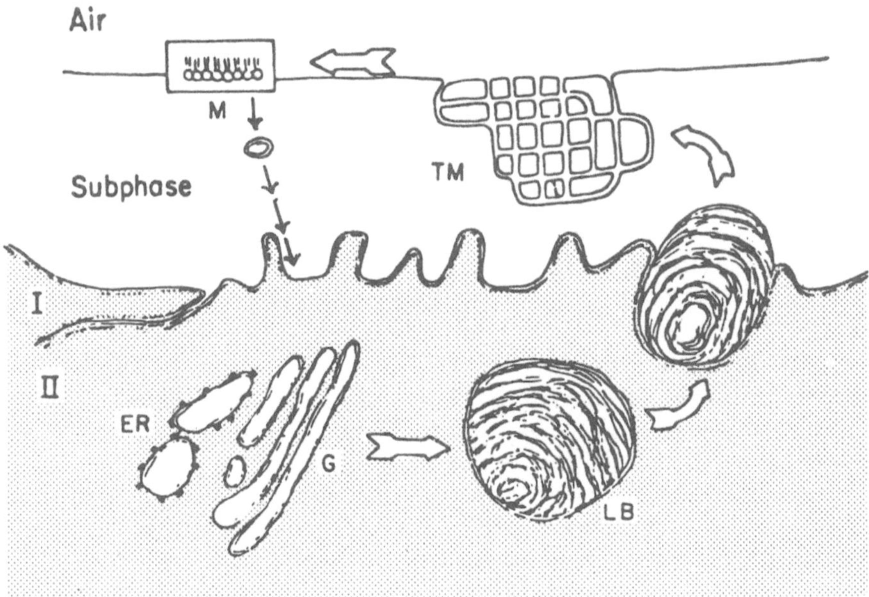

FIGURE 13.1. A schematic representation of surfactant production, extrusion, and reutilization. ER, endoplasmic reticulum; G, Golgi apparatus; LB, lamellar bodies; TM, tubular myelin, M, monolayer. Reprinted with permission from Shapiro et al.

TABLE 13.1. Calf lung surfactant extract.

Components	Percentage
Phosphatidylcholine (80% disaturated, mostly DPPC*)	79
Phosphatidylglycerol	6
Phosphatidylethanolamine	3
Phosphatidylinositol/phosphatidylserine	5
Sphingomyelin	2
Lysophosphatidylcholine	<1
Cholesterol and cholesterol esters	4
Protein	1

*DPPC, dipalmitoylphosphatidylcholine.
Reproduced by permission of *Pediatrics* **76,** 594, copyright 1985.

be an integral part of the surfactant, as it is present in the lamellar bodies as well as in the tubular myelin form.

To understand the action of surfactant it is necessary to understand the physiologic consequences of its loss in the lung as well as its biophysical and physicochemical properties. Lack of surfactant in the lung results in three clinical findings: (1) the lungs become stiff—they have low compliance, (2) there are areas of atelectasis, and (3) the alveoli are filled with proteinaceous fluid. Surfactant has four main properties that appear essential to its function as a surface active substance in the lung and prevent the consequences of surfactant loss: (1) It lowers surface tension, (2) it is rapidly adsorbed, (3) it rapidly spreads, and (4) it has the ability to vary surface tension during compression [11].

The concept of surface tension is best illustrated by the blowing of a soap bubble through a small plastic ring. The bubble produced has a tendency to collapse if the blowing pressure stops. This tendency to collapse is the result of surface tension on the radius of the bubble, trying to pull inward. The amount of tension is greater with small bubbles, and therefore they collapse more quickly. Surface tension for a bubble can be mathematically described by Laplace's equation:

$$\Delta P = \frac{4}{R} \sigma$$

In this equation ΔP is pressure across the surface, R is the radius, and σ is the surface tension. Therefore, the surface tension is inversely proportional to the radius and progressively increases as the radius decreases.

Another explanation of surface tension and surface tension-lowering substances is depicted in Figure 13.2. Water molecules under the surface of the water in a test tube have an attraction to each other in all directions. Water molecules located at the surface of the water are attracted in all directions except upward. This causes tension on the surface of the water, and a meniscus is formed. If we exchange the test tube for the alveolus and line up the water molecules in a layer as they are in reality (Fig. 13.3),

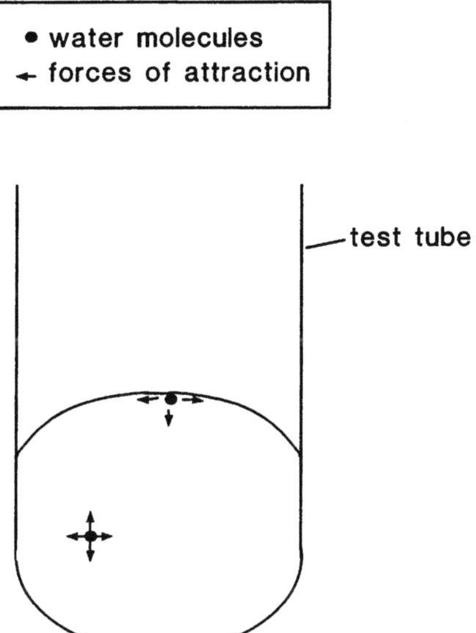

FIGURE 13.2. Water molecules form a meniscus because of forces of attraction.

the molecules in the subphase are equally attracted to each other and the molecules on the surface tend to pull together, trying to decrease the radius of the alveolus. If a bipolar molecule that is surface active, such as dipalmitoylphosphatidylcholine (DPPC), is added to the water it will line up with its hydrophilic end facing the subphase and its hydrophobic end

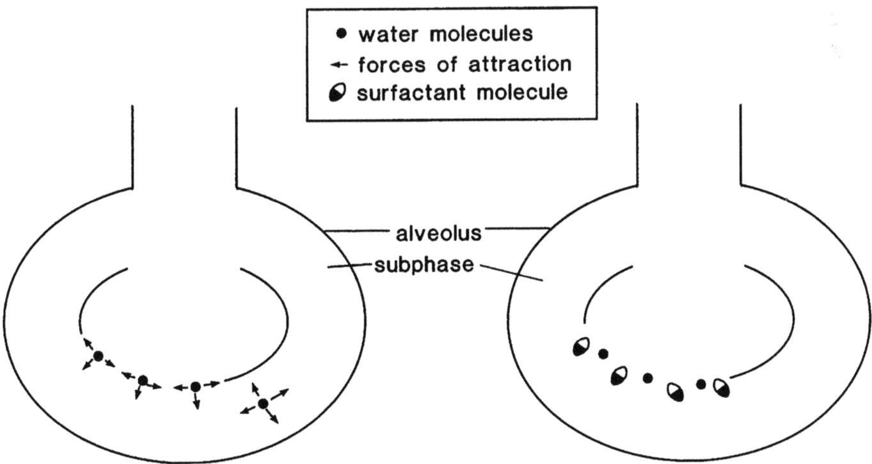

FIGURE 13.3. In a schematic alveolus, the forces of attraction between water molecules are broken by bipolar surfactant molecules.

facing the lumen. This will break the attraction between the water molecules and therefore stop the tendency to collapse. This property is known as lowering of the surface tension; it is the first property of surfactant.

The second property of surfactant is rapid adsorption. To adsorb is to be held on a surface. For surface active substances to change the surface tension they must be present on the surface of the substance and not just in solution. In the lung adsorption must be rapid in order to alter surface tension and allow respiration to occur rhythmically.

The third property of surfactant, rapid spreading, is necessary for the tubular myelin form of surfactant, which is thought to be extruded into the alveolus to change to the monolayer form and line the alveolus. Rapid spreading of a surface active substance can be illustrated by envisioning a greasy skillet with a thin layer of water added. When a drop of liquid soap touches the surface of the water, rapid spreading across the surface occurs as the soap breaks up the grease. If this type of spreading does not occur, the surfactant cannot cover the total alveolar surface area of the lung adequately.

As the lung expands and contracts, the surfactant spreads out and then concentrates in the monolayer on the alveolar surface. Because surface tension increases as the alveolus gets smaller (Laplace's law), the surfactant has to decrease the surface tension more in a small alveolus or the alveolus would collapse at expiration. This dynamic action of surfactant occurs with respiration.

As noted in Table 13.1, the main component of surfactant is DPPC. In the early 1960s single-component surface active substances were used in both animal and human trials to treat the lack of surfactant-respiratory distress syndrome [14,15]. These trials were unsuccessful, and at the time the cause for failure was not clearly understood. After much research into the biophysical properties of surfactant, it is now understood why these single-component surface active substances do not work in RDS. Single components have only a portion of the four properties necessary for surfactant to work. DPPC does lower surface tension very well and it does vary the surface tension during dynamic compression. It does not, however, adsorb or spread quickly, and therefore does not function in vivo.

Much research activity has focused on the function of the small amount of protein that is present in surfactant. The protein has been separated into three fractions—28 to 35 kD (kilodalton), 18 kD, and 5 kD [16]. These proteins have been found in lamellar bodies as well as in surfactant recovered from the lung by lavage. They are felt to help with the formation of the monolayer as well as in the reutilization of surfactant. Recent work indicates that these proteins may help with regulation of surfactant secretion [17] and with rapid adsorption of surfactant [18]. There is some evidence that surfactant reenters the cell and is repackaged and reexcreted in a type of recycling process. This reutilization process may also be enhanced by the presence of the proteins [19].

The presence of surfactant in the developing fetus is known to be developmentally as well as hormonally regulated [20]. Both types of regulation have been manipulated in the attempt to prevent serious RDS in infants. The use of steroids for the induction of enzymes has hormonally altered the appearance of surfactant in the fetus. Nature also contributes to this by stressing the fetus when prolonged rupture of the membranes or intrauterine growth retardation have occurred. The developmental process is presently being enhanced by Herron et al's strategy of preventing prematurity [8]. Now, with a better understanding of the action of surfactant and the development of exogenous sources, we will soon have the capability to treating infants in whom previously our obstetric attempts at prevention of RDS would have failed.

Surfactant Trials

In the last 6 years three types of exogenous surfactants have been used in clinical trials in infants—synthetic, human, and animal surfactants. In all of these studies the surfactant has been administered intratracheally. The trials have been generally implemented during two specific time periods: (1) immediately after delivery for very low birth weight prematures, and (2) after the disease has been established but usually before 12 hours of age in slightly larger prematures. This latter trial is called a rescue trial. The composition of each type of surfactant and the outcome of the clinical trials are presented below.

SYNTHETIC SURFACTANT TRIALS

The first trial using synthetic surfactant, done in 1967, failed [14]. This trial used dipalmitoyl lecithin alone, and there was no improvement noted in the infants. Recently a synthetic surfactant composed of 70% DPPC and 30% phosphatidylglycerol was used in two controlled randomized trials [21,22] after results of a pilot by Morley et al [23] appeared hopeful. Another randomized, controlled trial used a synthetic DPPC (70%) and high-density lipoprotein (30%) [24]. None of these three controlled trials demonstrated an improvement in the treated infants. One of the trials had a delivery room protocol and a rescue protocol. The other two trials were delivery room protocols only.

HUMAN SURFACTANT TRIALS

Human surfactant has been harvested from the amniotic fluid of women undergoing cesarean section [25]. After purification it was used in two controlled randomized trials in infants. One was a delivery room installation in 51 infants delivered at 24 to 29 weeks of gestation [26]; the other was a rescue study in 46 infants weighing less than 1,500 g with severe RDS who were enrolled by 10 hours of age [27]. In both trials significant improvement was noted in ventilatory requirements in the treated infants. There was also significant improvement in mortality in the treated group as well as a reduced incidence of bronchopulmonary dysplasia, pneumothorax, and pulmonary interstitial emphysema. The incidence of patent ductus arteriosus in all infants was the same. In both trials multiple doses of the human surfactant were given when the ventilatory indices began to decline. This decline, indicating a secondary lack of surfactant, appears to occur between 14 and 26 hours of age.

ANIMAL SURFACTANT TRIALS

The most extensive experience with exogenous surfactant has been with surfactant derived from animal sources. Generally it has been bovine in origin. The first trials, in infants treated by Fujiwara et al in Japan [28], were uncontrolled. The type of surfactant used was surfactant TA, which is from a bovine source. The drug appeared efficacious and no short-term sequellae were noted [28]. The only clinical problem appeared to be an increased incidence of patent ductus arteriosus at 36 hours of age, which responded to prostaglandin synthetase inhibitors [29]. Subsequently there have been four controlled, randomized trials of bovine surfactant. In three, calf lung lavage surfactant extract has been used in delivery room trials [13,30,31] and in one, surfactant TA has been used in a rescue trial [32]. Each of these trials revealed a significantly improved pulmonary course. Kwong et al [30] enrolled 27 infants 24 to 28 weeks of gestation; Endhorning et al [31] enrolled 72 infants less than 30 weeks of gestation; while Shapiro et al [13] enrolled 32 infants 25 to 29 weeks of gestation. Gitlin et al [32], using the rescue protocol, and enrolled 41 infants weighing between 1 and 1.5 kg with severe RDS. Endhorning et al had an improved incidence of pulmonary interstitial emphysema and Gitlin et al had an improved incidence of pneumothorax. None had any complications related to the treatment, and no other factors reached significance. None of the infants received a second dose of surfactant. Only one study mentions deterioration in a few infants between 24 and 48 hours, possibly indicating a need for a second dose of the drug [13].

Discussion

In order to speculate on the effect that use of exogenous surfactant may have on the morbidity and mortality of infants, I have combined the six controlled studies—human surfactant and animal surfactant—together into two groups—delivery room and rescue trials. This permits review of a larger sample and may allow better prediction of the alterations to be expected in the morbidity associated with prematurity and RDS. The only noted difference in the preparations in these studies appears to be a possible variation in the length of effectiveness. Human surfactant may have a shorter action than the presently used bovine sources, but since multiple doses of human surfactant were given, the studies may be comparable.

Taken together, an improvement in mortality is noted in both the delivery room and the rescue trials (Table 13.2). Pneumothorax and pulmonary interstitial emphysema improved in both protocols, and patent ductus arteriosus remained equal in incidence. Bronchopulmonary dysplasia and intraventricular hemorrhage may demonstrate a trend toward improvement, but the groups are not large enough to draw conclusions. A large multicenter trial is to be reported early in 1988 using surfactant TA in trials supported by Ross Laboratories. The morbidity aspects of this therapy may be answered at that time because of the size and controlled nature of the study.

Treatment with exogenous surfactant has been reported for the synthetic surfactant [21,33] as having no adverse effect after 2 years. Two-year follow-up on one of the bovine preparations has been reported, revealing no long-term side effects, particularly allergic, but also no long-term beneficial effect except for an improvement in incidence of early neonatal death [34]. The major concern of most investigators is the possibility that there may be some sensitization to the protein component of the surfactant derived from human or animal sources.

The trial by Enhorning et al [31] documents duration of intermittent mandatory ventilation and length of stay in neonatal intensive care with no statistical difference between the groups. Merritt et al [26], however, did show statistical significance for the length of stay in neonatal intensive care, 70.25 $\pm$ 25 days in the treated group versus 122.5 $\pm$ 33.5 days in the controls ($p <.015$). To calculate the possible impact of this change on neonatal intensive care units, let us look at the data from Merritt et al

TABLE 13.2. Effect of exogenous surfactant on morbidity and mortality of premature infants.*

	Delivery room trials		Rescue trials	
	Treated	Controls	Treated	Controls
Total	84	75	40	47
Died	8	24	6	12
Patent ductus arteriosus	48	47	29	28
Pneumothorax	14	25	4	20
Pulmonary interstitial emphysema	4	27	4	16
Bronchopulmonary dysplasia	33	40	6	15
Intraventricular hemorrhage	35	45	26	32

*Combined data from controlled neonatal surfactant trials, references 13, 25, 26, 30, 31, and 32.

[26] differently. Using their survival rate times the length of stay in the treated versus untreated groups, the total number of patient days is increased in the treated group—1,820 days versus 1,680 days in the untreated group. This is because many more infants survived in the treated group, even though they remained hospitalized a shorter time.

The effect of surfactant therapy on future bed needs in neonatal intensive care units remains difficult to interpret and predict. The number of patient days may be increased with surfactant therapy, but the infants may be less sick and able to be transferred to intermediate care earlier, rather than remaining on a ventilator and in a maximum care unit.

REFERENCES

1. Avery ME, Mead J: Surface properties in relation to atelectasis and hyaline membrane disease. *Am J Dis Child* **97**:517–523, 1959.
2. Potter EL: Pulmonary pathology in the newborn. *Adv Pediatr* **6**:157–189, 1953.
3. Gregory GA, Kitterman JA, Phibbs RH, et al: Treatment of idiopathic respiratory distress syndrome with continuous positive airway pressure. *N Engl J Med* **284**:1333–1340, 1971.
4. Usher RH: Reduction of mortality from respiratory distress syndrome of prematurity with early administration of intravenous glucose and bicarbonate. *Pediatrics* **32**:966–975, 1963.
5. Ferrell PM, Wood RE: Epidemiology of hyaline membrane disease in the United States: Analysis of national mortality statistics. *Pediatrics* **58**:167–176, 1976.
6. Liggans GC, Howie RN: A controlled trial of antepartum glucocorticoid treatment for prevention of the respiratory distress syndrome in premature infants. *Pediatrics* **50**:515–525, 1972.
7. Collaborative Group on Antenatal Steroid Therapy: Effect of antenatal dexamethasone administration on the prevention of respiratory distress syndrome. *Am J Obstet Gynecol* **141**:276–286, 1981.
8. Herron MA, Katz M, Creasy RK: Evaluation of a preterm birth prevention program: Preliminary report. *Obstet Gynecol* **59**:452–456, 1982.
9. Goerke J: Lung surfactant. *Biochem Biophys Acta* **344**:241–261, 1974.
10. Possmayer F, Yu SH, Weber JM, et al: Pulmonary surfactant. *Can J Biochem Cell Biol* **62**:1121–1133, 1984.
11. Notter RH, Finkelstein JN: Pulmonary surfactant: An interdisciplinary approach. *J Appl Physiol: Respir Environ Exer Physiol* **57**(6):1613–1624, 1984.
12. Sanders RL: Lung development: Biological and clinical perspectives. In Ferrell PM (Ed): New York: Academic Press, 1982, pp. 192–210.
13. Shapiro DL, Notter RH, Morin FC, et al: Double-blind, randomized trial of calf lung surfactant extract administered at birth to very premature infants for prevention of respiratory distress syndrome. *Pediatrics* **76**:594–599, 1985.
14. Chu J, Clements JA, Cotton EK, et al: Neonatal pulmonary ischemia: Clinical and physiological studies. *Pediatrics* **40**:709–782, 1967.
15. Robillard E, Dagenais-Perusse AY, et al: Microaerosol administration of synthetic beta-gamma-dipalmitoyl L lecithin in the respiratory distress syndrome:

A preliminary report. *Can Med Assoc J* **90**:55–57, 1964.

16. Hagwood S, Schlueter MA, Brown CL, et al: Effects of phospholipids (PL), recombinant human surfactant glycoprotein (SP28-36) and human surfactant proteins (SP5, SP18) on the pulmonary mechanics of premature rabbits. *Pediatr Res* **21**(4):454A, 1987.

17. Nogee LM, Rice WR, Whitsett JA: Role of distinct pools of surfactant protein (SAP-35) in regulation of surfactant secretion. *Pediatr Res* **21**(4):461A, 1987.

18. Glasser SW, Korfhagen TR, Weaver LTE: Cloning and predicted structure of hydrophobic surfactant protein SPL (Phe). *Pediatr Res* **21**(4):361A, 1987.

19. Snyder JM, Rodgers HR, O'Brian JA, et al: Uptake of the major surfactant aproprotein by neonatal lung tissue. *Pediatr Res* **21**(4):222A, 1987.

20. Ballard PL, Hawgood S, Wellenstein GA, et al: Surfactant protein of 18,000 dalton (SP 18) in human fetal lung. *Pediatr Res* **21**(4):442A, 1987.

21. Wilkinson A, Jenkins PA, Jeffrey JA: Two controlled trials of dry artificial surfactant: Early effects and later outcome in babies with surfactant deficiency. *Lancet* **2**:287–291, 1985.

22. Milner AD, Vyas H, Hopkins IE: Effect of exogenous surfactant on total respiratory system compliance. *Arch Dis Child* **59**:369–371, 1984.

23. Morley CJ, Bangham AD, Miller N: Dry artificial lung surfactant and its effect on very premature babies. *Lancet* **1**:64–68, 1981.

24. Halliday HL, McClure G, McReid M, et al: Controlled trial of artificial surfactant to prevent respiratory distress syndrome. *Lancet* **1**:476–478, 1984.

25. Hallman M, Merritt TA, Schneider H, et al: Isolation of human surfactant from amniotic fluid and a pilot study of its efficacy in respiratory distress syndrome. *Pediatrics* **71**:473–482, 1983.

26. Merritt TA, Hallman M, Bloom BT, et al: Prophylactic treatment of very premature infants with human surfactant. *N Engl J Med* **315**:785–790, 1986.

27. Hallman M, Merritt TA, Jarvenpaa AL: Exogenous human surfactant for treatment of severe respiratory distress syndrome: A randomized prospective clinical trial. *J Pediatr* **106**:963–969, 1985.

28. Fujiwara T, Meata H, Chica S, et al: Artificial surfactant therapy in hyaline membrane disease. *Lancet* **1**:55–59, 1980.

29. Fujiwara T: Surfactant replacement in neonatal RDS. In Robertson B, VanGolde LMG, Batenburg JJ (Eds): *Pulmonary Surfactant*. Amsterdam: Elsevier Science Publishers, 1984, pp. 479–503.

30. Kwong MS, Egan E, Notter RH, et al: Double-blind clinical trial of calf lung surfactant extract for the prevention of hyaline membrane disease in extremely premature infants. *Pediatrics* **76**:585–592, 1985.

31. Enhorning G, Shennan A, Possmayer F, et al: Prevention of neonatal respiratory distress syndrome by tracheal installation of surfactant: A randomized clinical trial. *Pediatrics* **76**(2):145–152, 1985.

32. Gitlin JD, Soll RF, Parad RB, et al: Randomized controlled trial of exogenous surfactant for the treatment of hyaline membrane disease. *Pediatrics* **79**(1):31–37, 1987.

33. Halliday HL, McClure G, Reid M: Growth and development two years after artificial surfactant replacement at birth. *Early Hum Devel* **13**:323–327, 1986.

34. Dunn MS, Shennan AT, Hoskins EM, et al: Two year follow-up of infants enrolled in a randomized trial of surfactant supplementation. *Pediatr Res* **21**(4):359A, 1987.

14
When Conventional Mechanical Ventilation Fails

Jay P. Goldsmith, Rodney B. Steiner, and Robert M. Arensman

The modern era of assisting neonatal ventilation dates back approximately 3 decades. During this time, numerous advances in diagnosis, ventilatory equipment, technique, adjunctive pharmacologic therapy, nutritional support, and understanding and treatment of cardiovascular aspects of respiratory pathology have helped to dramatically reduce morbidity and mortality from neonatal respiratory failure. Initial experience with neonatal assisted ventilation was far from encouraging in the treatment of respiratory distress syndrome (RDS) and other causes of ventilatory failure. The first major series reported only one long-term survivor in 18 infants affected with RDS [1]. Another early series reported that only 7 of 20 babies survived [2]. In a large group of ventilated infants ($n = 196$) treated at Stanford University from 1962 to 1969 for various causes of respiratory failure, only 33% survived [3]. Swyer's [4] survey of intensive care units in 1969 revealed only a 39% survival of infants with RDS who required assisted ventilation. Results were so poor in the first decade of experience with conventional mechanical ventilation that Behrman [5] concluded in a 1970 editorial that there was no proof that assisted ventilation was superior to oxygen therapy alone in premature infants and mechanical ventilation was not "the established treatment for hyaline membrane disease."

Today in most level III centers, the major causes of death in ventilated infants are intraventricular hemorrhage and sepsis rather than mechanical problems, pulmonary hypertension, and/or barotrauma complications. Although recent large series are rare and comparisons between institutions are difficult, survival in the last few years has dramatically improved over the early efforts with this technique. In one of the largest reported series, Schreiner and co-workers [6] analyzed 909 infants treated with mechanical ventilation between 1976 and 1978. They reported 68.3% of their patients were successfully weaned from assisted ventilation with large variations in outcome dependent upon birth weight, disease process, and barotrauma. Survival generally improved in each year studied and also improved with each incremental birth weight category (except for infants weighing more than 2,500 g). The complication of pneumothorax decreased survival from 75 to 60% in RDS, from 83 to 67% in persistent pulmonary hypertension of the newborn, and from 76 to 45% in meconium aspiration syndrome. At Ochsner Foundation Hospital, we now achieve an overall survival rate of 89% in infants placed on assisted ventilation (all infants weighing more than 500 g at birth, excluding those with lethal congenital anomalies). Of 100 consecutive inborn infants born between 1981 and 1986 weighing 1,000 to 1,500 g, 97 survived with the aid of mechanical ventilation. Of 342 outborn infants of the same birth weight born during this same period, 93% survived with assisted ventilation.

Even "successful" weaning from ventilatory support is not without a real incidence of short- and long-term complications. Pulmonary sequelae range from minimal bronchial hyperreactivity, which resolves within weeks, to crippling bronchopulmonary dysplasia (BPD), which may make the patient oxygen dependent for years. In their multicenter review, Markestad and Fitzhardinge [7] reported an incidence of BPD of 4 to 38% following assisted ventilation in various hospitals, with a resulting mortality in affected patients of 23 to 39%. Thus, the patient who survives assisted ventilation consisting of extremely high inflating pressures only to develop oxygen-dependent BPD and possibly succumb a year later to pneumonitis and/or cor pulmonale may be listed as a survivor in a neonatal intensive care unit report, but should not be considered a therapeutic success.

Despite increasing survival and decreasing morbidity rates over the past few years, investigators have attempted to develop new techniques that can improve outcome even further. The small but nevertheless substantial morbidity and mortality that still accompany assisted ventilation today make it essential to look beyond our current conventional applications. Two recent therapies undergoing experimental trials are high-frequency ventilation and extracorporeal membrane oxygenation. Both therapies are quite controversial and, despite relatively good outcomes in their short histories (especially when compared with early trials of assisted ventilation), neither has gained wide acceptance.

There are three critical questions in the application of both new techniques: (1) Should these therapies be used initially or as "rescue" treatment? (2) What is maximal conventional therapy, and when should extraordinary therapy be instituted? (3) Which patients can be helped? Most investigators have used these therapies as rescue techniques rather than treatments of first choice (initial therapies). The criteria for instituting these therapies have not been consistent among institutions, thus leading to doubts that the therapies were necessary and the suspicion that patients might have survived with conventional ventilation alone. It is interesting to note that these same problems of entry criteria plagued initial evaluations of mechanical ventilation for RDS [5].

This chapter reviews some of the methods and indices for predicting failure of mechanical ventilation and then briefly describes current modes of high-frequency ventilation and extracorporeal membrane oxygenation with a summary of recent outcome data.

Predictive Scoring Systems

If we could correctly predict with a high degree of sensitivity and specificity which patients would not survive assisted ventilation and which patients would develop unacceptable complications, the institution of experimental and possibly more dangerous therapies could proceed rationally. However, predictions are fraught with problems. Most predictive systems are retrospectively based on results obtained in past years, when techniques of ventilation were less well developed. A scoring system that has a positive predictive value of 80 to 90% mortality in one institution may not predict similar mortality in another. However, if patients are allowed to become moribund before qualifying for these experimental therapies, the new modalities will not be tested fairly.

Criteria for determining failure of conventional mechanical ventilation fall into three categories: (1) death, (2) failure to oxygenate (unacceptably low Po_2), or (3) failure to ventilate (unacceptably high Pco_2). To avoid the first category, death, we must determine criteria in the second and third categories, which allow us to move on to new therapies before the patient is beyond help.

FAILURE TO OXYGENATE

Failure to oxygenate (hypoxemia) is usually a complication of respiratory failure in near-term, term, or postterm infants. It is a direct result of persistent pulmonary hypertension of the newborn (PPHN), which is primary or secondary to numerous pathologic processes (e.g., meconium aspiration syndrome [MAS], asphyxia, group B streptococcal pneumonitis, large-baby RDS, and congenital diaphragmatic hernia [CDH]). Persistent hypoxemia may also be secondary to pulmonary hypoplasia resulting from extreme immaturity, oligohydramnios sequence, CDH, or other causes. In the latter cases, failure to oxygenate will also be accompanied by severe hypercapnia.

The original entry criteria for extracorporeal membrane oxygenation (ECMO) developed by Bartlett and co-workers [8] and Wetmore and colleagues [9] used a combination of factors including barotrauma, unacceptable blood gas determinations, and a scoring system termed the neonatal pulmonary insufficiency index (NPII). This index was based on measurements of blood gas pH (i.e., acidosis) and inspired oxygen concentration (Fio_2) over time and was calculated on a graph (Fig. 14.1). The values obtained by counting boxes when the Fio_2 was greater than the

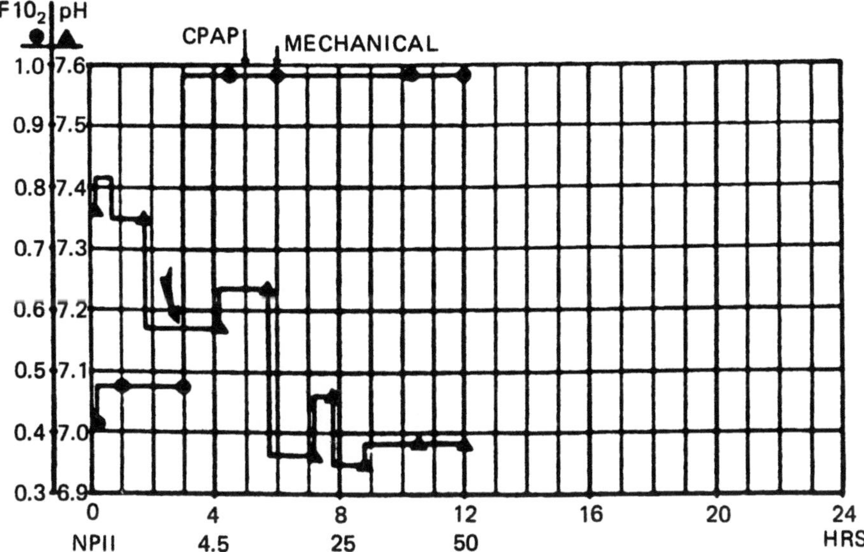

FIGURE 14.1. Neonatal pulmonary insufficiency index (NPII). Time zero is birth. In a normal infant, the value for inspired oxygen (FiO$_2$) is at the bottom, and the pH nearer the top. As pulmonary failure increases, the lines converge (at arrow). The squares are counted whenever the FiO$_2$ line is above the pH line, and the cumulative total of squares is the NPII. From Wetmore et al [9], used with permission.

pH (on the Y axis) over time (on the X axis) were compared with values of other patients with the same disease treated at that institution to predict percentage of expected mortality. However, since most institutions now treat patients suffering from PPHN with hyperventilation protocols using induced alkalosis (pH greater than 7.55), points cannot be attained in the box scoring system and thus the NPII has been discarded by most investigators [10].

Probably the most commonly used predictor of mortality in patients who cannot be oxygenated is the alveolar-arterial oxygen gradient ([A-a]DO$_2$). This calculation gives an estimate of how much oxygen crosses from the alveolae (A) into the bloodstream (a), thus estimating shunt. The equation is expressed as:

$$(A\text{-}a)DO_2 = P_AO_2 - PO_2$$
$$\text{where } P_AO_2 = \text{alveolar oxygen tension}$$
$$PO_2 = \text{arterial oxygen tension}$$

The PO$_2$ is measured directly from an arterial blood sample and P$_A$O$_2$ can be calculated from the alveolar air equation. However, when the FiO$_2$ is

1.0 during maximal ventilatory therapy, and assuming the alveolar carbon dioxide tension is equal to arterial carbon dioxide tension (P_{CO_2}) and the respiratory exchange ratio is 1.0, the calculation of this equation can be greatly simplified to:

$$(A\text{-}a)D_{O_2} = (P_{ATM} - P_{H_2O}) - (P_{O_2} + P_{CO_2})$$

where
$$P_{ATM} = \text{atmospheric pressure } (= 760 \text{ mm Hg at sea level})$$
$$P_{H_2O} = \text{water vapor pressure (47 mm Hg)}$$
$$P_{O_2} = \text{arterial oxygen tension}$$
$$P_{CO_2} = \text{arterial carbon dioxide tension}$$

Thus [11]:

$$(A\text{-}a)D_{O_2} = 713 - (P_{O_2} + P_{CO_2})$$

Several retrospective studies have used $(A\text{-}a)D_{O_2}$ as a predictor of mortality in large babies with respiratory failure secondary to PPHN or pulmonary hypoplasia (Table 14.1) [10,12–14]. In one report, an $(A\text{-}a)D_{O_2}$ of 620 torr or greater for 12 consecutive hours predicted 100% mortality despite the use of maximal conventional support and pulmonary vasodilators [12]. An $(A\text{-}a)D_{O_2}$ greater than 600 torr for 12 consecutive hours predicted 94% mortality in the same institution [13]. Beck and co-workers [14] reviewed 30 term infants with PPHN and found that an $(A\text{-}a)D_{O_2}$ of 610 torr for 8 consecutive hours would predict a 79% mortality rate. All of these infants were treated with hyperventilation and alkalinization. Moreover, an $(A\text{-}a)D_{O_2}$ of 605 torr or more for 4 hours with a peak inflating pressure (PIP) greater than or equal to 38 cm H_2O predicted an 84% mortality rate in this same institution [14]. However, Cook and co-workers [15] found that the $(A\text{-}a)D_{O_2}$ criteria of 610 torr for 8 hours or greater than 605 torr for 4 hours with a PIP greater than 38 cm H_2O predicted only a 55% mortality rate in their institution. Moreover, these and other investigators argued that by using hyperventilation for the treatment of PPHN and lowering the P_{CO_2} to the 15- to 35-torr range, a patient may meet $(A\text{-}a)D_{O_2}$ predictive mortality criteria when the P_{O_2} is in a very acceptable range by traditional standards (78–98 torr).

A more recent predictor that incorporates oxygenation ability with ven-

TABLE 14.1. Alveolar-arterial oxygen gradient ($[A\text{-}a]D_{O_2}$) criteria for extracorporeal membrane oxygenation.

Criteria	Study	Predicted Mortality (%)
$(A\text{-}a)D_{O_2}$ >620 torr ≥12 hours	Ormazabal et al [12]	100
$(A\text{-}a)D_{O_2}$ >600 torr ≥12 hours	Krummel et al [13]	94
$(A\text{-}a)D_{O_2}$ >610 torr ≥8 hours	Beck et al [14]	94
$(A\text{-}a)D_{O_2}$ >605 torr ≥4 hours + PIP* >38 cm H_2O	Beck et al [14]	84

*PIP, peak inflating pressure.

tilatory support is called the oxygen index [16]. This index attempts to determine how much damage is being inflicted on the lung (by measuring mean airway pressure) in the achievement of adequate oxygenation. If the mean airway pressure ($P_{\overline{aw}}$) to PO_2 ratio is greater than or equal to 0.4 on four consecutive blood gas measurements over a 3-hour period, an 80% mortality rate is predicted.

FAILURE TO VENTILATE

Failure to ventilate is usually a complication of respiratory failure in premature infants as a direct result of severe RDS or barotrauma. Occasionally, large babies with pulmonary hypoplasia will be hypercapnic with associated severe hypoxemia despite maximal ventilatory support.

Predictive criteria in this group of infants are based on combinations of data on birth weight, ventilatory support, barotrauma, and resultant blood gas values. Kimble and co-workers [17] looked retrospectively at 38 infants weighing less than 1,500 g at birth to predict mortality. They combined birth weight, presence or absence of pneumothorax, and mean airway pressure in a mathematical model to predict the probability that the infant would not survive tertiary care. The calculation was made as follows:

$$\text{Mean airway pressure (age 7 days)} - 7 + \text{pneumothorax}$$
$$(\text{yes} = 9, \text{no} = 0) + \text{birth weight}$$

Points for birth weight are given in chart A, Table 14.2. The probability of not surviving is derived from chart B of Table 14.2. Although these investigators looked at early neonatal events in attempting to design their model (i.e., Apgar scores, first mean airway pressure, first pH, inborn versus outborn status), these factors did not have significance in predicting outcome.

More recently Gaylord and co-workers [18] developed the "Z" score for predicting mortality in infants of very low birth weight with pulmonary interstitial emphysema (PIE). They retrospectively analyzed 70 infants to construct their predictive formula, which foretold mortality in this group:

$$Z = \text{birth weight} - (27 \times \text{highest PIP on day 1})$$

If the Z value was less than 393, the infant had an 81% probability of not surviving (Fig. 14.2).

Finally, Bohn and colleagues [19] examined the "ventilator index" (mean airway pressure $\times$ respiratory rate) in conjunction with PCO_2 in order to predict survival in infants with CDH. In reality this system can probably be applied to all severe forms of pulmonary hypoplasia. These investigators studied 66 infants with CDH in the first 6 hours of life and determined a predictive system based on a ventilatory index greater than 1,000 in conjunction with the PCO_2 value. Infants with CDH with a pre-

TABLE 14.2. Probability of infant not surviving through end of tertiary care.

Score:

Mean airway pressure − 7 (round to nearest integer)	____
Pneumothorax (yes = 9, no = 0)	____
Birth weight (points from chart A)	____
TOTAL	____
Probability of not surviving (from chart B)	____

Chart A

Birth weight (g)	Points	Birth weight (g)	Points
500	11	1,050	5
550	10	1,100	4
600	10	1,150	4
650	9	1,200	3
700	9	1,250	3
750	8	1,300	2
800	8	1,350	2
850	7	1,400	1
900	7	1,450	0
950	6	1,500	0
1,000	5		

Chart B

Points	Probability	Points	Probability
< 8	<.01	22	.62
8	.01	23	.70
9	.02	24	.77
10	.02	25	.82
11	.03	26	.87
12	.04	27	.90
13	.06	28	.93
14	.09	29	.95
15	.12	30	.96
16	.16	31	.98
17	.21	32	.98
18	.28	33	.99
19	.36	34	.99
20	.44	>34	>.99
21	.53		

operative P_{CO_2} greater than 40 torr had a 77% mortality rate. If the ventilatory index was greater than 1,000 to achieve a P_{CO_2} less than 40 torr before surgery, the mortality rate was still 50% (Fig. 14.3a). Postoperatively, if the P_{CO_2} could be ventilated to less than 40 torr, only 1 of 31 infants died. Conversely, only 2 of 27 infants survived if the P_{CO_2} was greater than 40 torr following surgery (Fig. 14.3).

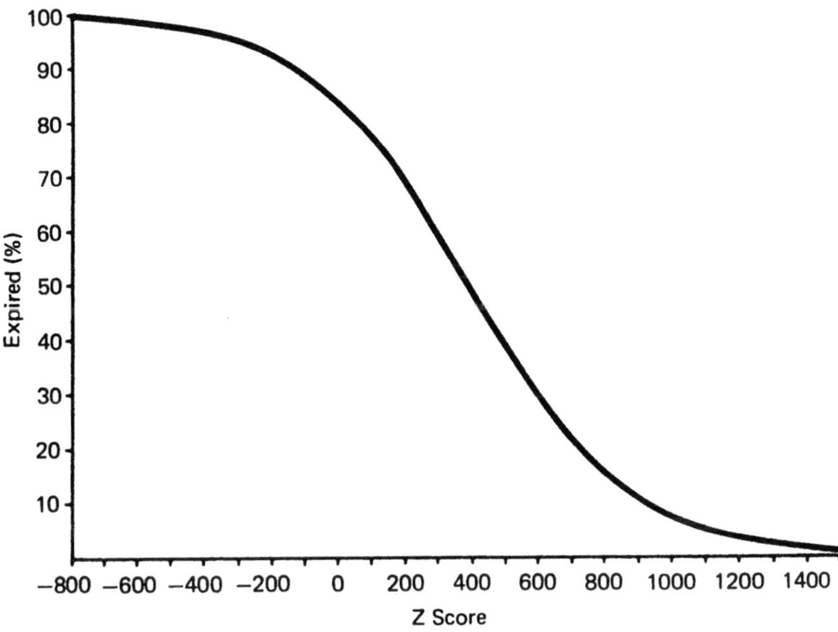

FIGURE 14.2. Relationship of Z score to mortality. Reproduced by permission of *Pediatrics* **76,** 219, © copyright 1985.

As we have seen, there are numerous predictive systems, all contro-versial and all individualized to distinct disease processes, birth weight groups, and individual institutions. Our experience with high-frequency jet ventilation and ECMO at Ochsner Foundation Hospital indicates that the Z number is probably the best predictor for infants less than 2,000 g birth weight with RDS, especially those with complicating PIE. In infants greater than 2,000 g birth weight, the 12-hour $(A-a)Do_2$ criteria work best for MAS and PPHN. However, the Bohn criteria (ventilation index versus Pco_2) most reliably predict survival in all forms of pulmonary hypoplasia.

High-Frequency Ventilation

In 1983, O'Rourke and Crone [20] described high-frequency ventilation (HFV) as "a pattern of ventilation using relatively high respiratory rates and small tidal volumes that are either less than or approximate to the patient's dead space volume" (p. 2845). Generally, rates of HFV are at least four times greater than the patient's normal respiratory rate. The Food and Drug Administration defines HFV as a rate of ventilation of 150 breaths per minute to 3,000 events per minute [21].

Three types of HFV have evolved (Table 14.3). The first is high-fre-quency positive pressure ventilation (HFPPV). This is basically conven-

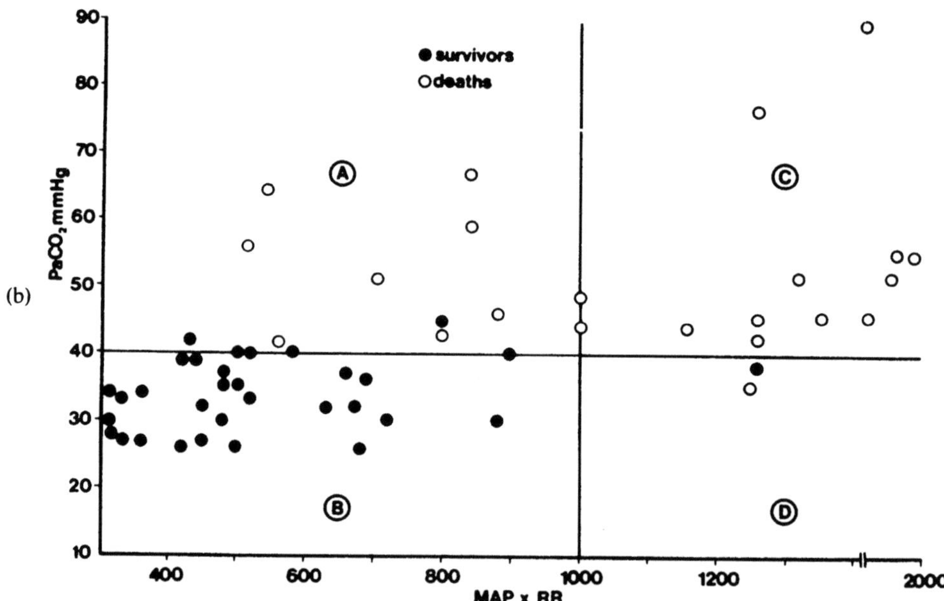

FIGURE 14.3. P_{CO_2} values correlated with ventilatory index (VI) (VI = mean airway pressure [MAP] × respiratory rate [RR]). a. In 58 patients before repair of congenital diaphragmatic hernia. Control of P_{CO_2} (<40 mm Hg) accurately predicted survival where VI was <1,000 (group B). Mortality was 100% in group C and 50% in group D. b. In 54 patients after surgical repair of congenital diaphragmatic hernia. All patients with P_{CO_2} <40 mm Hg and VI <1,000 survived (group B). All patients in group C died. From Bohn et al [19], used with permission.

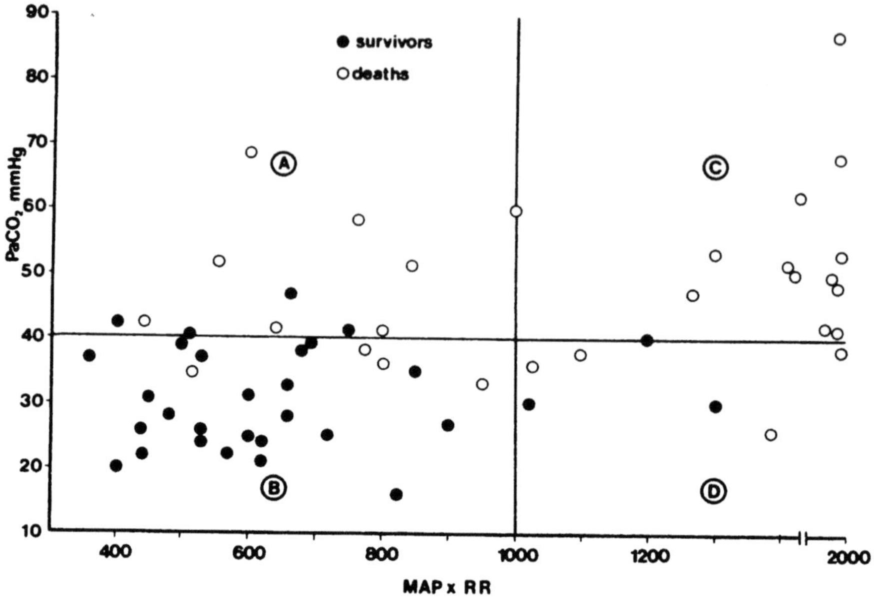

TABLE 14.3. Comparison of high-frequency ventilators.

Variable	HF positive pressure	HF jet	HF oscillatory	
			True oscillators	Flow interrupters
Delivery system	Conventional infant ventilator	High-pressure, source-regulator injector	Pistons, diaphragms	Rotating ball valves
Frequency range (breaths/minute)	60–150	100–900	400–2,400	400–2,400
Expiratory phase	Passive	Passive	Active	Active
Tidal volume	Tidal volume ↓ as frequency ↑	≥Anatomic dead space (increased by entrainment)	<Anatomic dead space	<Anatomic dead space
Inspiratory/ expiratory ratio	Variable	Variable	Variable or constant	Constant
Clinical experience	Yes	Yes	Yes	Yes
Controlled trials in neonates	No	Yes	No	Yes
Airway damage	Secondary to ET* tube	Necrotizing tracheobronchitis	Similar to CMV[†]	Similar to CMV

*ET, endotracheal tube.
[†]CMV, conventional mechanical ventilation.

tional mechanical ventilation at very fast rates. In neonates these rates are approximately 75 to 150 breaths per minute. Tidal volumes are small, but some of the HFV "physiology" (i.e., enhanced diffusion) must be operative for this technique to work. Most conventional ventilators now have rate adjustments to 150 breaths per minute, although few were designed with these high frequencies in mind. However, Boros and colleagues [22] have warned that tidal volume may drop to an inadequate amount in certain ventilators when rates above 75 breaths per minute are used, and patients may deteriorate when ventilated in this "unconventional" fashion.

HIGH-FREQUENCY JET VENTILATORS

High-frequency jet ventilators (HFJV) (Fig. 14.4) deliver rapid pulses of pressurized gas through a narrow-bore cannula, a jet injector inside the trachea, or a specially designed endotracheal tube. The injector requires very high driving pressures and can operate effectively at rates from 150 to 900 cycles per minute. The high velocity of the injected gases produces a Venturi effect, creating areas of negative pressure proximal to the injector site, which entrains ambient gases in the airway [24]. Inspiration and expiration are determined by a pneumatic or solenoid valve that interrupts gas flow to the injector. Expiration is passive. Tidal volumes are difficult to measure, but are assumed to be equal to or slightly more than anatomic dead space.

Generally, patients requiring HFJV are connected simultaneously to conventional mechanical ventilation for "sighs" at 4 to 10 breaths per minute. A recently developed triple-lumen endotracheal tube incorporates

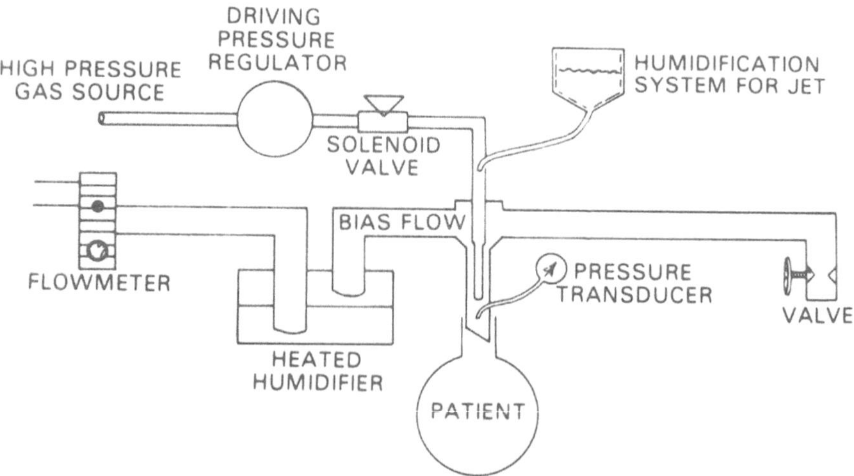

FIGURE 14.4. Diagram of a high-frequency jet ventilator. From Bancalari and Goldberg [23], used with permission.

the jet injector port and a monitoring port at the proximal end in a standard-sized neonatal tube [25]. Patients who meet entry criteria are generally started on HFJV peak inflating pressures 25 to 33% below the pressure settings on CMV with rates from 300 to 500 cycles per minute and an inspiratory time of 0.02 seconds. Mean airway pressures resulting from these settings are generally 20 to 25% less than those on conventional mechanical ventilation prior to initiating jet ventilation. This reduction in airway pressures makes HFJV attractive for patients with RDS complicated by barotrauma, especially PIE.

Disadvantages of HFJV include problems with humidification and reports of "necrotizing tracheobronchitis" [26,27]. Recently developed humidification systems may have solved many of these problems. Moreover, endotracheal tube resistance is increased because of the injector and pressure cannulae. Expiration in HFJV is passive, which increases the risk of air trapping if airway resistance or inspiratory time is increased [28]. Early reports of increased barotrauma and especially of pneumopericardium dampened some of the initial enthusiasm for this modality [29].

HIGH-FREQUENCY OSCILLATORY VENTILATORS

High-frequency oscillatory ventilators (HFOV) (Fig. 14.5) are essentially airway vibrators. They operate at rates ranging from 400 to 3,000 cycles per minute. Two types of HFOV are classified according to the way in which gas is delivered to the patient. True "oscillators" move gas toward

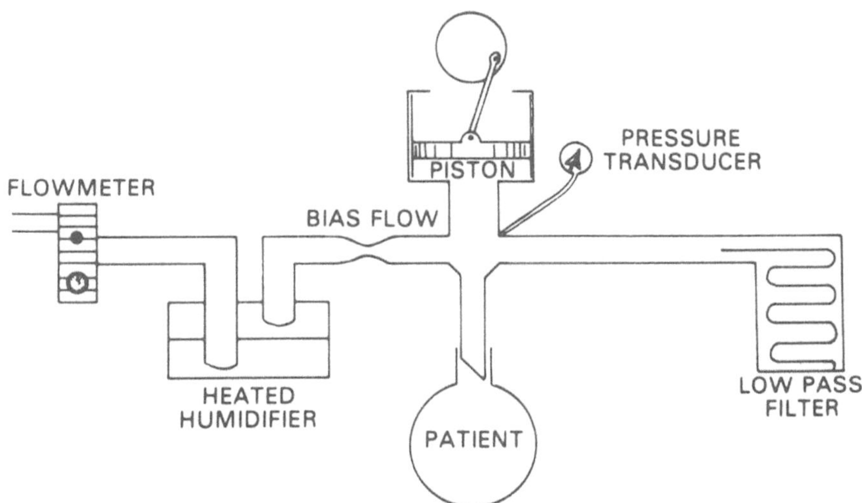

FIGURE 14.5. Diagram of high-frequency oscillatory ventilator. From Bancalari and Goldberg [23], used with permission.

and away from the patient by piston pumps or vibrating diaphragms. "Flow interrupters" are machines that intermittently interrupt a constant uni-directional flow of gas via a rotating ball valve. In both systems there is little, if any, bulk gas delivery [25]. The airway also must be connected to a source of continuous fresh gas flow or bias flow in order to provide the necessary inspired oxygen and eliminate carbon dioxide. This bias flow is eliminated through a controlled leak or low-pass filter which acts as a variable resistance, permitting adjustment of the mean airway pressure [23].

HFOV may be used in combination with conventional ventilation. The expiratory phase is active, thus generating less risk of gas trapping [27]. Most oscillators have constant inspiratory/expiratory (I/E) ratios. Warming and humidification of gases can be effectively accomplished via the bias flow. Measurement of HFOV pressures has been difficult, and the validity of such measurements has come under question. Development and avail-ability of these types of machines are extremely limited [25].

EXPERIENCE IN NEONATES

Most experience with true HFV in neonates has been "rescue" trials for short periods in small (less than 2,000 g) infants with RDS. Attempts to ventilate larger babies (term and near-term) with these devices have gen-erally been less successful.

In 1980, Bland and co-workers [30] used high rates (60 to 110 breaths per minute) on a conventional ventilator, treating infants with RDS to demonstrate that low-pressure, small-tidal-volume ventilation at faster than normal rates could maintain effective blood gases while decreasing the complications of barotrauma. Frantz and co-workers [31] used HFOV (frequencies up to 1,800 cycles per minute) in 10 infants for 1 hour and noted improvement in gas exchange at lower tracheal pressures. Another five patients with severe PIE were treated with HFOV for 2 to 26 days. No adverse effects of the ventilator were noted, and all patients had at least temporary radiologic and clinical improvement. Marchak and co-workers [32] supported these findings in the treatment of eight neonates with severe RDS. Oxygenation improved with lower tracheal pressures than those treated by conventional mechanical ventilation, but the patients were ventilated for only 67 to 233 minutes.

HFJV was used by Pokora and co-workers [33] to treat 10 neonates with respiratory failure. These infants had a variety of disease pathologies, a large weight range (700 to 4,030 g) and gestational age range (26 to 40 weeks), and variable outcomes. Of nine infants with barotrauma compli-cations in this group, seven had decreased gas leakage. Three of six infants treated for longer than 20 hours developed thick secretions leading to tra-cheal obstructions, which the authors postulated were due to inadequate humidification.

Boros and co-workers [29] used HFJV in 23 infants with life-threatening pulmonary air leaks over a 4-year period. Seventeen patients improved and nine ultimately survived.

HFJV was compared with conventional mechanical ventilation by Carlo and colleagues [34] in 12 preterm infants (birth weight $1,900 \pm 600$ g) for a short period (1–3 hours). These investigators demonstrated that HFJV produced a 30% decrease in average inflating pressures, a 29% decrease in mean airway pressure, and a decrease in Pco_2, but no change in oxygenation. They recently followed up this study with a similar comparison of HFJV and conventional mechanical ventilation in 41 infants (mean birth weight 1,447 g) for 48 hours [35]. The blood gas and airway pressure findings were comparable to those in the shorter study. The incidence of barotrauma, progression of intraventricular hemorrhage (IVH), and mortality were similar in the two groups. They concluded that HFJV can maintain adequate ventilation and oxygenation with lower mean airway pressures for 48 hours during the acute stages of RDS without increasing the incidence of complications.

Studies in the treatment of pulmonary hypoplasia and PPHN with HFV have been less encouraging. Reports by Karl et al [36], Boros et al [29], Bohn et al [37], and Harris et al [38] have shown temporary improvement but poor survival in the treatment of CDH with HFV. These reports describe a total of 25 infants with left-sided CDH. Eleven of these patients were treated with HFJV; 14 were placed on HFOV. In most patients, blood gas values improved temporarily at lower mean airway pressures. However, only two of these patients ultimately survived. Moreover, at Ochsner Foundation Hospital, we attempted to use HFJV in 10 term infants ages 12 to 86 hours who met criteria for ECMO. These infants all had PPHN secondary to asphyxia, MAS, and/or CDH. Despite improvement in Pco_2 in all patients, and transient improvement of Po_2 (in 8 of 10 patients), 7 of 10 patients eventually deteriorated (after a mean HFJV time of 6.7 hours) and had to be placed on ECMO. Six of these seven survived. Of the three infants not placed on ECMO, one survived. Thus, in our experience, 1 of 10 term infants survived after HFJV treatment alone.

In summary, it seems that a pattern is slowly emerging. HFV may ventilate small babies with RDS at lower airway pressures than conventional mechanical ventilation, and thus may produce less barotrauma if used as the initial therapy. As a rescue treatment for small infants with RDS complicated by barotrauma (especially severe PIE), the lower pressures of HFV may allow salvage of infants who previously were unresponsive to treatment. However, the use of HFV in large babies with PPHN, MAS, and especially pulmonary hypoplasia (e.g., CDH) has been less encouraging and may be futile. As of this date, multiple equipment and airway problems remain and this modality is still considered experimental [25].

Extracorporeal Membrane Oxygenation

Prolonged extracorporeal membrane oxygenation (ECMO) using a membrane oxygenator has been successfully used in several centers to treat infants with severe respiratory failure [8–10, 39–41]. The membrane lung is the key component of this procedure. It has two compartments divided by a gas-permeable membrane of silicone polymer separating the gas phase on one side from the blood phase on the other. Once the membrane lung and circuit become coated with a protein monolayer, blood is no longer in contact with the thrombogenic foreign surface, and gas exchange can continue for days without excessive hemolysis.

BYPASS PROCEDURE

ECMO has been successfully performed in over 1,000 patients using either venoarterial or venovenous bypass. The majority of patients have undergone the former type of bypass, and this now seems to be the preferred route. Previous problems with vascular access because of the use of small leg or umbilical vessels have been solved with the use of the internal jugular vein and common carotid artery for access into the central circulation. Venous outflow is established from the right atrium/superior vena cava via the right internal jugular vein with a 10-16 French cannula. Blood is returned to the aortic arch via an 8-12 French cannula positioned in the right common carotid artery. This route allows support of cardiac function as well as enhanced oxygenation; thus, this is the procedure of choice, especially in infants with hypoxic cardiomyopathy [42].

Placement of ECMO cannulae is generally performed in the neonatal intensive care unit. After appropriate analgesia, the vessels are isolated and the patient is anticoagulated with heparin, 100 to 200 units/kg of body weight. When the cannulae are in place, they are connected to the circuit (which has been previously preassembled, sterilized, and primed with packed cells, fresh frozen plasma, and platelets). Flow is started slowly to allow a gradual mixing of the prime solution with the patient's blood. Cannulae positions are confirmed by chest roentgenograms.

Once the bypass circuit is operational, deoxygenated blood travels by gravity from the right atrium through the polyvinyl tubing to a small venous bladder (capacity of 50 cc). In the event of inadequate venous return, the bladder collapses, causing the pump to shut off. Blood then travels to a 5-inch roller pump that propels it in a nonpulsatile manner through the membrane lung (SciMed 0.4 m^2 or SciMed 0.8 m^2). Blood is then routed through a heat exchanger, where it is rewarmed before being returned to the aortic arch via the arterial cannula. Anticoagulation is required to prevent clotting in the circuit. By means of continuous heparin infusion, the whole blood clotting time is maintained at 180 to 250 seconds, the platelet and fibrinogen levels being maintained near normal. Multiple ports can be incorporated into the tubing system for blood sampling and infusion. Using this bypass circuit, approximately 85% of venous return can be diverted away from the heart and lungs (Fig. 14.6) [42].

Once bypass is established, ventilator parameters are decreased to nontoxic levels using an inspired oxygen concentration of 0.21 to 0.40, breath rates of 20 to 40 per minute, and only enough mean airway pressure to avoid pulmonary atelectasis. Activated clotting times are determined hourly and maintained at two to three times normal by varying the rate of the heparin infusion. Transfusions of packed red blood cells and fresh frozen plasma maintain the hematocrit between 40 and 45%. Platelet counts are determined every 8 hours, and infusions of platelet concentrates are given to keep the platelet count above $125,000/mm^3$. Standard hyperalimentation protocols are used for nutritional support, including amino acid solutions, lipids, trace elements, and multivitamins. Standard antibiotics are given prophylactically but altered according to daily culture reports. Respiratory therapy consisting of lavage, suctioning, cupping, and postural drainage is done frequently to promote alveolar recruitment and maintain a patent airway. The infants are allowed to recover from paralysis, and normocapnia is maintained to promote respiratory muscle tone and coordination [43].

Flow through the bypass circuit controls the mixed arterial P_{O_2} by vary-

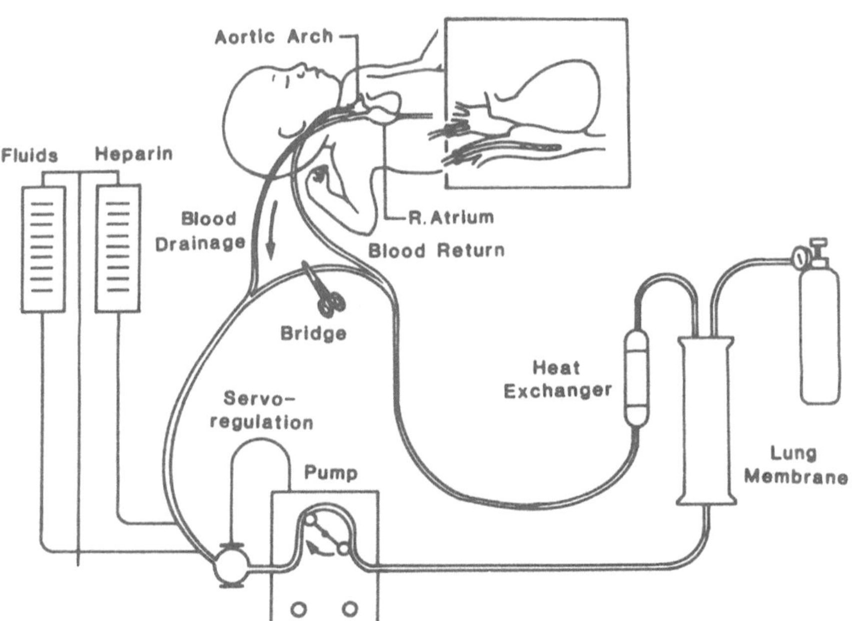

FIGURE 14.6. Schematic of venoarterial extracorporeal membrane oxygenation circuit. From Redmond et at [42], used with permission.

ing the relative contributions of the pump and the infant's heart and lungs. The arterial Po_2 sampled from the umbilical artery catheter represents a mixture of oxygenated blood from the ECMO circuit (saturation greater than 95%) and the partially oxygenated blood that has traversed the infant's pulmonary circuit. Initial flow rates are set at approximately the cardiac output calculated for the infant on bypass. At any given ECMO flow rate, as the umbilical artery catheter Po_2 increases, this additional oxygen can only come from the lungs. This indicates cardiopulmonary recovery, and the ECMO flow rate can be reduced. This process continues until flow is negligible (50 cc/min). The infant is then allowed to idle for a few hours by exclusion from the circuit, to make sure there are no setbacks.

The cannulae can then be removed. Both the carotid artery and internal jugular vein are permanently ligated to avoid the risk of thrombosis and embolization. Despite carotid artery ligation, digital subtraction angiography in 10 infants has demonstrated symmetrical blood flow in the intracranial vasculature [44]. Time on bypass ranges from 4 to 14 days, averaging 5.3 days in our patients. Once off bypass, patients are placed back on CMV, but usually can be extubated within 48 to 72 hours.

COMPLICATIONS

ECMO is an extremely invasive and highly technical procedure. Complications are most often secondary to bleeding, a result of the anticoagulation necessary for the procedure. Excessive bleeding may occur from surgical wounds, intraabdominal hemorrhage after CDH repair, intrapulmonary bleeding, or hemorrhage in the germinal matrix/intraventricular area. The latter complication may necessitate removal from bypass, although some institutions have maintained infants on ECMO with decreased anticoagulation in the face of minor intracranial hemorrhage. Other complications may occur from equipment failure, air embolism in the circuit, or accidental decannulation [45]. Many of the technical problems can be avoided by the continuous attention of a specially trained technician. These individuals may be physicians, perfusionists, nurses, or respiratory therapists. All ECMO personnel should have specific training in the procedure as well as suitable animal laboratory experience in prolonged perfusion before attempting ECMO in a clinical setting. Before an ECMO program is begun, manpower needs must be established and commitments made by the personnel involved. Insufficient planning, preparation, laboratory experience, or manpower will place patients at increased risk during this procedure.

PATIENT SELECTION

Entry criteria for ECMO are controversial. As a "rescue" therapy, the goal is to accurately select patients who will fail mechanical ventilation before they are moribund. Predictive indices discussed earlier are best individualized to the disease state and the institution. At Ochsner Foundation Hospital, we have found the single best predictor for primary and secondary PPHN to be the $(A-a)DO_2$. However, for pulmonary hypoplasia (i.e., CDH), the $(A-a)DO_2$ and Bohn's ventilator index are both used.

Contraindications to ECMO are conditions that preclude a quality outcome or a successful bypass run [45]. All patients must weigh more than 2,000 g or have a gestational age greater than 35 weeks. The high incidence of intraventricular hemorrhage in infants less than 35 weeks of age or 2,000 g in weight precludes these patients from ECMO therapy. A preexisting intracranial hemorrhage in any infant is also usually a contraindication. Therefore, all patients must have cranial ultrasonography before cannulation for bypass. Any congenital and/or neurologic abnormalities that would preclude quality of survival are also contraindications. Sometimes this determination is quite difficult to make in asphyxiated infants, especially when historical information is in doubt. The patient must also have reversible pulmonary disease indicated by a maximum of 7 to 10 days of previous conventional ventilatory support. After aggressive treatment for this length of time, chronic lung disease may make the pulmonary process irreversible and bypass is of no avail.

Outcome

As of October 1987, the National ECMO Registry in Ann Arbor, Michigan, has recorded 978 infants treated in 25 centers nationwide with 789 (80.7%) survivors. Survival has depended on the disease process (MAS, RDS, and PPHN have better survival rates than CDH) and the experience of the ECMO center. Centers with fewer than 10 cases have higher mortalities. Intracranial hemorrhage occurred in 13.5% of the registered patients with an associated mortality of 55%.

The only prospective randomized study of ECMO, by Bartlett and colleagues [46], caused great controversy because of the statistical method employed. Using the "play the winner" rule of Wei and Durham [47], Bartlett et al assigned patients to conventional or ECMO therapy in a manner analogous to a balls-in-urn selection process. One pair of treatment balls was placed in a jar, one ball marked "ECMO therapy" and the other ball marked "conventional therapy." The protocol called for the addition of one ECMO ball for each ECMO survivor or conventional therapy death and vice versa. Randomization was stopped when 10 balls of one therapy were added. In Bartlett's study, the first infant was randomized to ECMO and survived. The next infant was randomized to conventional therapy and died. The next nine infants were all randomized to ECMO and all survived. Assuming the entry criteria predicted 90% mortality, this study demonstrated a 98% probability that ECMO was a superior form of therapy for patients meeting the entry criteria.

Results at Ochsner Foundation Hospital are comparable to the national data. Since October 1983, physicians at Ochsner Foundation Hospital have treated 87 neonates with ECMO (Table 14.4). MAS accounted for nearly one half (41) of the patients in this group. Only 1 of the 87 patients was inborn; the rest were transferred for tertiary care or specifically for ECMO therapy. Overall survival of ECMO patients was very encouraging (81%), but there was a variance in survival according to the primary cause of respiratory failure. Survival for MAS was 87% and for primary PPHN was 89%. In the CDH group, a 66% survival was achieved, including four patients who required patch repair of the diaphragm.

Five patients were placed on ECMO who had congenital heart anomalies. Four had been evaluated with 2D echocardiography by at least one and sometimes two pediatric cardiologists before cannulation. The diagnosis of total anomalous pulmonary venous return was missed in four cases, and the patients were placed on ECMO for treatment of refractory pulmonary hypertension. After several days on bypass, the lack of substantial improvement in oxygenation led the team to catheterize the patients in order to arrive at a correct diagnosis. Three of these four patients survived operative repair.

The vast majority of neonates (86 of 87) undergoing ECMO at Ochsner have been outborn. Many have been successfully transported over 1,000 miles by jet in severely hypoxic condition. The extended geographic distribution of our patient population makes the task of neurologic follow-up very difficult. However, even the earliest reports of ECMO survivors reported that 75% of patients were neurologically normal at 7 to 10 years' follow-up [48]. These reports are encouraging, as are more recent short-term follow-up data, but more follow-up information is necessary to properly evaluate this therapy. However, it will be difficult to separate the etiologic factors responsible for poor neurologic outcome in ECMO patients, because nearly all infants are profoundly hypoxic before ECMO is initiated.

TABLE 14.4. Results of extracorporeal membrane oxygenation in neonates at the Ocshner Foundation Hospital, October 1983–October 1987.

Diagnosis	Number	Survivors	Percent survival
Acute respiratory failure			
Meconium aspiration syndrome	41	36	87
Primary persistent pulmonary hypertension of newborn	18	16	89
Respiratory distress syndrome	4	3	75
Sepsis	3	3	100
Nonimmune hydrops fetalis	1	0	0
Congenital heart disease			
Total anomalous pulmonary venous return	4	3	75
Coronary camarel fistula	1	0	0
Congenital diaphragmatic hernia	15	10	66
Total	87	71	82

Conclusions

Conventional mechanical ventilation for neonatal respiratory failure has improved remarkably over the past three decades. However, a small percentage of patients (5–30%) still succumb or have severe morbidity. Early selection of these patients for alternative therapies is now being attempted through a variety of predictive indices, which are controversial and vary from institution to institution. They must continually be reassessed in light of improvements in ventilator management and pharmacologic therapy (i.e., surfactant therapy). The goal is to ensure optimal management and minimal risk for each patient.

Over the last several years, high-frequency ventilation and extracorporeal membrane oxygenation have been developed in an attempt to rescue patients who fail conventional mechanical ventilation. However, with additional experience HFV may become the initial treatment of choice in premature infants with RDS. The two therapies (HFV and ECMO) seem complementary. It appears now that HFV may be more appropriate for premature infants with unrelenting hypercapnia, such as premature infants with RDS and pulmonary interstitial emphysema. Experience with HFV for treatment of hypoxic conditions such as persistent pulmonary hypertension of the newborn (PPHN) and pulmonary hypoplasia has not been encouraging. On the other hand, ECMO seems best suited to problems of oxygenation (such as PPHN and congenital diaphragmatic hernia [CDH]), and is confined at this time to infants weighing more than 2,000 g.

Currently, experience with each modality is limited to relatively few medical centers. Both therapies are considered extraordinary, and neither has gained widespread acceptance. Both therapies are highly technical, requiring advanced training of many skilled people. Neither should be instituted as an emergency procedure in an unprepared setting. Hospitals without facilities for HFV or ECMO may wish to develop their own predictive criteria for patients who will fail conventional mechanical ventilation and transport suitable candidates to centers with ongoing HFV and/or ECMO programs, to ensure the best possible treatment for their patients.

REFERENCES

1. Thomas DV, Fletcher G, Sunshine P, et al: Prolonged respirator use in pulmonary insufficiency of newborns. *JAMA* **193**:183–190, 1965.
2. Delivoria-Papadopoulos M, Levison H, Swyer P: Intermittent positive pressure respiration as a treatment in severe respiratory distress syndrome. *Arch Dis Child* **40**:474–479, 1965.
3. Johnson JD, Malachowski BA, Grobstein R, et al: Prognosis of children surviving with the aid of mechanical ventilation in the newborn period. *J Pediatr* **84**:272–276, 1974.

4. Swyer PR: Assessment of artificial ventilation in the newborn. In Lucey JF (Ed): *Problems of Neonatal Intensive Care Units.* Columbus, OH: 59th Ross Conference on Pediatric Research, 1969, pp. 25–35.

5. Behrman RE: Commentary: The use of assisted ventilation in the therapy of hyaline membrane disease. *J Pediatr* **76**:169–173, 1970.

6. Schreiner RL, Kisling JA, Evans GM, et al: Improved survival of ventilated neonates with modern intensive care. *Pediatrics* **66**:985–990, 1980.

7. Markestad T, Fitzhardinge PM: Growth and development in children recovering from bronchopulmonary dyplasia. *J Pediatr* **98**:597–602, 1981.

8. Bartlett RH, Gazzaniga AB, Jefferies R, et al: Extracorporeal membrane oxygenation (ECMO) for cardiopulmonary support in infancy. *Trans Am Soc Artif Intern Organs* **22**:80–93, 1976.

9. Wetmore N, McEwen D, O'Connor M, et al: Defining indications for artificial organ support in respiratory failure. *Trans Am Soc Artif Intern Organs* **25**:459–461, 1979.

10. Krummel TM, Greenfield LJ, Kirkpatrick BV, et al: Alveolar-arterial oxygen gradients versus the neonatal pulmonary insufficiency index for prediction of mortality in ECMO candidates. *J Pediatr Surg* **19**:380–384, 1984.

11. Krass AN: Ventilation-perfusion relationships in neonates. In Thibeault DW, Gregory GA (Eds): *Neonatal Pulmonary Care.* Menlo Park, CA: Addison-Wesley, 1979, p. 54.

12. Ormazabal MA, Kirkpatrick BV, Muller DG: Alteration of alveolar-arterial 0_2 gradient (A-a)DO$_2$ in response to tolazoline^T as a predictor of outcome in neonates with persistent pulmonary hypertension (PPH). (Abstract) *Pediatr Res* **14**:607, 1980.

13. Krummel TM, Greenfield LJ, Kirkpatrick BV, et al: Clinical use of an extracorporeal membrane oxygenator in neonatal pulmonary failure. *J Pediatr Surg* **17**:525–531, 1982.

14. Beck R, Anderson KD, Pearson GD, et al: Criteria for extracorporeal membrane oxygenation (ECMO) in a population of infants with persistent pulmonary hypertension of the newborn (PPHN). *J Pediatr Surg* **21**:297–302, 1986.

15. Cook LN, Wilkerson SA, Marsh TD, et al: Extracorporeal membrane oxygenation qualifying criteria. (Abstract) *Clin Res* **35**:75A, 1987.

16. Bartlett RH, Toomasian JM, Nixon C: *Extracorporeal Membrane Oxygenation Technical Specialist Manual.* 8th ed. Ann Arbor, MI: University of Michigan Press, 1986.

17. Kimble KJ, Ariagno RL, Stevenson DK: Predicting survival among ventilator-dependent very low birth weight infants. *Crit Care Med* **11**:182–185, 1983.

18. Gaylord MS, Thieme RE, Woodall DL, et al: Predicting mortality in low birth weight infants with pulmonary interstitial emphysema. *Pediatrics* **76**:219–224, 1985.

19. Bohn D, Tamura M, Perrin D, et al: Ventilatory predictors of pulmonary hypoplasia in congenital diaphragmatic hernia, confirmed by morphologic assessment. *J Pediatr* **111**:423–431, 1987.

20. O'Rourke PP, Crone RK: High frequency ventilation: A new approach to respiratory support. *JAMA* **250**:2845–2847, 1983.

21. Slutsky AS, Brono WR, Lehr J, et al: High frequency ventilation: A promising new approach to mechanical ventilation. *Med Instrum* **15**:229–233, 1981.

22. Boros SJ, Bing DR, Mammel MC, et al: Using conventional infant ventilators at unconventional rates. *Pediatrics* **74**:487–492, 1984.
23. Bancalari E, Goldberg RN: High frequency ventilation in the neonate. *Clin Perinatol* **14**:581–597, 1987.
24. Harris T: Physiologic principles. In Goldsmith JP, Karotkin EH (Eds): *Assisted Ventilation of the Neonate*. 2nd ed. Philadelphia: WB Saunders, 1988, pp. 22–69.
25. Boros SJ, Mammel MC: High frequency ventilation. In Goldsmith JP, Karotkin EH (Eds): *Assisted Ventilation of the Neonate*. 2nd ed. Philadelphia: WB Saunders, 1988, pp. 190–199.
26. Tolkin J, Kirpalani H, Fitzhardinge P, et al: Necrotizing tracheobronchitis: A new complication of neonatal mechanical ventilation. (Abstract) *Pediatr Res* **18**:391A, 1984.
27. Ophoven JP, Mammel MC, Coleman JM, et al: Necrotizing tracheal bronchitis: A new complication of neonatal mechanical ventilation. (Abstract) *Lab Inves* **52**:49A, 1985.
28. Bancalari A, Gerhardt T, Bancalari E: Gas trapping with high frequency ventilation: Jet versus oscillatory ventilation. *J Pediatr* **110**:617–622, 1987.
29. Boros SJ, Mammel MD, Coleman JM, et al: Neonatal high frequency ventilation: Four years' experience. *Pediatrics* **75**:657–663, 1985.
30. Bland RD, Kim MH, Light MJ, et al: High frequency mechanical ventilation in severe hyaline membrane disease. *Crit Care Med* **8**:275–284, 1980.
31. Frantz ID, Werthammer J, Stark AR: High frequency ventilation in premature infants with lung disease: Adequate gas exchange at low tracheal pressures. *Pediatrics* **71**:483–488, 1983.
32. Marchak BE, Thompson WK, Duffy P, et al: Treatment of RDS by high frequency oscillatory ventilation: A preliminary report. *J Pediatr* **99**:287–292, 1981.
33. Pokora T, Bing D, Mammel M, et al: Neonatal high frequency jet ventilation. *Pediatrics* **72**:27–32, 1983.
34. Carlo WA, Chatburn RL, Martin RJ: Decrease in airway pressure during high-frequency jet ventilation in infants with respiratory distress syndrome. *J Pediatr* **104**:101–107, 1984.
35. Carlo WA, Chatburn RL, Martin RJ: Randomized trial of high frequency jet ventilation versus conventional ventilation in respiratory distress syndrome. *J Pediatr* **110**:275–282, 1987.
36. Karl SR, Ballantine TVN, Snider MT: High frequency ventilation at rates of 375 to 1800 cycles per minute in four neonates with congenital diaphragmatic hernia. *J Pediatr Surg* **18**:822–828, 1983.
37. Bohn D, Tamura M, Bryan C: Respiratory failure in congenital diaphragmatic hernia: Ventilation by high frequency oscillation. (Abstract) *Pediatr Res* **18**:387A, 1984.
38. Harris TR, Christensen RD, Matlak ME, et al: High frequency jet ventilation treatment of neonates with congenital left diaphragmatic hernia. (Abstract) *Clin Res* **32**:123A, 1984.
39. Bartlett RH, Toomasian JM, Roloff DW, et al: Extracorporeal membrane oxygenation (ECMO) in neonatal respiratory failure: 100 cases. *Ann Surg* **204**:236–244, 1986.
40. Kirkpatrick BB, Krummel TM, Muller DG, et al: Use of extracorporeal mem-

brane oxygenation for respiratory failure in term infants. *Pediatrics* **72**:872–876, 1983.

41. Loe WA, Graves ED, Ochsner JO, et al: Extracorporeal membrane oxygenation (ECMO) for newborn respiratory failure. *J Pediatr Surg* **20**:684–688, 1985.

42. Redmond CR, Goldsmith JP, Sharp MJ, et al: Extracorporeal membrane oxygenation for neonates. *J La State Med Soc* **138**:40–45, 1986.

43. Redmond CR, Loe WA, Bartlett RH, et al: Extracorporeal membrane oxygenation. In Goldsmith JP, Karotkin EH (Eds): *Assisted Ventilation of the Neonate.* 2nd ed. Philadelphia: WB Saunders, 1988, pp. 200–212.

44. Voorhies TM, Tardo CL, Starrett AL: Evaluation of the cerebral circulation in neonates following extracorporeal membrane oxygenation. (Abstract) *Ann Neurol* **18**:380, 1985.

45. Short BL, Miller MK, Anderson KD: Extracorporeal membrane oxygenation and management of respiratory failure in the newborn. *Clin Perinatol* **14**:737–747, 1987.

46. Bartlett RH, Roloff DW, Cornell RG, et al: Extracorporeal circulatory support in neonatal respiratory failure: A prospective randomized study. *Pediatrics* **76**:479–487, 1985.

47. Wei LJ, Durham S: A randomized "play the winner" rule in medical trials. *J Am Stat Assoc* **73**:840–843, 1978.

48. Towne BH, Lott IT, Hicks DA, et al: Long term follow up of infants and children treated with extracorporeal membrane oxygenation (ECMO): A preliminary report. *J Pediatr Surg* **20**:410–414, 1985.

15
Surfactant: Its Role in the Therapy of Respiratory Distress Syndrome

Vivek Ghai, Lucky Jain, and Dharmapuri Vidyasagar

Over the past 2 decades major gains have been made in the area of the management of hyaline membrane disease [1–3]. Surfactant replacement therapy is probably the most exciting therapeutic milestone. It is expected that the introduction of this therapy will alleviate many of the complications associated with the classic therapeutic measures. Although surfactant is yet to be released for clinical use, this chapter summarizes the available literature and presents the results to the reader.

Pulmonary Surfactant

Bubbles are inherently unstable and have a tendency to collapse. The strength of the tendency to collapse is determined by the force of the surface tension operating across the bubble.

The pulmonary alveolus can be regarded as a bubble with a tendency to collapse if a distending pressure is not maintained from within to oppose this tendency. This relation is expressed mathematically by Laplace's equation:

$$P = \frac{2T}{R}$$

where P = pressure across the surface necessary to prevent collapse
R = radius of curvature of the bubble
T = force of surface tension

Obviously, during expiration, and at low lung and alveolar volumes (and thus low R values), if T were to remain constant an enormous intraalveolar pressure would be required to keep the alveolus open. Nature has obviated this by providing a substance—pulmonary surfactant—that maintains alveolar stability at low lung volumes by decreasing the force of the surface tension operating across the alveolus.

The existence of such a surface active material was first hypothesized by Von Neergard [4] in 1929 on the basis of differences in pressure volume characteristics of fluid-filled and air-filled lungs. It was seen that during lung inflation, work needs to be done against both the tissue elastic force (fluid-filled lung) and the force of surface tension. A major portion of the work is needed to overcome the force of surface tension. The difference in the pressure-volume curves between the inspiratory (inflation) or expiratory (deflation) phases (hysteresis) indicates that the surface tension must constantly change during any given cycle, and that on deflation (end expiration) the surface tension must be very low compared with the tension in saline or biologic fluids.

This observation went unheralded until the 1950s when Pattle [5] and Clements et al [6] showed that alveolar fluid stabilized small bubbles and that it did so in vivo by forming an insoluble film at the air-liquid interface of the alveolus. This film modifies the surface tension of this interface in proportion to the change in alveolar surface area. It was later demonstrated that this surface activity resided in the lipid fraction of pulmonary preparations [7], specifically in the dipalmitoylphosphatidylcholine (DPPC) fraction.

A few years earlier Avery and Mead [8] had demonstrated that RDS was due to a relative deficiency of pulmonary surfactant. This observation led, in the mid 1960s, to attempts by Robillard et al [9] and Chu et al [10] to treat hyaline membrane disease with aerosolized DPPC. These early trials met with little success. The issue of surfactant replacement therapy remained dormant until Enhorning and Robertson [11] showed that deposition of natural surfactant into the trachea of preterm rabbits improved their pressure volume *(P-V)* relationships and lung volumes. This set the stage for the successful clinical trials by Fujiwara et al in 1980 [12], who instilled a bovine surfactant preparation suspended in saline into the lungs of infants with hyaline membrane disease. Much work, both clinical and experimental, has been done since then. The purpose of our review is to present the relevant aspects of surfactant therapy in RDS.

Composition of Natural Surfactant

Surfactant as recovered by alveolar lavage varies from batch to batch in its composition depending on the methodology of separation used. Nevertheless there is enough consistency to discuss its composition. Natural surfactant differs little in its lipid or protein composition across mammalian species. It comprises phospholipids (85% by weight), neutral lipids and cholesterol (5% by weight), and protein (10% by weight) [13].

DPPC, the major constituent of surfactant, is thought to be the "effector" of its surface tension-lowering properties. Pure DPCC, however, is an ineffective surfactant. At temperatures below 41°C it exists in a gel (solid) state, with little or no capability to form monolayers or to spread rapidly across the alveolar lining. At temperatures above 41°C the stable form is a liquid crystalline form that exists in a bilayer. Conversion of this bilayer to the functionally active monolayer form is required. Other surfactant components (proteins, lipids) may facilitate and make possible DPPC's surfactant function in a variety of ways that are not completely understood at present.

Phosphatidylglycerol (PG) has received a considerable attention in the past as a functional component of surfactant. It is present in high concentrations in surfactant phospholipid [13], as unique from membrane and other tissue lipids in the body. During fetal lung development its appearance in the surfactant fraction indicates mature production and function. It is conspicuously absent from the surfactant of infants with the respiratory distress syndrome. It has been postulated that it may affect surface properties [14], help stabilize surfactant's physical structure, or help spreading [15] and adsorption [13]. It has recently been recognized that animals with surfactant deficient in PG are asymptomatic [16] and that surfactant deficient in PG has normal surface properties [17,18]. The roles of the other surfactant lipids (cholesterol, free fatty acids, neutral lipids, phosphatidylinositol, etc.) are even less defined.

The protein constituents (10%) of natural surfactant are mainly contaminating serum proteins. These can generally be removed by further purification. After removal of contaminants two specific proteins are left behind.

The major surfactant-associated protein (SP) (variously called SP-A (35 kd apoprotein A) is a glycoprotein rich in glycine and hydroxyproline and contains regions homologous to collagen. The other surfactant apoprotein (SP-B) (molecular weight 6 to 14 kD) is a very hydrophobic (lypophilic) protein that is closely associated with the surfactant phospholipids. The emerging consensus is that SPs are important for regulatory, structural, and biophysical attributes of surfactant.

Types of Exogenous Surfactant for Clinical Use

On the basis of extensive laboratory investigation and studies in animal models, a large number of exogenous surfactants have been tested in human infants. The general categories of surfactants and their chemical composition are shown in Table 15.1.

Natural Surfactants

Natural surfactants have their origin from animal lung wash (heterologous) or human amniotic fluid (homologous) [12,19]. Simple centrifugation and filtration procedures are used to recover the large surface active aggregates

TABLE 15.1. Types of exogenous surfactant.

Natural surfactant
Homologous: human amniotic fluid surfactant
Heterologous: lipid extract of bovine lung lavage
Modified natural surfactant
Lipid extract + DPPC + PG
Lipid extract + DPPC + palmitic acid + tripalmitoylglycerol
Artificial surfactant
DPPC
DPPC + PG (7:3)
DPPC + HDL (10:1)
Synthetic natural surfactant

DPPC, dipalmitoylphosphatidylcholine; PG, phosphatidylglycerol; HDL, High-density lipoprotein.

of surfactant. Calf lung alveolar wash has been the main source of heterologous surfactant, although other animals have been employed [20]. Homologous surfactant is derived from amniotic fluid collected at the time of cesarean section. Because of the differences in isolation techniques, quality of natural surfactants may vary considerably, making some modification necessary [21,22]. The goals of such modifications have been to enhance surface properties, decrease protein content, and improve stability. Modified natural surfactants are usually recovered by lipid extraction, followed by selective addition or removal of compounds [23,24].

ARTIFICIAL SURFACTANTS

Artificial surfactants, on the other hand, are a mixture of synthetic compounds like DPPC and PG. Some investigators have employed additional compounds like lexadecanol and tyloxapol [25].

Efforts are being made to reconstruct synthetic "natural surfactant" in vitro from specific apoproteins using molecular biologic techniques [26].

Surfactant Therapy in RDS

EXPERIMENTAL STUDIES

A variety of animal models have been used by investigators to study the physiologic effects of surfactant replacement therapy. The first demonstration of the efficacy of surfactant in the therapy of RDS (or hyaline membrane disease [HMD]) was provided by Enhorning and colleagues in a premature rabbit model for hyaline membrane disease [11]. In this study, natural surfactant was instilled into the trachea prior to the first breath. Surfactant instillation prevented alveolar collapse and promoted alveolar expansion to the extent seen in term animals.

From available evidence it is quite clear that instillation into the trachea of a sonicated aqueous solution of surfactant is better then administration of a nebulized form of surfactant. This was first demonstrated by Ikegami et al in a rat model [27]. In preterm lambs with HMD, Ikegami et al demonstrated that the maximal response to surfactant occurs with an administered dose of 40 to 60 mg of surfactant lipid per kilogram of body weight [28]. Metcalf et al [29] showed that the extent of improvement in pressure-volume curves in their preterm rabbits was proportional to the administered dose, up to a dose of around 40 mg/kg. Higher doses had no further effect on the P-V curves, suggesting that beyond this point structural immaturity of the lung was the limiting factor. On the basis of some of these data and the early clinical experience of Fujiwara's group, most investigators have used doses ranging from 25 to 200 mg/kg of surfactant phospholipid in clinical practice. We have used and obtained good results with a dose of 100 mg/kg in both animal [30] and clinical studies [31]. Most investigators have used single-dose administration of surfactant. However, Walther, et al [32] have demonstrated in premature lambs that repetitive treatment may be potentially useful.

The premature lamb with HMD has been the most extensively studied model for HMD. Jobe et al [33] have demonstrated prolonged survival and improved pulmonary function in lambs. They also demonstrated that treatment given after the development of respiratory failure would improve pulmonary status ("rescue" therapy) [34,35]. This effect was not, however, sustained and was attributed by the authors to bronchioepithelial injury and respiratory failure leading to leakage of serum proteins into the alveolar space. These serum proteins may function as inhibitors of surfactant function. Enhorning et al [36] used premature rhesus monkeys as a model for study. In their studies, animals were sacrificed by 6 hours of age and the evaluation was thus short term.

In the last 4 years our group has developed a premature baboon model for HMD. These baboons, delivered at 75% gestation, developed radiologic, biochemical, physiologic, and histologic evidence of HMD. Surfactant-treated baboons showed marked improvement in inspired oxygen concentration (FiO_2), arterial-alveolar (a/A PO_2), mean airway pressure, and lung compliance compared with controls (Fig. 15.1). These changes were well sustained until sacrifice at age 16 hours. Radiologic features also showed marked improvement [30]. The baboons treated with surfactant, however, showed a higher incidence of patent ductus arteriosus. On histopathologic study, the control baboon demonstrated typical changes of hyaline membrane disease, whereas the surfactant-treated baboons showed complete alveolar expansion. Pressure-volume curves on isolated lungs following sacrifice demonstrated improvement in lung mechanics, for example, better deflation curve and hysteresis of the P-V loop. In further studies we demonstrated that while both early (within 10 minutes of birth) and late (2 hours of age) recipients demonstrated good response

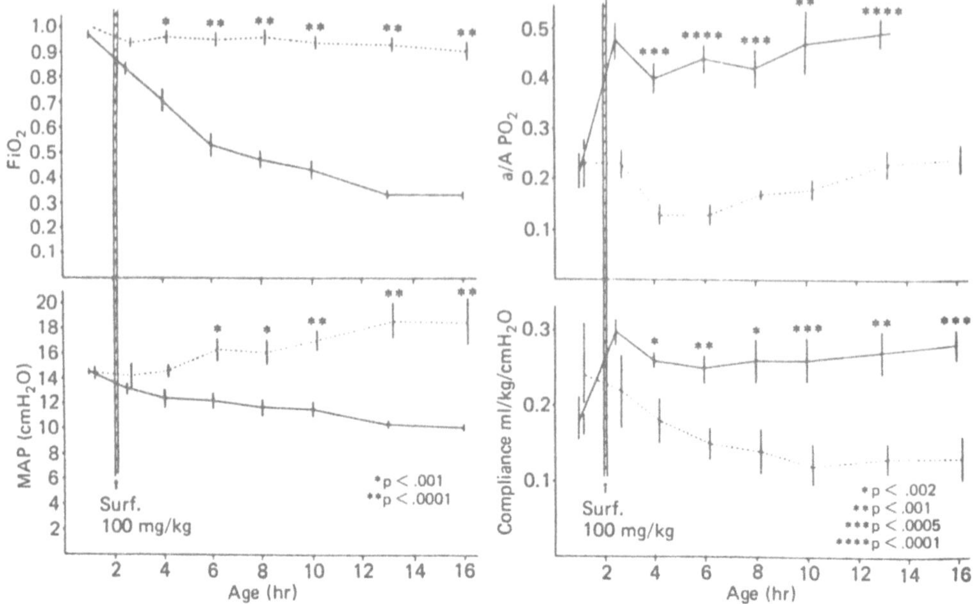

FIGURE 15.1. Sequential values of inspired oxygen (FiO₂), mean airway pressure (MAP), arterial-alveolar oxygen ratio (a/A PO₂), (from birth to 16 hours of age) in premature baboons. All values shown are mean ± SE. The surfactant-treated group is shown by a solid line and the control group by a dotted line. The arrow indicates the time of surfactant instillation. Reproduced by permission of *Pediatrics* **75**, 1132, © copyright 1985.

to surfactant therapy, response was better with early treatment [37], suggesting that delivery room (prophylactic) treatment may be preferable. However, other studies have indicated that early treatment in the delivery room may lead to considerable overtreatment.

We have also conducted long-term survival studies on our model. We were able to successfully maintain the baboon on assisted ventilation with and without surfactant therapy for up to 8 days. It was shown that surfactant therapy may prevent residual lung disease [38].

In most studies, surfactant-treated animals developed a symptomatic patent ductus arteriosus (PDA) soon after treatment, probably resulting from the lowering of pulmonary vascular pressure secondary to improved lung mechanics and oxygenation. However, despite the PDA the surfactant-treated animals did consistently better than the control animals.

Animal studies have thus increased our understanding of the pathophysiology of hyaline membrane disease and surfactant therapy and have made clinical trials and clinical use feasible.

CLINICAL TRIALS

The use of surfactant for prevention of RDS has been reported in a large number of studies. Although there has been considerable variation in patient population, methodology, and type of surfactant employed by various investigators, most clinical trials have been well designed and executed. Depending on whether surfactant has been used immediately after birth or later after development of signs and symptoms of RDS, clinical trials can be grouped as "prophylactic" or "rescue."

Prophylactic Treatment

Prophylactic treatment involves administration of surfactant, ideally prior to the infant's first breath and definitely before signs and symptoms of RDS have appeared. Several methods of administration have been employed for prophylactic studies [39,40]. Nasopharyngeal administration of surfactant has been used with varying results. Endotracheal administration gives more consistent results; it involves injection of surfactant solution through a feeding tube placed in the endotracheal tube followed by ventilation. To ensure even distribution, the infant is rocked from side to side and cephalad to caudad; or alternatively, one-fourth of the total amount is instilled into each of the four lung quadrants with the infant turned to a different position each time. The dose of surfactant employed has been empirical, varying from 20 to 150 mg/kg of surfactant phospholipid. Dry powders and saline suspensions have been employed.

Artificial surfactants were the first to be employed for prophylactic therapy. Initial attempts were aimed at administration of aerosols of DPPC to spontaneously breathing preterm infants. Investigators employed a 7:3 mixture of DPPC and PG or DPPC and high density lipoprotein (HDL). The first reports were, however, not very encouraging. Robillard et al [9] reported no improvement in clinical status following aerosol administration, although a slight change in compliance of lungs was noticed. Morley et al [39], employing a single 25-mg dose of DPPC and PG blown into the airways of infants in the delivery room, reported comparable oxygen requirements but lower ventilatory pressures at 6 hours of age and a lower mortality rate in the surfactant treated group. Milner, et al [41], Wilkinson et al [42], and Halliday et al [43] used various forms of artificial surfactant but were unable to demonstrate any beneficial effect. In a recent multicenter trial of artificial surfactant, Morley's [44] 10-center study group has reported some decrease in ventilatory support and a reduction in mortality rate from 27 to 14% in surfactant-treated infants.

Human amniotic fluid surfactant has been recently employed by Merritt et al [45] for prophylactic treatment of infants born to mothers with documented immature lecithin/sphingomyelin (L/S) ratio and absence of PG, indicating deficiency of surfactant. There were significantly fewer deaths in the treated group and a lower incidence of complication.

Enhorning et al [46] have reported prophylactic use of lipid extract of bovine lung lavage in 72 preterm infants with better oxygenation and lower incidence of pulmonary interstitial emphysema. Shapiro et al [42], using a similar study design, reported a reduction in severity of respiratory distress in treated infants at 12 to 26 hours of age, but such differences were not evident at 48 to 72 hours. Kwong et al [40] have also reported beneficial effect with the prophylactic use of modified natural surfactant.

Table 15.2 summarizes some of these studies.

"Rescue" Treatment

In contrast to prophylactic treatment, where surfactant is employed in the delivery room prior to the first breath in premature infants at high risk for developing RDS, "rescue" treatment implies its use in infants who have developed the full-blown picture of hyaline membrane disease. In the trials reported so far, most investigators have employed this mode in infants manifesting moderately severe RDS. Although study design and methodology remain the same as with the prophylactic group, certain differences exist. Infants were at least 4 hours old and were intubated at the time of treatment. Most investigators have employed a single dose of saline suspension of surfactant deposited into the lung via the endotracheal tube, but multiple treatments have also been tried.

There are only a few reports on the use of artificial surfactant in rescue treatment. Milner et al [48] and Wilkinson et al [42] failed to demonstrate improvement after use of artificial surfactant in infants with established RDS.

Hallman et al [49,50] have employed human amniotic fluid surfactant in treatment of premature infants with RDS. They showed marked reduction in the severity of RDS.

Modified natural surfactants have been employed in a large number of rescue trials. In their historic trial reported in 1980, Fujiwara et al [12] employed reconstituted bovine surfactant for treatment of RDS in infants who were several hours old. A dramatic improvement in ventilatory status was reported within minutes after administration of surfactant. The authors have subsequently published numerous reports confirming their initial results [51,52].

Raju et al [31] from our institution have recently reported results of a randomized controlled trial of bovine surfactant (surfactant TA) in infants with severe RDS. Infants with birth weight of 750 to 1,750 g who had clinical and radiologic evidence of severe RDS were enrolled at 6 hours of age. Sick infants were on assisted ventilation and required more than 50% inspired oxygen concentration. They had a mean airway pressure of 8 cm H_2O or greater with evidence of poor oxygenation (arterial-alveolar oxygen gradient of 0.24 or less). Infants were assigned to either surfactant

TABLE 15.2. Summary of prophylactic treatment trials.

Surfactant type		Enhorning et al [76]	Halliday et al [44]	Kwong et al [41]	Merritt et al [46]	Morley [45]
		Lipid extract of bovine lung lavage	DPPC + HDL	Lipid extract of bovine lung lavage	Human amniotic fluid	DPPC + PG (70:30)
No. of infants	c	33	51	13	29	149
	s	39	49	14	31	159
Gestational age	c	27.4	31.0	26.7	26.8	27.6
(weeks) ($\bar{x}$)	s	27.2	30.3	26.2	26.7	27.6
Birth Weight	c	974	1,486	892	964	1,070
(g) ($\bar{x}$)	s	976	1,591	971	938	1,093
Dose (mg/kg)		75–100	20–30	100	60	100
Results		↓ RDS, ↑ Fio$_2$, ↓ MAP	No improvement	↓ RDS, ↑ Fio$_2$, ↓ MAP	↓ RDS, ↑ Fio$_2$, ↓ MAP	No improvement
Mortality (%)	c	21	43	15	52	27
	s	3	6	7	16	14
Bronchopulmonary	c	81	16	82	64	—
dysplasia*	s	58	19	46	19	—
(%)						
Patent ductus	c	58	14	31	83	23
arteriosus*	s	46	24	50	74	26
(%)						
Pneumothorax*	c	33	NA	15	24	NA
(%)	s	18	NA	29	7	NA

DPPG, dipalmitoylphosphatidylcholine; PG, phosphatidylglycerol; HDL, c, controls; s, study subjects; RDS, respiratory distress syndrome; Fio$_2$, inspired oxygen concentration; MAP, mean airway pressure.
*In survivors.

or placebo group using a stratified randomization scheme based on infant sex and on birth weight intervals of 250 g. A single dose of surfactant TA, 100 mg/kg in 3.3 saline, was sonicated and administered via the endotracheal tube. Infants in the placebo group received 1 ml/kg (maximum 1 ml) of sterile normal saline. The treated group showed an early and significant improvement in oxygenation and required considerably less ventilatory support. The combined incidence of death and severe bronchopulmonary dysplasia was 17.6% in the surfactant-treated group as opposed to 69.2% in the placebo group. Air leak syndromes (pneumothorax and pulmonary interstitial emphysema) occurred less frequently in the treated group, although the incidence of hemodynamically significant patent ductus arteriosus was higher in this group. Overall, our study demonstrated considerable beneficial effect from a single dose of surfactant TA. Gitlin et al [53] have recently reported similar results. Table 15.3 summarizes some rescue studies.

Effect of Surfactant on Course and Complications of RDS

Most controlled trials have reported a significant reduction in complications of RDS with surfactant therapy. Surfactant treatment reduces the occurrence of air leak syndromes. Initial trials with surfactant had reported a higher incidence of patent ductus arteriosus in treated infants [12,24,50], but most prophylactic treatment trials have shown no difference in incidence of this condition between control and treated groups. Although data on incidence of other major complications associated with prematurity and RDS have not been reported consistently, no significant difference is noticeable between the two groups. Most recent studies have reported a marked reduction in mortality in surfactant-treated infants. In the treated infants followed up so far, despite the reduction in acute complications, the incidence of bronchopulmonary dysplasia has not registered any consistent decline.

There are concerns regarding the long-term effects of the foreign protein present in exogenous surfactant as well as the possibility of transmission of infections with administration of surfactant. Experience thus far provides no foundation for these concerns.

Summary

From data published so far, surfactant therapy has proved to be effective in reducing the incidence and severity of RDS. Its use has not been associated with any short-term untoward effects. Long-term follow-up studies are still awaited. Surfactant is not available commercially at present

TABLE 15.3. Summary of rescue trials.

	Fujiwara et al [52]	Gitlin et al [54]		Hallman et al [51]	Raju et al [31]
Surfactant type	Surfactant TA	Surfactant TA		Human amniotic fluid	Surfactant TA
No. of infants	41	23 ep 18	c	23	13
	50		s	22	17
Gestational age (weeks) ($\bar{x}$)	29.0	29.0	c	27.2	27.6
	28.8	29.0	s	27.0	28.4
Birth weight (g) ($\bar{x}$)	1,267	1,214	c	1,056	1,096
	1,261	1,258	c	987	1,119
Dose (mg/kg)	106			60	100
Age at therapy	6–8 hr			5 hrs	5 hr
Results	↓ Fio$_2$, ↓ MAP	↓ Fio$_2$, ↓ MAP		↓ Fio$_2$, ↓ MAP	↓ Fio$_2$, ↓ MAP, ↓ RDS
Mortality (%)	20	26	c	26	46
	12	17	s	14	12
Bronchopulmonary	30	41	c	35	57
dysplasia* (%)	11	27	s	14	60
Patent ductus arteriosus*	37	39	c	83	23
(%)	46	44	s	95	71
Air leak syndrome	44	57	c	30	46
(PIE + PTX)* (%)	6	17	s	5	15

c, controls; s, study subjects; Fio$_2$, inspired oxygen concentration; MAP, mean airway pressure; RDS, respiratory distress syndrome; PIE, pulmonary interstitial emphysema; PTX, pneumothorax.
*In survivors.

because of federal testing requirements. Considering the ease of administration and relative low cost, it can be expected that exogenous surfactant will be available routinely in the delivery room or neonatal intensive care unit for the prevention of RDS.

REFERENCES

1. Farrell PM, Avery ME: Hyaline membrane disease. *Am Rev Respir Dis* **11**:657, 1975.
2. Inselman LS: Respiratory distress syndrome. *Pediatr Ann* **7**:34, 1978.
3. Kamper J: Longterm prognosis of infants with severe idiopathic respiratory distress syndrome. 1. Neurological and mental outcome. *Acta Pediatr Scand* **67**:61, 1978.
4. Von-Neergaard K: Neue Auffassungen uber einen Grundbegriff der Atemechanic. *Z Ges Exptl Med* **66**:373–394, 1929.
5. Pattle RE: Properties, function and origin of the alveolar lining layer. *Nature* **175**:1125, 1955.
6. Clements JA, Brown ES, Johnson RP: Pulmonary surface tension and the mucous lining of the lung: Some theoretical considerations. *J Appl Physiol* **12**:262–268, 1958.
7. Klause MH, Clements JA, Havel RJ: Composition of surface active material isolated from beef lungs. *Proc Natl Acad Sci (USA)* **47**:1858–1859, 1961.
8. Avery ME, Mead J: Surface properties in relation to atelectasis and hyaline membrane disease. *Am J Dis Child* **97**:517, 1959.
9. Robillard E, Alarie Y, Dagenais-Perusse P, et al: Microaerosol administration of synthetic B-dipalmitoyl-L-lecithin in the respiratory distress syndrome: A preliminary report. *Can Med Assoc J* **90**:55, 1964.
10. Chu J, Clements JA, Cotton EK, et al: Neonatal pulmonary ischemia. *Pediatrics* **40**:709, 1967.
11. Enhorning G, Robertson B: Lung expansion in the premature rabbit after tracheal deposition of surfactant. *Pediatrics* **50**:58, 1972.
12. Fujiwara T, Chida S, Watabe Y, et al: Artificial surfactant therapy in hyaline membrane disease. *Lancet* **1**:55–59, 1980.
13. King RJ, MacBeth MC: Interaction of lipid and protein components of pulmonary surfactant: Role of phosphatidyl glycerol and calcium. *Biochim Biophys Acta* **647**:159–168, 1981.
14. Hallman M, Gluck L: Phosphatidyl glycerol in lung surfactant. III. Possible modifier of surfactant function. *J Lipid Res* **17**:257–262, 1976.
15. Bangham AD: Lung surfactant: How it does and does not work. *Lung* **165**:17–25, 1987.
16. Beppu OS, Clements JA, Goerke S: Phosphatidyl glycerol-deficient lung surfactant has normal properties. *J Appl Physiol. Respirat, Environ Exer Physiol* **55**(2):496–502, 1983.
17. Hallman M, Enhorning G, Possmayer F: Composition and surface activity of normal and phosphatidyl deficient lung surfactant. *Pediatr Res* **19**:286–292, 1985.
18. Suzuki Y: Effect of protein, cholesterol and phosphatidyl glycerol on the surface activity of the lipid protein complex reconstituted from pig pulmonary surfactant. *J Lipid Res* **23**:62–69, 1982.

19. Hallman M, Merrit TA, Schneider H, et al: Isolation of human surfactant from amniotic fluid and a pilot study of its efficacy in respiratory distress syndrome. *Pediatrics* **71**:473–482, 1983.

20. King RJ, Clements JA: Surface active materials from dog lung: Composition and physiological correlation. *Am J Physiol* **223**:715–726, 1972.

21. Keough KMW, Farrell E, Cox M, et al: Physical, chemical and physiological characteristics of isolates of pulmonary surfactant from adult rabbits. *Can J Physiol Pharmacol* **63**:1043–1051, 1985.

22. Benson BJ, Williams MC, Sueishi K, et al: Role of calcium ions in the structure and function of pulmonary surfactant. *Biochem Biophys Acta* **793**:18–27, 1984.

23. Whitsett JA, Ohning BL, Ross G, et al: Hydrophobic surfactant associated protein in whole lung surfactant and its importance for biophysical activity in lung surfactant extracts used for replacement therapy. *Pediatr Res* **20**(5):460–467, 1986.

24. Fujiwara T: Surfactant replacement in neonatal RDS. In Robertson B, Van Golde LMG, Batenburg JJ (Eds): *Pulmonary Surfactant*. Amsterdam: Elsevier Science Publishers, 1984, pp. 479–503.

25. Durand DJ, Clyman RI, Heymann MA, et al: Effects of a protein free synthetic surfactant on survival and pulmonary function in preterm lambs. *J Pediatr* **107**:775–780, 1985; *Fed Proc* **45**:1014, 1986.

26. Floros J, Phelphs DS, Taeusch HW: Biosynthesis and in vitro translation of the major surfactant associated protein from human lung. *J Biol Chem* **260**:495–500, 1985.

27. Ikegami M, Hesterberg T, Nozaki M, et al: Restoration of lung pressure-volume characteristics with surfactant: Comparison of nebulization versus instillation and natural versus artificial surfactant. *Pediatr Res* **11**:178–182, 1977.

28. Ikegami M, Adams FM, Tower B, et al: The quantity of natural surfactant necessary to prevent the respiratory distress syndrome in premature lambs. *Pediatr Res* **14**:1082–1085, 1980.

29. Metcalf IL, Burgoyne R, Enhorning G: Surfactant supplementation in the preterm rabbit: Effects of applied volume on compliance and survival. *Pediatr Res* **16**:834–839, 1982.

30. Vidyasagar D, Maeta H, Raju TNK, et al: Bovine surfactant (surfactant TA) therapy in immature baboons with hyaline membrane disease. *Pediatrics* **75**:1132–1142, 1985.

31. Raju TNK, Vidyasagar D, Bhat R, et al: Double blind controlled trial of single dose treatment with bovine surfactant in severe hyaline membrane disease. *Lancet* **1**(8534):651–655, 1987.

32. Walther FJ, Blanco CE, Houdijik M, et al: Single versus repetitive doses of natural surfactant for treatment of respiratory distress syndrome in premature lambs. *Pediatr Res* **19**:224–227, 1985.

33. Jobe A, Ikegami M, Glatz T, et al: Duration and characteristics of treatment of premature lambs with natural surfactant. *J Clin Invest* **67**:320–325, 1981.

34. Jacobs H, Jobe A, Ikegami M, et al: Premature lambs rescued from respiratory failure with natural surfactant: Clinical and biophysical correlates. *Pediatr Res* **16**:424–429, 1982.

35. Enhorning G, Hill D, Sherwood G, et al: Improved ventilation of prematurely delivered primates following tracheal deposition of surfactant. *Am J Obstet Gynecol* **132**:529–536, 1978.

36. Cutz E, Enhorning G, Robertson B, et al: Hyaline membrane disease: Effect of surfactant prophylaxis on lung morphology in premature primates. *Am J Pathol* **92**:581–594, 1978.

37. Maeta H, Vidyasagar D, Raju T, et al: Comparison of early and late surfactant treatments in baboon HMD model. *Pediatrics* **81**:277–283, 1988.

38. Maeta H, Vidyasagar D, Raju T, et al: Pathologic finding in surfactant treated and control animals after prolonged ventilation. *Pediatr Res* **20**:435A, 1986.

39. Morley CJ, Miller N, Bangham AD: Dry artificial lung surfactant and its effect on very premature babies. *Lancet* **1**:64–68, 1981.

40. Kwong MS, Egan EA, Notter RH, et al: Double blind clinical trial of calf lung surfactant extract for prevention of hyaline membrane disease in extremely premature infants. *Pediatrics* **76**:585–592, 1985.

41. Milner AD, Vyas H, Hopkin IE: Effect of exogenous surfactant on total respiratory system compliance. *Arch Dis Child* **59**:369–371, 1984.

42. Wilkinson A, Jenkins PA, Jeffrey JA: Two controlled trials of dry artificial surfactant: Early effects and later outcome in babies with surfactant deficiency. *Lancet* **2**:287–291, 1985.

43. Halliday HL, Reid M, Meban C, et al: Controlled trial of artificial surfactant to prevent respiratory distress syndrome. *Lancet,* March 3: 476–478, 1984.

44. Morley CJ: Ten-centre trial of artificial surfactant (artificial lung expanding compound) in very premature babies: Ten centre study group. *Br Med J* **294**:991–996, 1987.

45. Merritt TA, Hallman M, Bloom BT, et al: Prophylactic treatment of very premature infants with human surfactant. *N Eng J Med* **315**:785–790, 1986.

46. Enhorning G, Shennan A, Possmayer F, et al: Prevention of neonatal respiratory distress syndrome by tracheal instillation of surfactant: A randomized clinical trial. *Pediatrics* **76**:145–153, 1985.

47. Shapiro DL, Notter RH, Morin FC, et al: Double blind randomized trial of calf lung surfactant extract administered at birth to very premature infants for prevention of respiratory distress syndrome. *Pediatrics* **76**:593–599, 1985.

48. Milner AD, Vyas H, Hopkin IE: Effects of artificial surfactant on lung function and blood gases in idiopathic respiratory distress syndrome. *Arch Dis Child* **58**:458–460, 1983.

49. Hallman M, Merritt TA, Schneider H, et al: Isolation of human surfactant from amniotic fluid and a pilot study of its efficacy in respiratory distress syndrome. *Pediatrics* **71**:473–482, 1983.

50. Hallman M, Merritt TA, Jarvenpaa AL, et al: Exogenous human surfactant for treatment of severe respiratory distress syndrome: A randomized prospective clinical trial. *J Pediatr* **106**:963–969, 1985.

51. Fujiwara T, Konishi M, Nanbu H, et al: Surfactant replacement therapy in neonatal respiratory distress syndrome: A collaborative randomized controlled trial. *Jap J Pediatr* **40**:549–568, 1987.

52. Fujiwara T, Konishi M, Chida S, et al: Exogenous surfactant therapy in infants with RDS: Comparison of early versus late treatment. *Pediatr Res* **18**:353A, 1984.

53. Gitlin JD, Sell RF, Parad RB, et al: Randomized controlled trial of exogenous surfactant for treatment of hyaline membrane disease. *Pediatrics* **97**:31–37, 1987.

16
Perinatal Factors and Intraventricular/Subependymal Hemorrhage in the Very-Low-Birth-Weight Infant

ARTHUR A. STRAUSS

Background

INCIDENCE

Intraventricular/subependymal hemorrhage (IVH/SEH) in the very-low-birth-weight (VLBW, ≤ 1,500 g) infant is a both common and potentially devastating event. Bleeding occurs in approximately 40% of VLBW infants, with major hemorrhaging occurring in up to half of these infants [1,2]. Bleeding usually occurs in the first 3 days after birth. Major hemorrhages have been associated with abnormal neurologic outcome in at least 50% of affected infants [2–5].

GRADING

The grading system described by Papile et al [5] has been most frequently used as a means of uniform communication among researchers. A more descriptive approach has been advocated by some authors [3,6]. Minor hemorrhages consist of isolated subependymal/choroid plexus bleeding (grade 1 IVH/SEH) or of intraventricular hemorrhage without ventricular dilatation (grade 2 IVH/SEH). Major hemorrhages involve ventricular dilatation (grade 3 IVH/SEH) or intraparenchymal bleeding (grade 4 IVH/SEH). Parenchymal bleeding has been observed without an intraventricular component. The presence of periventricular leukomalacia (increased non-vascular density or cystic changes in the periventricular area) should also be noted [6,7].

PATHOGENESIS

Anatomic and physiologic developmental characteristics of the germinal matrix and choroid plexus areas of the preterm infant's brain are said to make this group of newborn infants vulnerable to a variety of perinatal events [2,4,8]. These characteristics include persistence of the germinal matrix area, relative hyperemia of the periventricular area versus the cerebral cortex, periventricular capillary tenuosity, and impairment of vascular autoregulation [8]. Hypoxic-related effects (increase in cerebral blood flow, further impairment of vascular autoregulation, increase in venous pressure, and endothelial injury) that directly or indirectly involve the immature central nervous system make this region prone to capillary rupture with subsequent injury [2,8]. Adverse perinatal events stated to be related to IVH/SEH include perinatal asphyxia, labor and its duration, mode and presentation of delivery, immediate neonatal management, and subsequent neonatal complications [9,10].

Perinatal Factors

FETAL DISTRESS

Current literature regarding IVH/SEH is divided over whether the predominant factors in the pathogenesis of this lesion are intrapartum or postnatal in origin [9–12]. One group has postulated that prepartum events may be related to subsequent IVH/SEH in some infants as well [13].

The immature fetus is at a disadvantage in the face of fetal compromise related to either uteroplacental insufficiency or umbilical cord compression. Abnormal fetal heart rate (FHR) patterns in the immature fetus have the following characteristics:

1. They progress more rapidly to severe heart rate abnormalities than do those in the term infant.
2. Late decelerations are associated with a higher incidence of neonatal depression and metabolic acidosis compared with the term fetus.
3. Abnormal patterns and acidosis are correlated with adverse neonatal outcomes [14–17].

Few studies have addressed the specific role of fetal distress objectively measured with either physiologic or biochemical means in relation to IVH/SEH. Ominous FHR patterns (late or moderate-to-severe variable decelerations, decreased heart rate variability) have been related to both direct (ultrasound documentation of major IVH/SEH [18]) and indirect (elevated brain-specific creatinine kinase, metabolic acidosis, adverse neurologic outcome) evidence of IVH/SEH by some authors [17,19,20]. Preliminary data suggesting that the presence of ominous FHR patterns correlate with a high incidence of IVH/SEH, extent of bleeding, and mortality rate could not be confirmed by more recent studies, including additional observations in our center (unpublished data) [13,21]. The low incidence of severe IVH/SEH in these latter studies may have been responsible for the inability of FHR pattern analysis to serve a predictive function, as was hypothesized earlier [18]. Alternatively, the poor correlation of abnormal FHR patterns and neonatal death may be related to expeditious delivery in those cases with ominous periodic FHR or decreased baseline variability [15]. The same explanation may be made for severe IVH/SEH.

OTHER OBSTETRIC FACTORS

While various authors have related presence and duration of labor, mode and presentation of delivery, and pregnancy complications (toxemia, bleeding, amnionitis) to IVH/SEH, such studies have suffered from retrospective data collection or small numbers of patients [9,10]. Brain-specific creatine kinase elevations have not been related to either mode of delivery or presence of labor in the limited investigations reported to date [20,22,23]. At this time, there are no convincing data that identifiable obstetric factors, independently of fetal distress/acidosis and premature delivery, contribute to IVH/SEH in VLBW infants [12,13,18,21,23].

Neonatal Factors

Neonatal factors reported to be associated with neonatal intracranial hemorrhage (other than birth weight less than 1,800 g and gestational age less than 34 weeks) have included hyaline membrane disease, hypercerbia, hypoxia, hypotension/hypertension, assisted ventilation, air leaks (pneumothorax, pulmonary interstitial emphysema), use of muscle relaxants or sodium bicarbonate, volume expansion, coagulopathy, and mode of closure of patent ductus arteriosus [2,8,15,18]. Neonatal complications related to prematurity and its management have been felt to be of primary importance in the evolution of IVH/SEH by some authors [12]. More research is needed to identify those postnatal events (or combination of events) that contribute to IVH/SEH.

Possibilities for Prevention

The extent, rather than the incidence, of intracranial hemorrhage is of critical importance with respect to the neurobehavioral development of surviving VLBW infants [2–5]. Intraparenchymal hemorrhages, in particular, have been found to be associated with profound alteration of cerebral blood flow [24]. Conversely, in the absence of major central nervous system hemorrhage, the majority of VLBW infants appear to have a relatively good prognosis [5]. The condition of the infant at birth, that is, asphyxiated, acidotic, depressed, and requiring assisted ventilation beyond immediate delivery room resuscitation, may be a more significant factor in determining the degree of IVH/SEH when it occurs in the early postpartum period than a variety of obstetric variables [18]. Avoidance of these conditions, if possible, may result in a minimal incidence of severe IVH/SEH. Not surprisingly, use of surfactant to modify respiratory distress syndrome has not been shown to decrease the risk or severity of IVH/SEH [25]. Attempts at prevention of fluctuations in blood pressure and air leaks, selective use of sedation and/or paralysis in the infant exhibiting asynchronous respirations during assisted ventilation [26], and gentle resuscitation technique (early intubation, avoidance of routine volume expansion, and use of hyperosmolar agents) may decrease the incidence of IVH/SEH in the sicker infants [18]. Attempts at prophylaxis via pharmacologic means (i.e., phenobarbital), have yielded mixed results, with potentially severe complications [27–29]. Maternal transport and delivery of the VLBW infant in a perinatal center may contribute to a decreased incidence of IVH/SEH compared with transported infants [18]. The ultimate prevention of IVH/SEH, obviously, would be to identify preventable factors that lead to premature delivery and to make an educational and economic commitment to this problem.

Conclusion

Despite suggestions that perinatal events may be of paramount importance with regard to IVH/SEH in the VLBW infant, there are no consistent data that reveal what markers could serve as reliable predictive indicators of potential risk for major IVH/SEH (i.e., fetal distress, creatine phosphokinase isoenzyme, acid-base balance) other than premature delivery associated with respiratory distress. Delivery in a perinatal center with modern neonatal intensive care techniques may keep the incidence of severe IVH/SEH at a minimum, thereby optimizing neurologic outcome for these at-risk infants. The issue of ischemic lesions independent of IVH/SEH, which may not be preventable or identifiable shortly after birth and which have similar effects to major IVH/SEH, is an area of active research at the present time.

REFERENCES

1. Papile L, Burstein J, Burstein R, et al: Incidence and evolution of subependymal and intraventricular hemorrhage: A study of infants with birth weights less than 1,500 grams. *J Pediatr* **92**:529–534, 1978.
2. Volpe JJ: Neonatal intraventricular hemorrhage. *N Engl J Med* **304**:886–891, 1981.
3. Palmer P, Dubowitz LM, Levene MI, et al: Developmental and neurological progress of preterm infants with intraventricular hemorrhage and ventricular dilatation. *Arch Dis Child* **57**:748–753, 1982.
4. Shinner S, Molteni RA, Gammon K, et al: Intraventricular hemorrhage in the premature infant. *N Engl J Med* **306**:1464–1468, 1982.

5. Papile L, Munsick-Brown G, Schaefer A: Relationship of cerebral intraventricular hemorrhage and early childhood neurologic handicaps. *J Pediatr* **103**:273–277, 1983.
6. DeVries LS, Dubowitz V, Long S, et al: Predictive value of cranial ultrasound in the newborn baby: A reappraisal. *Lancet* **2**:137–140, 1985.
7. Levene MI, Wigglesworth JS, Dubowitz V: Hemorrhagic periventricular leukomalacia in the neonate: A real-time ultrasound study. *Pediatrics* **71**:794–797, 1983.
8. Volpe JJ: *Neurology of the Newborn.* Philadelphia: WB Saunders, 1981, pp. 262–298.
9. Horbar JD, Pasnick M, McAuliffe, et al: Obstetric events and risk of periventricular hemorrhage in preterm neonates. *Arch Dis Child* **137**:678–681, 1983.
10. Worthington D, Davis LE, Grausz JP, et al: Factors influencing survival and morbidity with very low birth weight delivery. *Obstet Gynecol* **62**:550–555, 1983.
11. Levene MI, Fawer C, Lamont RF: Risk factors in the development of intraventricular hemorrhage in the preterm neonate. *Arch Dis Child* **57**:410–417, 1982.
12. Rayburn WF, Donn SM, Kolin MG, et al: Obstetric care and intraventricular hemorrhage in the low birth weight infant. *Obstet Gynecol* **62**:408–413, 1983.
13. Hameed C, Tejani N, Tuck S, et al: Correlation of fetal heart rate monitoring and acid-base status with periventricular/intraventricular hemorrhage in the low birthweight neonate. *Am J Perinatol* **3**:24–27, 1986.
14. Martin CB Jr, Siassi B, Hon BH: Fetal heart rate patterns and neonatal death in low birth weight infants. *Obstet Gynecol* **44**:503–510, 1974.
15. Bowes WA, Gabbe SG, Bowes C: Fetal heart rate monitoring in premature infants weighing 1500 g or less. *Am J Obstet Gynecol* **137**:791–796, 1980.
16. Zanini B, Paul RH, Huey JR: Intrapartum fetal heart rate: Correlation with scalp pH in the preterm fetus. *Am J Obstet Gynecol* **136**:43–47, 1980.
17. Westgren M, Holmquist P, Svenningsen NW, et al: Intrapartum fetal monitoring in preterm deliveries: A prospective study. *Obstet Gynecol* **60**:99–106, 1982.
18. Strauss AA, Kirz D, Modanlou HD, et al: Perinatal events and intraventricular/subependymal hemorrhage in the very low-birth weight infant. *Am J Obstet Gynecol* **151**:1022–1027, 1985.
19. Westgren M, Holmquist P, Ingemarsson I, et al: Intrapartum fetal acidosis in preterm infants: Fetal monitoring and long-term morbidity. *Obstet Gynecol* **63**:355–359, 1984.
20. Feldman RC, Tabsh KM, Shields, WD: Correlation of ominous fetal heart rate patterns and brain-specific creatine kinase. *Obstet Gynecol* **65**:476–480, 1985.
21. Rayburn WF, Johnson MZ, Hoffman KL, et al: Intrapartum fetal heart rate patterns and neonatal intraventricular hemorrhage. *Am J Perinatol* **4**:98–101, 1987.
22. Shields WD, Feldman RC: Serum CK-BB isoenzyme in preterm infants with periventricular hemorrhage. *J Pediatr* **100**:464–468, 1982.
23. Speer ME, Ou C, Buffone GL, et al: Creatinine phosphokinase BB isoenzyme in very-low-birth-weight infants: Relationship with mortality and intraventricular hemorrhage. *J Pediatr* **103**:790–793, 1983.

24. Volpe JJ, Herscovitch P, Perlman JM, et al: Position emission tomography in the newborn: Extensive impairment of regional cerebral blood flow with intraventricular hemorrhage and hemorrhagic intracerebral involvement. *Pediatrics* **72**:589–601, 1983.
25. Hallman M, Merritt TA, Jarvenpaa A, et al: Exogenous human surfactant for treatment of severe respiratory distress syndrome: A randomized prospective clinical trial. *J Pediatr* **106**:963–969, 1985.
26. Perlman JM, Goodman S, Krosser KL, et al: Reduction in intraventricular hemorrhage by elimination of fluctuating cerebral blood-flow velocity in preterm infants with respiratory distress syndrome. *N Engl J Med* **312**:1353–1357, 1985.
27. Goldstein GW, Donn SM: Further observations on the use of phenobarbital to prevent neonatal intracranial hemorrhage. *Pediatrics* **70**:1014–1015, 1982.
28. Porter FL, Marshall RE, Moore J, et al: Effect of phenobarbital on motor activity and intraventricular hemorrhage in preterm infants with respiratory disease weighing less than 1,500 grams. *Am J Perinatol* **2**:63–66, 1985.
29. Kaufman RE: Therapeutic interventions to prevent intracerebral hemorrhage in preterm infants. *J Pediatr* **108**:323–325, 1986.

17
Delivery of an Infant with an Unanticipated Birth Defect

MARY F. HAIRE

The onset of pregnancy involves the couple in a reorganization of relationships, including a critical review of friends and relatives in an attempt to determine the possible effect a child will have on close relationships. Pregnancy and postpregnancies, therefore, are periods of destabilization [1]. Such destabilization is a recognized part of the growth process. However, for the couple delivering a child with a birth defect, especially if that birth defect was unanticipated, the postpregnancy period is one of special stress.

A couple's beliefs and expectations regarding childbearing are influenced by a number of factors, such as past experiences with children, cultural influences, and family expectations [2]. Americans, in particular, place a high importance on beauty, perfection, and success. These expectations are usually established long before the pregnancy and may be seriously tested by the delivery of a child with a birth defect. Many people see the child as a reflection of the parents' ability to reproduce and (eventually) to raise a child [3,4]. There is often an unconscious belief that reproduction is natural and therefore easy. Complications are not an acknowledged part of most people's fantasies regarding childbearing.

Additionally, fears during pregnancy may be unvoiced or unacknowledged [4,5]. These fears may be based on a general lack of knowledge. For instance, few couples know prior to pregnancy that the incidence of serious birth defects is as high as 2 to 4% in the general population. Thus they are often unprepared for even the possibility of a child who is not perfect. When a child is born with a birth defect, the stress of dealing with the complications related to that defect are added to the stress of attending to the needs of any newborn baby. We know that stress is necessary for continued growth; however, if the stressful event overwhelms the parents' coping skills, the disequilibrium may be prolonged or complete [3,6]. The individual's perception of stress depends on (1) past experience with handling stress, (2) past ability to adapt successfully to stress, (3) other stressors ongoing in the person's life, and (4) support available from family and professionals [5,7]. The birth of a child with a serious defect requires, in many instances, considerable alterations in life-style [8]. Such a child affects the time the parents have to spend with other children and the time they have to spend together alone. Having a child with a birth defect can often alter their social life drastically, since it is difficult to find sitters willing to care for such an infant. If it becomes necessary for the mother to stay home to care for the child, the financial status of the family may be further burdened.

Denial

Often, the initial response of parents to being told that their child has a major birth defect is shock [9]. They are unable to absorb detailed medical information. Facts need to be repeated several times before the parents can assimilate the information. Simple honest answers, given when the parents show readiness to hear the information, is the best approach during this first phase [3,10].

Denial is an attempt to maintain affective equilibrium [11]. Failure on the part of health professionals to recognize the parents' need for some degree of denial may precipitate or reinforce despair [3]. Parents need time to mobilize their defenses and coping behaviors. However, denial should not be allowed to continue for any long period of time.

Acceptance

Parents signal their readiness to move from denial to acceptance by asking questions or by expressing anger. Anger can provide a strong stimulus to combat despair. Our insistence, either overtly or covertly, on maintaining a positive mood therefore trivializes the parents' distress. Anger may be due to their recognition of the cost of care now and in the future, the burden that such care may place on their other children, and the necessary alterations in their life-style [8]. Therefore, anger is to be encouraged and attempts should be made to channel that anger into constructive activities. Cues that may indicate parents' inability to absorb information include restless body movements, unexpressive gestures, and questions unrelated to the conversation. Other evidence of maladaptive coping behaviors includes devotion of all energies and resources into caring for the one child to the exclusion of others, or conversely, rejection of the affected child totally and failure to develop any kind of positive relationship [4,11].

Treatment Issues

Treatment issues are often very difficult for both parents and health care professionals. In deciding on treatment versus nontreatment, professionals should remember that parents are the true risk takers [12]. They must ultimately bear the burden of choice of treatment or nontreatment. It is the parents who must speak for the involved child, other children in the family, and other family members. It is the parents who must live with the responses of family and friends to the choices made. Their need for adequate honest information at appropriate times and for professional support is considerable.

Frequently the outcome for a child with a serious birth defect is uncertain. That uncertainty adds to the parents' difficulties in adapting to their child's condition. Certainly the parents have concerns over the future appearance of the child and the child's level of functioning, areas that are sometimes difficult for us to determine or predict at the time of birth [8,13]. They have very legitimate concerns over the duration of illness, the number of hospitalizations that may be expected, and the helplessness of the child, all of which add to the sense of powerlessness for the parents and the professionals caring for the child [8,10,14].

Should separation from the infant be necessary at birth for medical reasons, parents should be reassured that normal attachment can still occur. Parental motivation and involvement in caretaking activities and decision making are of equal importance to early contact in the delivery room [10,15,16].

When the child's condition is so severe that termination of treatment is being considered, professionals should keep in mind that decisions to terminate treatment require (1) sufficient time for the parents to accurately observe and assess the baby's condition, (2) a mature assessment of available options, and (3) parental involvement in the decision, which may be influenced by publicity or other media coverage and by the knowledge of advances in neonatal technology.

Support by Professionals

When the birth defect is uncorrectable, parents must learn to deal with chronic sorrow [8]. Chronic sorrow may be defined as the persistence of grieving behaviors stimulated by constant reminders of the child's defect, and the ongoing effect of that condition on family life. Chronic sorrow is resolved only by the death of the child or the parents [3,8]. Manifestations of chronic sorrow should not be interpreted as either helplessness or inability to function, or as lack of joy about the child [15].

There are many ways in which professional staff can work with parents to help them adapt to the child who has a serious birth defect. Acceptance of the parents' initial grieving behaviors allows them to express the intense emotions stimulated by the birth of the baby. Such acceptance sets up trust in the relationship, which can further promote the professional's ability to assist the parents [3,4]. Positive regard of the parents and their responses recognizes their worth as people and as parents at a time when their self-esteem may be very low. We can further promote positive self-esteem by teaching the parents how to care for their child, helping them to anticipate problems, and making referrals to community agencies, most especially to parent support groups [3,4,16,17]. With such interventions there is every reason to believe that parents can learn to appreciate the specialness of this child [6].

REFERENCES

1. O'Connell ML: Locus of control specific to pregnancy. *J Obstet Gynecol Nurs* **12:**161–164, 1983.
2. Harris R, Dombro M, Ryan C: Therapeutic uses of human figure drawings by the pregnant couple. *J Obstet Gynecol Nurs* **9:**232–237, 1980.
3. Floyd CC: A defective child is born. *J Obstet Gynecol Nurs* **6:**56–62, 1977.
4. Opirhory GJ: Counseling the parents of a critically ill newborn. *J Obstet Gynecol Nurs* **8:**179–182, 1979.
5. Cassidy JE: A nurse looks at childbirth anxiety. *J Obstet Gynecol Nurs* **3:**52–54, 1974.
6. Burden RL: Measuring the effects of stress on the mothers of handicapped infants: Must depression often follow? *Child Health Care Develop* **6:**111–125, 1980.
7. White M, Ritchie J: Psychological stressors in antepartum hospitalization: Reports from pregnant women. *Mat Child Nurs J* **13:**47–56, 1984.
8. McCleary CS: Needed: Earlier psychological support for "special-needs" parents. *J Calif Perinat Assoc* **3:**36–38, 1984.
9. Veach SA: Down's syndrome: Helping the special parents of a special infant. *Nursing 83,* September: 42, 1983.
10. Harkins-Walsh E: Dimensions of anxiety in parents of sick newborns. MCN: The American Journal of Maternal Child Nursing **5:**30–34, 1980.
11. Scupholme A: Who helps? Coping with the unexpected outcomes of pregnancy. *J Obstet Gynecol Nurs* **7:**36–39, 1981.
12. Drane JF: The defective child. *J Obstet Gynecol Nurs* **13:**148–154, 1984.
13. Shenna AT, et al: Perinatal factors associated with death or handicap in very preterm infants. *Am J Obstet Gynecol* **151:**231–237, 1985.
14. Jackson PL: When the baby isn't perfect. *Am J Nurs* **85:**396–399, 1985.
15. Chitwood L: A lesson in living. *Nursing 84,* January: 55, 1985.
16. Schraeder BD: Attachment and parenting despite lengthy intensive care. MCN: The American Journal of Maternal Child Nursing **5:**37–41, 1980.
17. Blackburn S: Fostering behavioral development of high-risk infants. *J Obstet Gynecol Nurs* **12:**76–86, 1983.

ADDITIONAL READING

1. Chinn PL (Ed): Attachment, loss, and change. ANS, July, 1981 (entire issue).
2. Haylor MJ: Human response to loss. Nurse Pract, **12:**63–66, 1987.
3. Horner MM, Rawlins P, Giles K: How parents of children with chronic con-

ditions perceive their own needs. MCN: The American Journal of Maternal Child Nursing **12:**40–43, 1987.

4. Humenick SS, Bugen LA: Parenting roles: Expectation versus reality. MCN: The American Journal of Maternal Child Nursing **12:**36–39, 1987.
5. Penticuff JF: Psychological implications in high-risk pregnancy. *Nurs Clin No Am* **17:**69–78, 1982.

18
Hemodynamically Significant Patent Ductus Arteriosus in Low-Birth-Weight Infants: Fact or Fiction?

CHARLES R. ROSENFELD

Both the ductus arteriosus and foramen ovale provide a means whereby blood flow in the fetus is diverted away from the high-resistance pulmonary vascular bed to the much lower resistance systemic circulation. At birth or soon thereafter the pulmonary vascular bed experiences a substantial degree of vasodilation and lowering of vascular resistance by mechanisms presently unknown, whereas systemic vascular resistance increases. The former occurs in order to permit the dramatic rise in pulmonary artery blood flow that is necessary for initiation of lung function and thus the exchange of respiratory gases, to replace the function of the placenta. In concert with these changes in lung function and pulmonary blood flow is the anatomic closure of the foramen ovale and the functional closure of the ductus arteriosus. However, in contrast to the foramen ovale, the ductus arteriosus generally remains patent for some time after birth. Whereas this patency is of little consequence to the well term infant [1], it may result in substantial problems in the preterm infant due to the magnitude of the left-to-right shunt that may occur. This chapter discusses the patent ductus arteriosus (PDA) in the preterm infant, pointing out present-day problems in our understanding of its role in neonatal illness and thus in the care and treatment of the preterm infant, in particular the infant of less than 1,500 g birth weight.

In early studies of the preterm infant with hyaline membrane disease (HMD), it was observed that neonatal death occurred more frequently in those infants without spontaneous closure of the PDA than in infants without evidence of a PDA, 71 versus 19%, respectively [2]. Moreover, when the PDA was surgically closed, death did not occur in infants without hyaline membrane disease (HMD), but did so in 60% of infants with a diagnosis of HMD. Thus, it appeared that the simultaneous occurrence of HMD and PDA substantially increased the risk for neonatal death. As survival of the low-birth-weight (LBW) infant (<1,500 g) rose in the early and mid-1970s, PDA was observed to be an increasingly common problem. For example, Siassi et al [3] reported that the incidence of PDA increased with decreasing gestational age and birth weight, occurring in 50% or more of infants under 32 weeks' gestational age and weighing 1,500 g or less at birth. In fact, it was observed to occur in 77% of infants from 28 to 30 weeks of gestation and 83% of those under 1,000 g birth weight. The number of infants evaluated, however, was quite small, 13 and 6, respectively.

When these investigators compared the incidence of HMD and that of PDA at the same gestational ages, the values were very similar, suggesting a close association between the two and the possibility that the presence of one might in fact affect the course and/or occurrence of the other. This of course is supportive of the observations by Edmonds et al [2]. In subsequent studies, Cotton and co-workers [4] reported similar relationships in a much larger population of infants less than 1,500 g birth weight ($n = 100$), that is, a hemodynamically significant PDA (sPDA) occurred in 69% of infants with HMD compared with 32% in infants without HMD, and the incidence of sPDA increased with decreasing birth weight, reaching 69% in infants weighing less than 1,000 g. Furthermore, they reported a higher mortality among infants with evidence of a sPDA, as well as a longer need for ventilatory support. Finally, Cotton et al [4] also noted that sPDA was generally evident within the first week after birth.

Similar observations have been reported by others [5]. Thus, sPDA might contribute not only to the mortality among LBW preterm infants, but also to their morbidity, especially in the presence of HMD.

In view of their own observations and those reported by others, Cotton and co-workers [6] sought to determine the effect of early aggressive medical management (i.e., fluid restriction, diuresis, etc., over 72 hours) plus surgical ligation on the outcome of LBW infants with sPDA. For their outcome variables they chose to examine the duration of intubation (i.e., the need for ventilatory support), the time in days to reach a reasonable oral caloric intake (80 cal/kg·day), mortality, and the cost of hospitalization. The incidence of sPDA was greater than 50% in their study population, which consisted of both inborn and transferred or outborn infants. Although there was no difference in the mortality between infants receiving medical therapy alone and those receiving medical plus surgical therapy, infants included in the latter group were observed to have the following characteristics: (1) They required a shorter duration of ventilatory support, (2) they reached an oral intake of 80 cal/kg·day sooner (13 ± 3 vs. 24 ± 4 days), and (3) their total cost of hospitalization was lower. Thus, they concluded from these findings that aggressive medical management, which included fluid restriction and diuretic therapy, should be used no more than 48 to 72 hours, and in the absence of significant improvement, as determined clinically, radiographically, or by echocardiogram, surgical ligation should be considered.

Since a potential advantage to early aggressive management of the sPDA was demonstrated in the above and other studies [6,7], the utility of early, prophylactic closure of the PDA prior to significant shunting was raised by a number of investigators. However, to design a study that would minimize the risks of early closure, either surgical or pharmacologic, and restrict the population studied, it would be necessary to predict with some accuracy which LBW infants are at highest risk of developing a sPDA. Therefore, Cotton et al [8] next sought to determine the characteristics of the LBW infants in their special care nursery who were at-risk for developing sPDA and to establish a discriminate function that would permit them to identify and include such neonates for subsequent therapeutic trials. One-hundred infants were studied, consisting again of both inborn and outborn neonates; the incidence of sPDA was 50% and the onset was at less than 7 days of age. Through the use of univariant analysis, five characteristics were identified that separated infants with and without sPDA: birth weight, presence or absence of HMD, presence or absence of intrauterine growth retardation, the use of continuous positive airway pressure (CPAP) or intermittent positive pressure breathing (IPPB), and the presence or absence of an acute perinatal "stress" (e.g., low Apgar score, hypovolemia, hypotension, etc). Infants with a sPDA were found to be smaller (1,078 vs. 1,215 g) but appropriate for gestational age, and more likely to have HMD (50% vs. 23%), require ventilatory support (86% vs. 45%), and have a history of perinatal "stress" (91% vs. 63%). Using these factors, a discriminant model was constructed that correctly predicted outcome in 80 of 100 (80%) infants—35 of 44 (80%) with subsequent sPDA and 45 of 56 (80%) without sPDA. When prospectively applied 1 year later to a similar population of neonates admitted to the institution, with a 51% (48/94) incidence of sPDA, 80% were correctly predicted— 44 of 48 (92%) with sPDA and 31 of 46 (67%) without sPDA. There was, however, no note in this report of the fluid therapy used, the extent of volume expansion in the first 24 hours after birth, or any differences that might have existed between the inborn and outborn infants, factors that potentially might have influenced the occurrence of sPDA. Nevertheless, it appeared that a tool was now available to facilitate the design of subsequent clinical studies related to the management of sPDA.

Because of the relatively high incidence (~50%) and early onset (<5– 6 days of life) of sPDA reported by the above investigators and those in numerous other institutions [1–5], and because of what seemed to be a rather infrequent occurrence and late onset of sPDA among infants in the Special Care Nursery at Parkland Memorial Hospital, Dallas, which is essentially a totally inborn population, we reviewed the charts of all infants of 1,500 g or less birth weight who survived more than 72 hours and were delivered over a 12-month period (June, 1978, through May, 1979). With the criteria of Cotton et al [6], only 5 of 81 infants (6.2%) had documentation in their chart of having a sPDA; furthermore, the mean age of onset was 20 (±9) days rather than 5 to 6 days of life. Twenty-eight other infants (35%) had evidence of a clinically evident PDA murmur, but were not considered to be symptomatic (i.e., the PDA was not hemodynamically significant); the age of onset in this group also was late, 14 days. In view of these obvious differences in the incidence (ours being actual incidence among all infants delivered in a single institution rather than among infants admitted to intensive care) and the age of onset, we designed a descriptive study similar to that of Cotton et al [6], utilizing their criteria for the diagnosis of sPDA (Table 18.1), in order to permit a reasonable comparison between the two populations. We also sought to determine the prognostic value of the M-mode echocardiogram obtained at 7 to 11 days of age, since sPDA did not occur until day 14 or thereafter. Furthermore, since fluid therapy had been reported to have a substantial effect on the occurrence of sPDA [9,10], we sought to determine the role of volume expansion in the first 24 hours after birth and of routine fluid therapy in the first day and week of life. Finally, we examined the role of birth weight, gestational age, Apgar score, acute perinatal "stresses," HMD, hypocalcemia (<7.5 mg%), and prolonged rupture of membranes (>24 hours) in the occurrence of sPDA.

Over an 11-month period, 120 consecutively born infants of 1,500 g or less birth weight and who had survived 72 hours or more were admitted to the study [11], the minimum number necessary to obtain statistical differences between infants with and without a sPDA if the incidence was 12 to 15%. Of the total group enrolled in the study, 19 (16%) developed a sPDA (Fig. 18.1) and 25 others (21%) had evidence of a PDA murmur but were not symptomatic. As illustrated in the figure, the incidence of sPDA was 12% for infants of 1,500 to 1,000 g and 26% for infants less than 1,000 g birth weight. The mean age of onset of sPDA was 15 (±3) days, with only four infants (21%) demonstrating a sPDA before 7 days of age. With univariant analysis, six perinatal factors were found to be either significantly different ($p <.05$) or of borderline significance ($.05< p <.1$) between infants with and without sPDA; they are listed in Table 18.2. Most of these items were consistent with observations in previous

TABLE 18.1. Criteria for the diagnosis of symptomatic or hemodynamically significant patent ductus arteriosus.

Clinical evidence of left-to-right shunt (four or more present)
Resting heart rate >150 bpm
Hyperdynamic precordium
Bounding pulses
Characteristic murmur
Cardiomegaly by chest x-ray
Shunt by echocardiogram (e.g., LA:AO, LV)
Clinical evidence of congestive heart failure (two or more present)
Gallop rhythm
Pulmonary edema
Hepatomegaly
Apnea and bradycardia
Hypercapnea (P_{CO_2} >50 mm Hg)

LA, left atrium; AO, aortic root; LV, left ventricle.

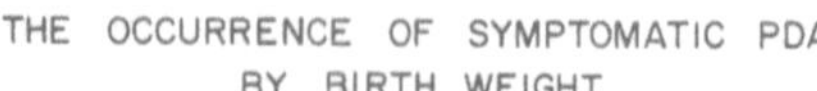

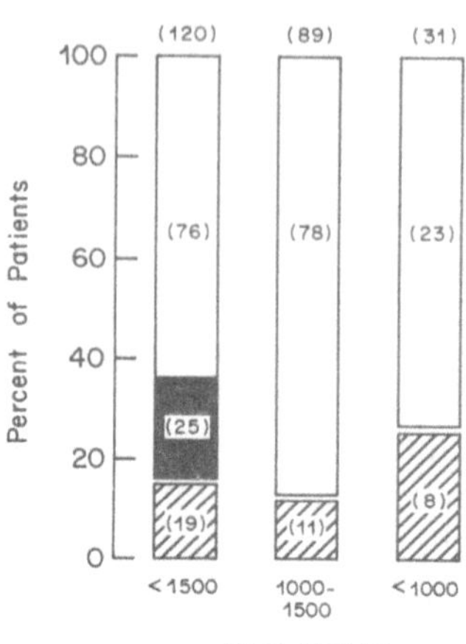

FIGURE 18.1. Incidence and distribution of symptomatic and asymptomatic patent ductus arteriosus in inborn infants of 1,500 g or less birth weight. Values in parentheses represent number of infants. From Furzan et al [11], used with permission.

reports. Of note, however, is the "new" observation that the use of volume expansion in the first 24 hours after life was a significant factor, occurring more than twice as often in infants with sPDA, whereas fluid therapy in the first 2 weeks was not important as an individual factor, increasing from 85 ml/kg·day on day 1 of life to 130 ml/kg·day on day 7 and to greater than 150 ml/kg·day by day 14. There was no difference in either neonatal mortality or the occurrence of necrotizing enterocolitis and intracranial hemorrhage.

Rather than use only those factors obtained by univariant analysis to establish a working discriminant function useful for the prediction of sPDA,

TABLE 18.2. Factors differing in infants with and without hemodynamically significant patent ductus arteriosus (sPDA), as determined by univariant analysis.

Variable	With sPDA	Without sPDA	p
No. of infants	19	101	
Birth weight (g)	1,048±247 (685–1,495)	1,189±223 (590–1,500)	<.05
Gestational age (weeks)	29.4±2.2	31.2±2.2	<.05
Use of volume expanders	10 (53%)	22 (22%)	<.05
Hyaline membrane disease	9 (47%)	30 (30%)	<.05
Hypocalcemia	18 (95%)	77 (76%)	>.05, <.1
Use of CPAP	12 (63%)	37 (37%)	>.05, <.1

as is frequently done, we performed a stepwise multivariant discriminant analysis, utilizing all of the factors evaluated, thus permitting the evaluation of interacting variables. From this analysis, four factors when taken together provided the best predictor for the occurrence of sPDA: the obstetric estimate of gestational age in weeks, race, the use of volume expanders, and fluid intake of more than 100 ml/kg·day in the first 24 hours after birth. With this model, the outcome in 95 of 120 infants (79%) was correctly predicted (similar to results of Cotton et al [8])—sPDA was correctly predicted in 15 of 19 infants (79%) and the absence of sPDA in 80 of 101 infants (79%). When Cotton's discrimination function was applied to our population of infants for reasons of comparison, 73% of all infants were correctly classified, 68% with sPDA and 73% without sPDA. However, in contrast to the experience of Cotton et al [8], when our model was applied to a similar population of infants delivered in our institution 1 year later, its ability to correctly predict sPDA was quite poor, reflecting the dramatic decrease in the use of volume expanders in our institution, from 27% of infants (32 of 120) to nearly zero, and the general use of 60 to 70 ml/kg·day of fluid therapy in the first day of life. This of course is reflective of our indications for the administration of volume expanders: delayed capillary filling (>3.0 s) and hypotension reflected by a systolic blood pressure of more than one standard deviation below the mean for age and weight as reported by Bucci et al [12]. Nevertheless, the mean age of onset and incidence of sPDA remained 2 weeks and 15%, respectively.

To the best of our knowledge, no other group of investigators has carefully examined the role of volume expansion in the occurrence of sPDA in low-birth-weight infants, even though available experimental data are supportive of a pathogenic role via stimulation of vasodilating prostaglandins [13]. It is of interest that even though our fluid therapy in the first day and week of life was similar to that reported by Lorenz et al [14], their reported incidence of sPDA was nearly twice that reported by us and the age of onset was less than 7 days. However, upon careful inspection of their data, it was observed that nearly all of their infants received some form of therapy with volume expanders in the initial 24 hours of life, that is, their infants received a mean of 7 to 8 ml/kg of blood products and some received as much as 30 ml/kg [14]. When a subpopulation of these infants was studied with serial echocardiography, they observed a 65% incidence of hemodynamically significant PDA within the first week after birth that was not related to apparant fluid therapy during that time [15]. As noted above, however, they did not control for the use of volume expanders or take such use into account when they analyzed their data. Because of the low incidence of sPDA and virtual absence of the use of volume expansion in our institution, we are unable to study this problem further; however, a properly designed study seems indicated in an institution where this mode of fluid therapy is commonly employed.

244   Charles R. Rosenfeld

We were able to obtain echocardiograms on 85 of 120 study infants
between 7 and 11 days of age, when a sPDA was not apparant either
clinically or radiographically, to determine usefulness of echocardiography
in predicting the occurrence of sPDA [11]. Since four infants had a sPDA
prior to 7 days of age, they were not included in this analysis. Significant
differences were found in left atrial size, left atrium/aortic root ratio, and
the indices of the left ventricle and left atrium to birth weight (Table 18.3).
Therefore it appears that infants who subsequently develop a sPDA have
echocardiographic data different from data in asymptomatic infants prior
to the onset of sPDA. When infants with HMD who developed sPDA
were compared with those who did not, they had significantly higher values, but they were not different from infants without HMD who developed
sPDA. These data and those noted above are suggestive that sPDA and
HMD might not necessarily occur together and that other factors might
actually influence this relationship, for example, the use of volume expansion and/or excessive intravenous fluid therapy in the first day of life.

These observations raise important questions regarding the need for
prophylactic closure of the PDA in the first day of life in all low-birth-
weight infants [16] as well as the hypothesis suggested by Jacob et al [17]
that infants weighing less than 1,200 g at birth have both sPDA and HMD,
with sPDA playing the major role in the course of their pulmonary disease.
In fact, Mahony et al [18] recently have reported that 80% of low-birth-
weight sick infants will never demonstrate signs of a hemodynamically
significant PDA, and although prophylactic therapy may decrease the incidence of sPDA, it does not alter morbidity, for example, duration of
ventilatory support or oxygen therapy. It should be pointed out, however,
that this differs from the observations of Dudell and Gersony [19], who
reported that more than 60% of sick infants of less than 1,500 g birth
weight continued to have evidence of sPDA on day 3 of life, as evidenced
by a contrast echocardiogram, and that heart failure and the need for PDA

TABLE 18.3. Echocardiographic data in infants with and
without subsequent development of hemodynamically
significant patent ductus arteriosus (sPDA).*

Variable	With sPDA	Without sPDA
No. of infants	15	70
Age (days)	8.2 ± 1.0	8.7 ± 1.2
Left atrium (cm)	0.83 ± 0.21[†]	0.72 ± 0.14
Left atrium/aortic root ratio	1.42 ± 0.30[†]	1.17 ± 0.26
Left ventricle (mm)/birth weight (g)	13.67 ± 3.1 [†]	11.13 ± 2.0
Left atrium (mm)/birth weight (g)	8.26 ± 2.44[†]	6.13 ± 1.3

*Values are mean ± SD.
[†]p <.05
Source: Furzan et al [11], used with permission.

closure occurred in 97% and 75%, respectively. Thus, it appears that the substantial variation in the occurrence of sPDA between institutions [20] is not fully understood and might actually be reflective of differences in clinical management in the first 24 hours of life, such as the use of volume expanders. Until this is made more clear, a recommendation for early prophylactic closure of the PDA in low-birth-weight infants cannot be made.

REFERENCES

1. Gentile R, Stevenson G, Dooley T, et al: Pulsed doppler echocardiographic determination of time of ductal closure in normal newborn infants. *J Pediatr* **98**:443–448, 1981.
2. Edmonds LH, Gregory GA, Heymann MA, et al: Surgical closure of the ductus arteriosus in premature infants. *Circulation* **58**:856–863, 1973.
3. Siassi B, Blanco C, Cabal LA, et al: Incidence and clinical features of patent ductus arteriosus in low-birth-weight infants: A prospective analysis of 150 consecutively born infants. *Pediatrics* **57**:347–351, 1976.
4. Cotton RB, Stahlman MT, Kovar I, et al: Medical management of small preterm infants with symptomatic patent ductus arteriosus. *J Pediatr* **92**:467–473, 1978.
5. Kitterman JA, Edmunds LH, Gregory GA, et al: Patent ductus arteriosus in premature infants: Incidence, relation to pulmonary disease and management. *N Engl J Med* **287**:473–477, 1972.
6. Cotton RB, Stahlman MT, Bender HW, et al: Randomized trial of early closure of symptomatic patent ductus arteriosus in small preterm infants. *J Pediatr* **93**:647–651, 1978.
7. Naulty GM, Horn S, Conry J, et al: Improved lung compliance after ligation of patent ductus arteriosus in hyaline membrane disease. *J Pediatr* **93**:682–684, 1978.
8. Cotton RB, Lindstrom DP, Stahlman MT: Early prediction of symptomatic patent ductus arteriosus from perinatal risk factors: A discriminant analysis model. *Acta Pediatr Scand* **70**:723–727, 1981.
9. Stevenson JG: Fluid administration in the association of patent ductus arteriosus complicating respiratory distress syndrome. *J Pediatr* **90**:257–261, 1977.
10. Bell EF, Warburton D, Stonestreet BS, et al: Effect of fluid administration on the development of symptomatic patent ductus arteriosus and congestive failure in premature infants. *N Engl J Med* **302**:598–604, 1980.
11. Furzan JA, Reisch J, Tyson JE, et al: Incidence and risk factors for symptomatic patent ductus arteriosus among inborn very-low-birth-weight infants. *Early Hum Devel* **12**:39–48, 1985.
12. Bucci G, Scalamandre A, Savignoni PC, et al: The systemic systolic blood pressure of newborns with low weight: A multiple regression analysis. *Acta Pediatr Scand* (Suppl) **229**:1–26, 1972.
13. Arant BS Jr: Nonrenal factors influencing renal function during the perinatal period. *Clin Perinatol* **8**:255–240, 1981.
14. Lorenz JM, Kleinman LI, Kotagal UR, et al: Water balance in very low-birth-weight infants: Relationship to water and sodium intake and effect on outcome. *J Pediatr* **101**:423–432, 1982.

15. Reller MD, Lorenz JM, Kotagal UR, et al: Hemodynamically significant PDA: An echocardiographic and clinical assessment of incidence, natural history, and outcome in very low birth weight infants maintained in negative fluid balance. *Pediatr Cardiol* **6:**17–24, 1985.
16. Mahony L, Carnero V, Brett C, et al: Prophylactic indomethacin therapy for patent ductus arteriosus in very-low-birthweight infants. *N Engl J Med* **306:**506–510, 1982.
17. Jacob J, Gluck L, DiSessa T, et al: The contribution of PDA in the neonate with severe RDS. *J Pediatr* **96:**79–87, 1980.
18. Mahony L, Caldwell RL, Girod DA, et al: Indomethacin therapy on the first day of life in infants with very low birth weight. *J Pediatr* **106:**801–805, 1985.
19. Dudell GG, Gersony WM: Patent ductus arteriosus in neonates with severe respiratory disease. *J Pediatr* **104:**915–920, 1984.
20. Ellison RC, Peckham GJ, Lang P, et al: Evaluation of the preterm infant for patent ductus arteriosus. *Pediatrics* **71:**364–372, 1983.

19
An Update on Genetic Prenatal Diagnosis

AMY A. LEMKE

Each year approximately 3 to 5% of live born babies, 150,000 children in the United States alone, are born with congenital anomalies [1]. Some of these conditions have hereditary or genetic causes. Only during the past 20 years has prenatal diagnosis of genetic conditions moved from a research orientation to a major clinical service. With all of the new developments in the field of medical genetics, it has become increasingly vital that physicians and health care specialists who work with families at risk for genetic disease be aware of the advances in prenatal diagnosis that may be important to their patient care. Therefore, this chapter reviews current methods of genetic prenatal diagnosis, as well as techniques of maternal screening.

Prenatal Diagnostic Techniques

Most often, prenatal genetic testing is used to look for conditions that would result in significant disability, handicap, or premature death. Although prevention of genetic disease is one reason for testing, a decision to terminate a pregnancy involving a detected abnormality is not a prerequisite for prenatal diagnosis. For many couples at risk of having a child with a prenatally diagnosable condition, the option of monitoring pregnancies and the availability of elective abortion allow parents to undertake pregnancies that they would otherwise forego. According to Thompson and Thompson [2], only about 2% of pregnancies for which prenatal diagnosis is undertaken are terminated, due to a detected genetic abnormality. More commonly the fetus is unaffected and the pregnancy continues.

AMNIOCENTESIS

Mid-trimester amniocentesis is the most widely used method of prenatal detection of genetic conditions. This procedure is usually performed 16 to 18 weeks after the last menstrual period. Ultrasound is used to confirm gestational age and estimates the placental and fetus location, as well as detects multiple pregnancies, missed abortions, or gross malformations. A needle is then inserted into the lower abdomen and 20 to 30 ml of amniotic fluid is aspirated. The cells shed from the amnion or fetus in the collected amniotic fluid are cultured and analyzed for chromosome abnormalities or other diagnosable conditions. At present, 2 to 4 weeks are often needed for results of chromosome studies, and roughly 3 to 6 weeks for results of biochemical and DNA studies. Besides the parental anxiety experienced during the wait for results, maternal complications can include cramping, spotting, or leaking of amniotic fluid. The main risk of the procedure is loss of the pregnancy. In the United States, the rate of spontaneous abortion following amniocentesis is approximately 0.5% [3]. Other complications, though rare, include infection, Rh immunization, and dimpling marks on the fetus from the needle.

With respect to procedural complications, a repeat amniocentesis may have to be performed in a small number of cases because there is either not enough amniotic fluid or there is failure of cell growth. Most established laboratories have less than 1% culture failure rates.

Indications

Chromosome Abnormalities

The majority of amniocenteses are performed for cytogenetic studies. A common indication is advanced maternal age. At age 35 there is a 0.25% risk of having a liveborn with trisomy 21 and a 0.49% risk of having a liveborn with any chromosomal abnormality. By age 45, the risk for trisomy 21 rises to 3.33% and is 5.26% for any chromosome abnormality [4]. In the United States the general age for women to be offered amniocentesis has been 35 or older at delivery, although this age requirement varies. A paternal age effect may also be a consideration when offering prenatal diagnosis.

Other couples offered amniocentesis are those who have had a previous live-born child or miscarriage with a chromosome abnormality. The most common chromosome abnormality in newborns is trisomy 21, or Down syndrome. It represents roughly one half of the abnormal chromosome results from amniocentesis. Once a couple has had a child with a numeric chromosomal abnormality such as Down syndrome, the risk of chromosomal abnormality in future pregnancies rises to approximately 1%. In cases where a normal parent is a known carrier of a balanced translocation or other chromosome rearrangement, the risk for having a child with a chromosomal abnormality or having a miscarriage may be much higher. It is important that chromosome studies be performed on all infants clinically suspected of having a chromosomal abnormality. The results can help predict the risk of the parents having another affected pregnancy.

Fetal sexing through karyotyping is important for X-linked diseases when there is not a more specific means of diagnosis. An example of such a case is Duchennes muscular dystrophy in families non-informative for DNA studies. With X-linked inheritance, a carrier female has a 50% chance of having affected sons and a 50% chance of having carrier daughters. Knowing that the fetus is female provides reassurance to the parents, because virtually all affected individuals are males. If the fetus is male, there is a 50% chance that the fetus will have the condition.

The fragile X syndrome, another probable X-linked condition, is estimated to be the second most common genetic cause of mental retardation in males, after Down syndrome. This condition can potentially be diagnosed prenatally by culturing amniotic fluid cells in a medium deficient in folic acid. Affected males show a portion of cells with the X chromosome having a fragile site near the end of the long arm (Xq27). Since fragile X syndrome appears to follow X-linked inheritance, women who are at risk to have a child with the fragile X syndrome can be offered prenatal testing for chromosome analysis. In some of these cases, fetal blood analysis may provide a more accurate prediction of fragile X.

Occasionally the cytogenetic findings from amniocentesis cannot be readily explained. In such cases, it may be helpful for the parents to have their chromosomes analyzed to rule out a normal familial variation.

Neural Tube Defects

Some of the most common congenital central nervous system abnormalities are neural tube defects, including spina bifida and anencephaly. In the United States Caucasian population, approximately 1 to 2 in 1,000 liveborn infants have such anomalies. Neural tube defects appear to be inherited in a multifactorial manner, and the recurrence risk after having one affected child is 2 to 4%. Couples who have had a child with a neural tube defect, and their siblings, are potential candidates for prenatal testing.

Prenatal diagnosis of open neural tube defects is possible by measurement of amniotic fluid alpha-fetoprotein. This protein is found in fetal serum and is normally excreted in fetal urine in small amounts into the amniotic fluid. When there is an open neural tube defect, alpha-fetoprotein leaks through the membrane covering the defect into the amniotic fluid, and a high alpha-fetoprotein concentration can be found. Elevated levels of amniotic fluid alpha-fetoprotein are detected in approximately 95% of cases of open neural tube defects. Increased amniotic fluid alpha-fetoprotein levels can also be caused by factors other than neural tube defects, including the presence of gastroschisis, omphalocele, cystic hygroma, and nephrosis. Measurement of acetylcholinesterase may provide additional confirmation for the presence of a fetal defect and also may reduce the incidence of false positive results based on increased amniotic fluid alpha-fetoprotein alone.

Limitations of testing for neural tube defects include the fact that closed or very small defects may not produce elevated alpha-fetoprotein levels and so escape detection. Also there is the problem of false-positive results and the unnecessary anxiety this causes the parents.

Inborn Errors of Metabolism

Human biochemical disorders, often called inborn errors of metabolism, are conditions in which a specific genetically determined enzyme defect produces a metabolic block that has pathologic consequences. Most inborn errors of metabolism follow autosomal recessive inheritance, and a few are X-linked recessive. These metabolic diseases usually result in currently untreatable, often progressively debilitating, conditions. In diseases where the responsible enzymes are expressed in amniotic fluid cells, prenatal diagnosis from measurement of the enzyme activity is possible. Testing is not usually of the actual defective gene, but of its gene product. There are many genetic metabolic disorders amenable to this type of prenatal testing including disorders of carbohydrate metabolism—galactosemia, lysosomal storage diseases—Tay Sachs disease, organic acidemias and urea cycle defects.

DNA Abnormalities

Techniques have recently become available to allow testing for the gene itself rather than the gene product. These methods have been developed to quantitate the number of genes in a cell, as in alpha-thalassemia. Messenger RNA for the alpha-globin chain is first isolated and radiolabeled DNA is synthesized to be used as a probe. DNA from the cell to be tested is denatured to single strand. The probe will hybridize to the alpha-globin genes in the single-stranded DNA and the new double-stranded DNA segments can be measured for radioactivity level. The amount of radioactivity corresponds to the number of alpha genes present. No hybridization is seen in homozygous alpha-thalassemia (all four genes absent), because the sequences are absent. Heterozygotes (carriers, one to three genes absent) show that 25 to 75% of the usual amount of DNA hybridizes.

Another technique to recognize DNA abnormalities is the use of restriction endonucleases. These enzymes are isolated from bacteria that use them to "digest" foreign DNA. These bacterial enzymes are used to recognize and cut DNA at specific nucleotide sequences. Sickle cell anemia and some beta-thalassemias have been demonstrated to be due to DNA mutations that are recognized by certain restriction endonucleases. Prenatal diagnosis of beta-thalassemia should be possible using amniocyte DNA.

For a few genetic conditions in which the exact gene abnormality is not known, the techniques utilizing linkage analysis can be used to indirectly deduce the gene causing the disorder. Benign genetic markers, called restriction fragment length polymorphisms, are used, which are closely linked to the gene(s) that result in disease. Examples of conditions for which such genetic markers have been located for linkage analysis are cystic fibrosis, certain muscular dystrophies, hemophilia A and B, some of the hemoglobinopathies, and Huntington's disease. Much of the X chromosome, and therefore X-linked recessive diseases, probably will be linked to specific markers in the very near future.

For each specific family seeking prenatal diagnosis, the size of the DNA fragment to which the disease gene is linked must be determined by DNA studies of family members, optimally *prior* to pregnancy. The gathering of this information can take a few weeks to months. Ideally, blood is obtained from known heterozygotes and at least one known homozygous normal or affected family member. Other family relatives may be included. Families must be "informative," for prenatal diagnostic studies to be performed. In informative cases, the carrier of a deleterious gene also is heterozygous for a closely linked marker. This linked marker can therefore be followed in the family. It should be noted that there are still technical limitations to this approach, but the number of genetic conditions for which linked markers are available will most certainly increase.

Chorionic Villus Sampling

Chorionic villus sampling (CVS) is a first-trimester technique of obtaining fetal cells for genetic analyses. The sampling is usually performed at approximately 8 to 10 weeks from the last menstrual period and in some cases is performed later in the pregnancy. Chorionic villi can be either aspirated transcervically through a flexible catheter or transabdominally, both under ultrasound guidance. Results are usually available in 1 to 10 days.

The indications for chorionic villus sampling include chromosome studies, metabolic assays, and restriction enzyme analysis. Alpha-fetoprotein (AFP) cannot be measured in the cells obtained by this technique, and therefore a maternal serum AFP screening is currently recommended at 16 weeks from the last menstrual period, to screen for neural tube defects.

Advantages in offering CVS include privacy, speed of results, and less risk from an earlier abortion if chosen. Because the procedure is new, the fetal loss rate and maternal risks are being tabulated by the National Institutes of Health from a multicenter study. Preliminary data indicates that the risk of miscarriage related to CVS is approximately 1–2%. Maternal infection has been reported in the transcervical approach and in both CVS approaches, some discomfort such as bleeding and nausea can occur in a small percentage of patients. There is a small chance (1–2%) that an abnormality will be found in the CVS sample which is not present in the fetus. An amniocentesis may be necessary to obtain more accurate information. There is also a small chance (less than 1%) that CVS results will be normal, but the baby may be born with a chromosomal abnormality.

ULTRASONOGRAPHY

With increasing experience gained by sonographers and the new sophistication of scanners and real-time units, an increasing number of congenital malformations can be detected by ultrasonography. This technique is not yet usable in early pregnancy for detection of most anomalies, but the resolution of ultrasound generally allows relatively good visualization of the fetus after 17 to 20 weeks. In addition to its use in prenatal diagnosis as a necessary tool in either amniocentesis or chorionic villus sampling, ultrasound is also indicated for suspicion of abnormal gestation size, the presence of oligohydramnios or polyhydramnios, abnormal alpha-fetoprotein levels, drug exposure during the pregnancy, or a family history of a specific genetic condition. Examples of conditions prenatally diagnosed by ultrasound include neural tube defects, limb defects, polycystic kidneys, diaphragmatic hernia, and duodenal atresia. Also, a more specialized form of ultrasound, fetal echocardiography, can detect certain congenital heart defects.

Risks associated with ultrasound are difficult to assess because of the relative newness of the procedure. Stark et al [5] found no biologically significant difference in physical, neurologic, and developmental parameters in 425 children, ages 7 to 12 years, who were exposed to ultrasound in utero compared with controls. It appears that ultrasound exposure to the fetus carries little risk, however, should be used only in pregnancies at risk or where it may benefit pregnancy management.

OTHER METHODS

Fetoscopy

Direct fetal visualization, usually performed at 17 to 20 weeks' gestation, utilizes a small-bore fiberoptic endoscope that is inserted in the uterus under local anesthesia. A separate channel may also be used for fetal skin or blood sampling. Indications for fetoscopy include pregnancies at risk for fetal structural abnormalities that are recognizable from viewing only a small area of the fetus. As part of known genetic syndromes, conditions involving major clefts, limb defects, extra digits, and malformed ears have been detected by fetoscopy. Fetal blood sampling has been done for pregnancies at risk for hemoglobinopathies and coagulation disorders. Indications for fetal skin biopsy include genetic conditions such as ectodermal dysplasia, Ehlers-Danlos syndrome, and epidermolysis bullosa. Few centers in the United States are experienced in performing fetoscopy, and there is an estimated 5 to 8% risk for fetal demise and early pregnancy loss from the procedure.

Percutaneous Umbilical Blood Sampling

Fetoscopy for fetal blood sampling may be used less as the experience with percutaneous umbilical blood sampling (PUBS) becomes a more widely used procedure for fetal assessment and therapy. Currently performed in the second and third trimester of pregnancy, this technique allows sampling of fetal blood from the umbilical cord by means of an ultrasound-guided needle. Indications can include chromosomal studies, isoimmune disorders, and nonimmune fetal hydrops. Advantages include rapid evaluation of chromosomes (48 to 72 hours) of equivocal amniocentesis results, diagnosis of fetal hematologic disorders for which DNA analysis can not be performed, and having access to a fetal blood sample to assess fetal infection or fetal antigen status. Also, the risk of PUBS appears to be much less than that of fetoscopy [6].

Radiography

Direct radiography after mid-trimester has allowed the prenatal diagnosis of malformation syndromes with skeletal abnormalities, such as certain types of dwarfism. Also, contrast radiography utilizing a water-soluble dye can show fetal swallowing and thus defects such as esophageal and duodenal atresia. Although sometimes helpful in prenatal diagnosis, radiography probably will be used less frequently as ultrasound techniques continue to improve.

Maternal Screening

MATERNAL SERUM ALPHA-FETOPROTEIN

Ninety to 95% of neural tube defects occur in families without a positive family history of similar problems. Even if amniocentesis were chosen in all families with a previously affected child, the disease incidence would be decreased by only 10%. Since AFP in the amniotic fluid enters the maternal circulation, the idea arose to measure serum AFP to predict which fetuses might have a neural tube defect. Since the maternal serum AFP (MSAFP) concentration increases rapidly from week 15 to week 24 of pregnancy, a correct estimation of the gestational age is important for diagnostic purposes. Optimal timing for measurement of MSAFP seems to be between 16 and 18 weeks from the last menstrual period.

Elevated MSAFP levels can indicate a neural tube defect, but can be "elevated" due to miscalculated gestational age, multiple gestation, or fetal demise. After a normal ultrasound examination that confirms an appropriately dated, single, viable fetus, the risk to the baby for a neural tube defect is approximately 10% if MSAFP levels are elevated. Also of importance is that low MSAFP levels have been associated with Down syndrome [7]. Abnormal AFP results may require further testing, including a repeat MSAFP, ultrasonography, and possibly amniocentesis.

Because measurement of MSAFP levels is only a screening test and not specifically diagnostic, it is important that the couple be informed about the possible meanings of an abnormal MSAFP, including a good chance that an abnormal result does not necessarily indicate the baby is abnormal.

CARRIERS AT RISK

Part of routine early obstetric care should include obtaining a family history to determine if the pregnant woman is at risk of being a carrier of a genetic condition. Genetic screening is offered to families having a significant history of a genetic disease, as well as to those from various ethnic backgrounds. Couples of Ashkenazi Jewish descent are at increased risk for carrying the Tay-Sachs gene (1 in 27); 8% of Black Americans are at risk for having sickle cell trait; and Greeks, Italians, and Southeast Asians are at increased risk for carrying the thalassemia gene. If carrier testing suggests that both parents are carriers of the same autosomal recessive disease, the chance for an affected pregnancy is 25%. Prenatal testing can be offered in many cases to determine if the fetus has the hereditary condition.

FETAL CELLS IN MATERNAL CIRCULATION

A recent development with potential implications for prenatal diagnosis is the discovery that fetal cells can be recovered in maternal serum during very early pregnancy [8]. Researchers have recovered nucleated fetal cells from maternal serum that could potentially be used to analyze fetal chromosomes [9] and possibly to detect inborn errors of metabolism, or to look for DNA markers. However, many technical obstacles must still be overcome before this type of maternal screening is feasible for prenatal diagnosis.

Future Therapy Considerations

One of the ultimate goals of prenatal testing is to treat the affected fetus to prevent sequelae of disease. Although treatment for the fetus is not often available after prenatal diagnosis of a genetic disease, a few conditions have been treated prenatally with success. These conditions include biotin-responsive multiple carboxylase deficiency and vitamin B_{12}-responsive methylmalonic acidemia. In pregnancies known to involve an affected fetus, mothers can be given large oral doses of biotin and vitamin

B_{12}, respectively. By and large, if actual gene therapy or specific enzyme replacement were possible, this would truly broaden the area of fetal therapy.

Some structural defects have been treated prenatally. Generally, treatment has been considered for those abnormalities that interfere with fetal organ development and those in which in utero correction would allow the fetus to grow normally. After detection by ultrasonography, two conditions for which in utero surgery has been performed are hydrocephalus and urethral obstruction. Treatment is not always beneficial, however, and surgery at term is still the preferred option if irreversible damage has not occurred.

It should be mentioned that attempts at "gene therapy," such as in the case of Lesch-Nyhan syndrome, seem to have raised some hope for treatment of genetic diseases, it appears that in the near future. However, such therapy is far from routine application.

Conclusion

Growth in the field of medical genetics and prenatal diagnosis has developed tremendously, in part because of the increased number of techniques available to diagnose various conditions. Certainly the use of restriction fragment-length polymorphisms and gene mapping will become applicable to more families who have a known genetic disease, and this will most likely fuel the demand for prenatal diagnosis. The continued responsibility of health care professionals will include being aware of not only the new genetic technologies, but also the psychological impact these developments can have on the families at risk. Finally, it cannot be ignored that a variety of ethical concerns have been raised with regard to genetic testing; these ethical concerns should be openly discussed with the family involved.

REFERENCES

1. Hill LM, Breckle R, Gehrking WC: The prenatal detection of congenital malformations by ultrasonography. *Mayo Clin Proc* **58**:805, 1983.
2. Thompson JS, Thompson MW: *Genetics in Medicine*, 4th ed. Philadelphia: WB Saunders, 1986, p. 291.
3. Simpson JL, Golbus MS, Martin AO, et al: *Genetics in Obstetrics and Gynecology*, New York: Grune and Stratton, 1982, p. 110.
4. Schreinemachers DM, Cross PK, and Hook, EB: Rates of trisomies 21, 18, 13 and other chromosome abnormalities in about 20,000 prenatal studies compared with estimated rates in livebirths. *Hum Genet* **61**:320, 322, 1982.
5. Stark CR, Orleans M, Haverkamp AD, et al: Short and long-term risks after exposure to diagnostic ultrasound in utero. *Obstet Gynecol* **63**:194, 1984.

6. Daffos F, Capella-Pavlosky M, Forestier F: Fetal blood sampling during pregnancy with the use of a needle guided by ultrasound: a study of 606 consecutive cases. *Amer J Obstet Gynecol* **153**:655, 1985.
7. Cuckle HS, Wald NJ, Lindenbaum RH: Maternal serum alpha-fetoprotein measurement: A screening test for Down syndrome. *Lancet* Vol. 1:926, 1984.
8. Covone AE, Johnson PM, Mutton D, et al: Trophoblast cells in peripheral blood from pregnant women. *Lancet* Vol. 2:841, 1984.
9. Elias S, Chandler RW, Wachtel S: Relative deoxyribonucleic acid content of interphase leukocytes by flow cytometry: A method for indirect diagnosis of chromosomal abnormalities with potential for prenatal diagnosis. *Amer Jr of Obstet/Gynecol,* April '88, p. 808.

20
The Effects of Nursing Care on Medical Malpractice*

MARY F. HAIRE

In any discussion of clinical practice today, the medicolegal climate is a frequent topic of concern. The issue of legality of practice is, in addition, often raised in the professional literature. However, over the years the basic relationships between nursing practice and the law have remained unchanged. Nurses are still responsible for their own practice, and documentation of that practice is still their best defense.

The role of the nurse in health care delivery is changing, however. Nursing salaries have increased. The number of nurses in private practice has increased. The number of nurses carrying individual malpractice insurance has increased, and we have insisted very vocally on recognition of the independent nature of our professional role. It is possible, therefore, that the increasing number of nurses named individually in lawsuits is a recognition of the independent identity of the nursing role.

While nursing is independent, it is not, except in rare instances, in competition with medicine. Medicine and nursing continue to be interdependent in health care delivery [1]. Instances of competition do exist where nurse midwives and obstetricians practice in the same setting, and where some nurse practitioners and family practice physicians offer similar services.

An awareness of the legal system and its expectations for professionals can assist nurses by allowing them to use the legal system as a protection rather than a punishment [2]. Failure to maintain such an awareness of the interrelationship between professional practice and the law can easily result in negligence or malpractice charges.

Professional Accountability

Professional accountability involves more than simply accepting responsibility for one's actions [3]. Accountability includes identification of those to whom the professional is accountable and recognition of the activities required to fulfill the professional role [4].

---

*Portions of this presentation were published as "Accountability in Nursing Practice" in Vanderbilt Medical Center *Nursing Notes*, April/May 1984.

Certainly the professional is accountable to the patient in several areas. Maintenance of the education and specialized skills that are part of the professional's role is necessary to protect the patient from harm from outmoded practices [2,5,6]. I believe the time will come when failure to participate in continuing professional education may be grounds for negligence if harm occurs to a patient through lack of current knowledge.

Accountability means recognition of the patient's right to know [7]. If questions are asked regarding the care that is being administered, they should be answered by the person who has the best understanding of the information. If the nurse has such understanding and is asked, she or he should have the freedom to answer the questions. If not, the nurse should accept responsibility for ensuring that the patient has access to the physician for such information. Needless to say, each professional has a responsibility not to interfere with other professionals' patient relationships. Both physician and nurse must be willing to accept the importance of a therapeutic relationship between the patient and the other practitioner.

Accountability to one's self is also part of the professional's responsibility. Each of us entered our profession with goals and aspirations we set for ourselves on the basis of our knowledge of the profession. Maintaining the image of a caring and competent professional requires continuing education and continued professional growth [8]. Perhaps one component of professional burnout involves unintentional neglect of one's accountability to personal growth.

We also are accountable to the profession of nursing. We should be actively involved in the setting of standards of care for our own practice. National standards are a means of drawing the profession together through the recognition of shared expertise. These standards provide a resource by which we can judge our level of practice against that of other nurses of comparable education and experience. In addition, hospital standards (which should reflect national standards) are the responsibility of all nurses on staff. Such responsibility can never be abdicated to administration, which may or may not understand the complexities of nursing care [2].

We should be equally involved in policing our own profession. It is the responsibility of professionals to protect both the public and other members of the nursing profession from those practitioners who consistently deliver care at a level below that which we would find acceptable if administered to our own family [2]. Involvement in such activities may reduce the likelihood of other professions interfacing with the practice of nursing.

As professionals, we also are accountable to our employers. A contract exists between the employer and employee whenever a salary has been accepted. In nursing the contract implies adequate knowledge to fulfill the role on the part of the nurse who accepts the position, and commitment to providing on-the-job training where needed in specialty areas on the part of the employer who hires the professional. It further implies a commitment to continuing education on the part of both the employer and the employee [4].

Accepting a salaried position also implies acceptance of the policies of the institution. Institutional policies should be consistent with the Nurse Practice Act of the individual state. These policies should reflect national standards of care, and it is the responsibility of both physicians and nurses to notify the hospital about outdated policies on the books [9].

Documentation of Care

Documentation of care continues to be the best means of protecting one's self against charges of negligence or malpractice [9]. There is no doubt that documentation takes time, time that often is needed in providing care. However, documentation need not occur at the exact time the care is given [10]. It may be a summary written after the event when the patient's condition no longer requires immediate attention. Documentation can occur at the bedside as easily as at the nurses' station.

Documentation of practice provides information about actions that were taken. It should indicate why a particular action was undertaken, the recipient of the action, the administrator, the treatment method and time, and a description of the patient's responses to treatment. Documentation protects the nurse's colleagues from errors of omission and of commission, and protects the patient from overtreatment or undertreatment [10]. Documentation provides a record on which future treatment may be ordered or discontinued. In addition it provides a legal document of the care rendered to a particular patient [11].

The patient records should reflect pertinent information. Negative findings are often as important as positive findings [10]. For instance, lack of progress in dilatation of the cervix should precede a note indicating that a cesarean section was performed for cephalopelvic disproportion. Such documentation is as important as the positive findings of fetal distress prior to emergency cesarean section.

Documentation of vital signs is often overlooked as being so routine that it is unimportant; however, evidence of fever, of tachycardia, or of uterine tenderness should be noted to explain the administration of antibiotics for endometritis. Evidence of elevations in blood pressure and/ or hyperreflexia should document the need for magnesium sulfate for treatment of preeclampsia.

Periodic reevaluations of patient condition indicate the alertness of the attending staff as well as documenting efforts made to protect the patient from unexpected harm [12]. For instance, a normal fetal heart rate tracing obtained throughout labor may serve as an excellent defense for allowing a vaginal delivery for a baby who later develops cerebral palsy. Nurses should remember that their own evaluations are of importance to the welfare of the patient. The courts consider that nursing care is not simply a response to medical orders, but includes evaluation of patient response to treatment and independent evaluations of patient condition [2,9].

Documentation need not be voluminous. It should, however, be consistent, conform to recommended guidelines, and be comprehensive enough to indicate why changes in management were undertaken or not undertaken. Periodic assessments of patient condition on the part of the nursing staff can provide the necessary documentation to support the medical decision. Failure to assess the patient on a periodic basis can be used to support charges of nursing negligence [10].

Areas of Malpractice Concern

Some general concerns apply equally well to all nurses. For instance, nurses have been successfully sued for:

1. Failure to observe and act on a patient's worsening condition, since nurses must use professional judgment and cannot rely solely on the physician for evaluation of patient condition.
2. Failure to report changes in patient condition for better or worse if those changes indicated a possible need for altered medical management.
3. Failure to recognize and act on improper or inappropriate medical actions [13,14].

USE OF OXYTOCIN

Areas of specific concern to obstetric nurses often center around oxytocin, since a significant number of perinatal claims are related to oxytocin use. The object of oxytocin use is to stimulate contractions comparable to spontaneous labor contractions. The nurse must therefore be competent in assessing labor and its effects on the fetus. Improper use of oxytocin is an area in which nurses and physicians bear joint responsibility. The nurse must understand the use of the medication, how to evaluate its effectiveness and safety for a particular patient, and when to stop or decrease the amount of medication being given [10,15]. The physician bears the additional responsibility for ordering the use of oxytocin on the basis of patient need and safety.

Standards are available in both medical and nursing literature to document the correct administration of oxytocin and the correct use of equipment to increase its safety [10,15]. Such equipment includes calibrated infusion pumps and fetal monitors to evaluate not only contraction activity but fetal heart rate response as well.

FETAL MONITORING

Another common area of investigation in perinatal law suits relates to the use of fetal monitors. The *NAACOG Standards* say, "Following specific orientation and education and in accordance with hospital policies and protocols the nurse may monitor and interpret uterine contractions and fetal heart rate" [15]. Unless the physician is at the bedside continuously, it is the responsibility of the nurse to observe and interpret fetal monitor changes. The nurse must continually observe, assess, and document such changes.

My belief is that late or variable decelerations are descriptive terms only. Whether they require a change in medical management is up to the doctor, but the nurse must know how to recognize and respond to the data. Nursing management when these abnormalities are seen may include position change, oxygen administration, and/or altered IV rates.

INFORMED CONSENT

The concept of informed consent is often a point of discussion when medicolegal implications are being addressed. "The purpose of an informed consent is to protect the provider from battery charges" [16]. The purpose is not to protect the provider from malpractice charges. Generally speaking, the person doing the procedure should do the *explanation* for consent [6,7]. The nurse, however, can get a signature from the patient on the consent form after confirming that the patient does understand. In that instance the nurse serves only to witness that the patient was informed and understood what would be done.

If the patient does not understand, the nurse should not have the patient sign the consent form [16]. He or she should notify the physician that this patient apparently needs further information. Failure to notify the physician of the patient's lack of understanding, or of the patient's withdrawal of consent, may result in filing of battery charges [16]. If the nurse fails to determine the patient's level of understanding prior to having the consent form signed, she or he may be listed as a coconspirator in a legal case if something goes wrong during the procedure.

If the nurse does undertake an explanation of the procedure for purposes of obtaining informed consent, he or she is held at the same level of competence in *explaining* the procedure as the physician would be. For that reason, in many hospitals, the nurse is prohibited from providing information for informed consent.

ABANDONMENT

The concept of abandonment has only recently been applied to nursing practice [13]. Abandonment may fall into one of three categories:

1. Leaving the patient inappropriately attended. For instance, family is not a substitute for the professional nurse in the second stage of labor. In many instances it is also inappropriate to leave an obstetric patient recovering from a general anesthetic with only an aid or technician to

care for her. Should complications arise during this recovery phase, professional care is indicated [13].
2. Failure to take the necessary precautions to protect the patient. For example, the failure to secure prompt and appropriate care for patients in emergency situations, or to adequately assess a patient to determine the level of care needed, could be considered abandonment. Another example would be failure to follow through when a physician does not respond to a call for help [13,14].
3. The *American Nurses' Association* Code for Nurses says the nurse is responsible for recognizing and pointing out questionable conduct on the part of other nurses and/or a physician [14]. Needless to say, such questionable conduct should be discussed tactfully and in private, not in front of the patient. Certainly, in such confrontations, the decision should be based on adequate, accessible, and objective information.

Conclusion

All of us have made errors in patient care, some of them serious. However, there is little excuse for inconsistency of care, or inadequacies based on outdated procedures. Good care requires very little effort. It does require a degree of compulsiveness on the part of the health care provider, an unwillingness to take shortcuts, and an unwillingness to compromise quality. Many of the high-risk factors in perinatal nursing could be avoided if we took the time to practice compulsively the things that we have been taught to protect patients.

REFERENCES

1. Driscoll V: Liberating nursing practice. *Nurs Outlook* **20**:24–27, 1972.
2. Harvey CK: Avoid legal problems by knowing your scope of practice. AORN *J* **32**:948–949, 1980.
3. Sigman P: Ethical choice in nursing. ANS **1**:37–52, 1979.
4. Carson FE, Ames A: Nursing staff bylaws. *Am J Nurs* **80**:1130–1134, 1980.
5. Hochman G: Mandatory continuing education: How will it affect you? *Nursing 78* **8**:105–113, 1978.
6. Southby JR: Legal considerations for nurse researchers. AORN *J* **33**:1278–1290, 1981.
7. Dickman RL: The ethics of informed consent. *Nurs Pract* **5**:25–26, 1980.
8. Rubenfeld MG, Donley R, Fralinski EG, et al: The nurse training act: Yesterday, today, and. . . . *Am J Nurs* **81**:1202–1204, 1981.
9. Wiley L: Liability for death: Nine nurses' legal ordeals. *Nursing 81* **11**:34–43, 1981.
10. Fiesta J: The law and liability. New York: Wiley Medical Publications, 1983.
11. Health Law Center: *Nursing and the Law*. Rockville, Md: Aspen Systems Corp., 1985.

12. Murchison I, Nichols TS, Hanson R: *Legal Accountability in the Nursing Process*. St. Louis: CV Mosby, 1982.
13. Cushing M: Expanding the meaning of accountability. *Am J Nurs* **83**:1202–1203, 1983.
14. Rhodes AM: Liability for the actions of others. *MCN: The American Journal of Maternal Child Nursing,* **11**:315, 1986.
15. NAACOG: *Standards for Obstetric, Gynecologic, and Neonatal Nursing.* 2nd ed. 1981.
16. Klein CA: Informed Consent. *Nurs Pract* **9**:56–62, 1984.

ADDITIONAL READING

1. Bullough B: Influences on role expansion. *Am J Nurs* **76**:9, 1976.
2. Chinn PL: Science and the politics of sexism. ANS 7:vii–viii, 1985.
3. Ciesla JH: Nurse practice acts. *Occ Health Nurs* **25**:13–17, 1977.
4. Creighton H: *Law Every Nurse Should Know*. Philadelphia: WB Saunders, 1970.
5. Creighton H: When can a nurse refuse to give care? *Nurs Manage* **17**:16–20, 1986.
6. Divoll MK: The role of the perinatal and neonatal nurse in risk management. *Perinat Neonatal Nurs* **1**(2):1–8, 1987.
7. Crabenstein J: Nursing documentation during the perinatal period. *Perinat Neonatal Nurs* **1**(2):29–38, 1987.
8. Kendellen R: The medical malpractice insurance crisis. *J Nurs-Midwif* **32**:4–10, 1987.
9. Kroner K: If you're moving into management. . . . *Nursing 80* **10**:105–114, 1980.
10. Regan WA: Can an employer block a nurse from acting as an expert witness? AORN *J* **32**:781, 1980.
11. Spitzer RB: Legislation and new regulations. *Nurs Manage* **14**:13–21, 1983.
12. Stein LI: The doctor-nurse game. *Arch Gen Psychiat* **16**:699–703, 1967.
13. Nosek JA: Expanded role liability in perinatal nursing. *Perinat Neonatal Nurs* **1**(2):39–48, 1987.

21
Advances in Diagnosis of Cardiac Disease in the Fetus and the Newborn

RABI F. SULAYMAN

Congenital heart disease continues to be a relatively common problem in the fetus and the newborn. In fact, recent reviews suggest that the incidence of congenital heart disease is probably on the rise in some groups of patients [1]. While the presence of heart disease may not produce any hemodynamic alterations in the fetus, it is associated with a significant increase in morbidity and mortality in the newborn [2]. Hence, any pregnancy in which the fetus is suspected of having cardiac disease must be considered a high-risk pregnancy and handled as such. This adds to the challenge facing perinatologists, neonatologists, and cardiologists today and creates the need for an early and definitive diagnosis.

Heart disease in the fetus and the newborn may be anatomic (congenital heart disease), structural (the cardiomyopathies), a disorder of cardiac rhythm, or a combination of all three problems. It may present with heart murmurs, cyanosis, arrhythmias, or even congestive heart failure. Congestive heart failure and arrhythmias may be detected in the fetus before birth. Prenatal diagnosis depends on the presence of a high degree of suspicion that heart disease exists and on the performance of technically adequate diagnostic procedures. In the past, such procedures were either unavailable or, if available, were crude, inaccurate, or unreliable. Recent advances, particularly in the fields of genetics, radiology, and ultrasound, have resulted in the development of newer, reliable diagnostic methods that allow for accurate diagnosis of cardiac disease in the fetus and the newborn. Early diagnosis and hence early intervention have significantly decreased the mortality and morbidity of the critically ill newborn.

To fully understand the capabilities of these procedures, when to use them, and the impact they may have on diagnosis of the heart with abnormal anatomy, structure, or functions, it is necessary to briefly review the anatomy, structure, and function of the normal fetal heart.

The Fetal Circulation and Cardiovascular Dynamics

The anatomy, structure, and function of the fetal heart differ significantly from those of the neonate. Adult norms are not established until months or even years after birth.

In the fetus, the right and left atria communicate through a gap between the septum primum, which forms from one of the endocardial cushions, and the septum secundum, which forms from the root of the atria. This gap is known as the patent foramen ovale. The pulmonary artery and the aorta also communicate, through the patent ductus arteriosus. The fetal right and left ventricles are hemispheric in cross section [3] and appear structurally to be similar in the infant, in whom the right ventricle is no longer hemispheric in shape. The right ventricle has larger volume than the left ventricle [4]. Both ventricles have relatively thick walls and are poorly compliant.

Highly oxygenated blood coming from the placenta returns to the right atrium via the inferior vena cava. This inferior vena cava blood streams preferentially across the patent foramen ovale into the left ventricle [5]. The left ventricle ejects into the ascending aorta, supplying the cerebral structures with this highly oxygenated blood.

Less oxygenated venous blood returns to the right atrium via the superior vena cava and, together with some of the inferior vena caval return, enters the right ventricle. The right ventricle ejects blood into the pulmonary trunk where it mostly proceeds to a widely patent ductus arteriosus and descending aorta to supply the chest, abdominal organs, and the extremities before returning to the placenta via the umbilical arteries.

Because of the extremely high pulmonary vascular resistance during fetal life, very little blood (less than 7% of the right ventricular cardiac output) flows into the lungs [6]. Consequently, the pulmonary venous return is also negligible. Figure 21.1 illustrates blood flow in the fetal circulation.

Because both ventricles eject into the systemic circulation with each stroke, their pressures are high and almost equal [5]. The ventricular outputs, however, are not similar, that of the right ventricle being greater than that of the left. In the fetal lamb, the right ventricular/left ventricular stroke volume ratio appears to be 60:40 [5]; in the human fetus, it is closer to 55:45 [7].

The fetal Po_2 is 30 to 35 torr in the umbilical vein, 20 to 22 torr in the umbilical artery. The fetal heart rate is normally between 120 and 160 beats per minute, and the fetal systolic blood pressure is about 40 mm Hg.

After birth a series of changes take place. The lungs expand, which dramatically decreases pulmonary vascular resistance, increases pulmonary blood flow, and correspondingly increases pulmonary venous return.

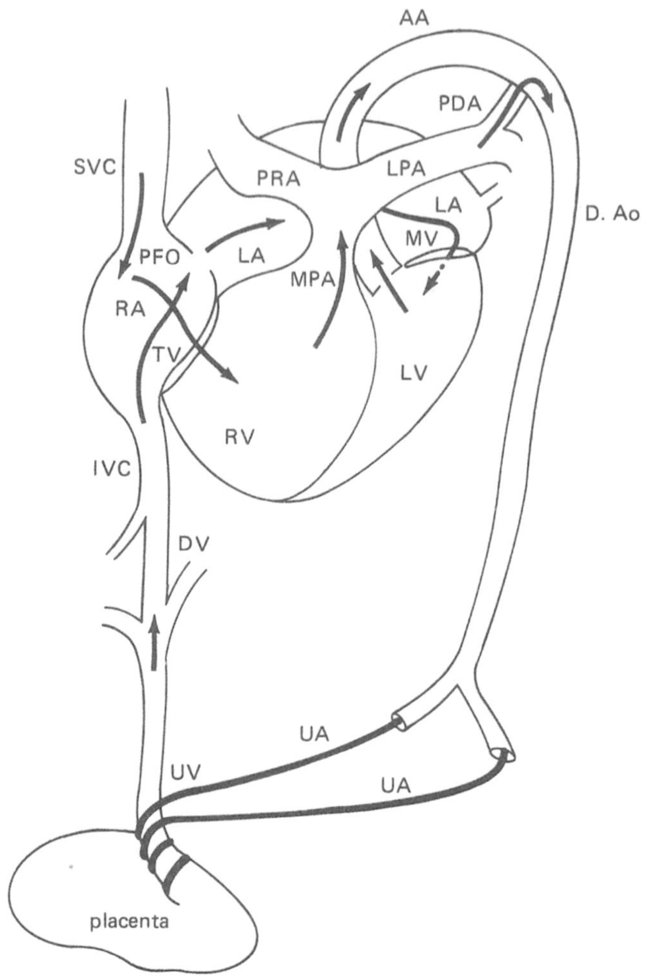

FIGURE 21.1. Schematic diagram of the fetal circulation. Arrows point toward the direction of blood flow. UV, umbilical vein; DV, ductus venosus; IVC, inferior vena cava; RA, Right atrium; SVC, superior vena cava; RV, right ventricle; MPA, main pulmonary artery; RPA, right pulmonary artery; LPA, left pulmonary artery; PDA, patent ductus arteriosus; AA, aortic arch; D.Ao, descending aorta; LA, left atrium; LV, left ventricle, PFO, patent foramen ovale; UA, umbilical artery.

TABLE 21.1. Normal values in the newborn.

	pH	Pco$_2$ (torr)	Po$_2$ (torr)	Heart rate/min	Hemoglobin (g %)	Pulse rate (internal)	Amplitude V i (mm)		Amplitude V6 (mm)		Blood pressure (mm Hg)
							R wave	S wave	R wave	S wave	
Premature 1–3 days											
<1,250 g birth weight	7.38	38	50	95–160	13.4	0.08–0.15					35–57 / 20–35 Mean = 42/23
>1,250 g birth weight	7.35	40	50	95–160	14.5	0.08–0.15					38–58 / 20–38 Mean = 47/26
Term infant											
Birth	7.27	54	55	93–154	16.5	0.08–0.16	5.6–26.1 (13.8)	0–22.7 8.5	0–11.1 4.2	0–9.6 (3.2)	50–73 / 28–48 Mean = 60/38
1 hour	7.30	39	65								
3 hours	7.34	38	65								
1–3 days	7.35	35	70	91–160	18.5	0.08–0.14	5.3–26.9 (14.4)	0–20.7 (9.1)	0–12.2 (4.5)	0–9.4 (3.0)	43–73 / 30–50 Mean = 70/40
1–3 weeks	7.37	36	70	102–182	16	0.07–0.14	3.2–20.8 (10.6)	0–10.8 (4.2)	2.6– 16.4) (7.6)	0–9.8 (3.4)	60–80 / 38–50 Mean = 70/43

PR = P-R interval on the Electrocardiogram

Po$_2$ & Pco$_2$ = Torr or mm Hg.

V1 & V6 are Leads V1 & V6 of the ECG

Amplitude = height of the ORS complex of the ECG measured in millimeters.

The sudden increase in the return into the left atrium results in increased left atrial pressure, and this forces the patent foramen ovale to become functionally closed.

Removal of the placenta eliminates that segment of the systemic circulation with an unusually low vascular resistance. Systemic vascular resistance is increased, and systemic venous return decreases. The left ventricle starts to undergo physiologic hypertrophy, and the right ventricle assumes a crescentic shape. The arterial P_{O_2} increases to 80 to 90 torr and the patent ductus arteriosus undergoes functional closure within hours to days after birth. The heart rate increases initially and then gradually decreases.

The cardiac output increases from 150 ml/kg/min in the left ventricle and 300 ml/kg/min in the right ventricle, to about 400 ml/kg/min in both. Table 21.1 shows the normal values for various variables in the newborn.

Clinical Correlations

From the above, it becomes very apparent that cardiac disease presents and manifests itself very differently in the fetus or newborn as contrasted to infants or children. Problems resulting in significant cardiac pressure or volume overload, to the extent that congestive heart failure may occur even before birth, are likely to present clinically as fetal ascites or pericardial effusion. Cardiac dilatation, if it occurs, is more likely to affect the right ventricle, whose output mostly proceeds to the low-resistance placental vascular bed. Anatomic anomalies, which traditionally present as cyanotic heart disease after birth due to obligatory right-to-left shunting and/or decreased pulmonary blood flow, cause no deleterious hemodynamic effects to the fetus. Should such a condition exist, however, it becomes critical to maintain the patency of the ductus arteriosus after birth to maintain an adequate pulmonary and/or systemic blood flows. The normal closure of the ductus in these conditions obviously is not desirable. It is also evident that premature closure of the ductus or foramen ovale before birth results in fetal death. Both conditions have been reported.

The high pulmonary vascular resistance and right ventricular pressures in the fetus and in the newborn up to age 8 weeks prevent significant left-to-right shunting across even large atrial or ventricular septal defects. The implications here are, of course, that if a fetus or newborn less than 8 weeks of age presents with evidence of volume overload and congestive heart failure, the likely cause is other than septal defect, unless accompanied by a premature drop in pulmonary vascular resistance. This may not be the case in the prematurely born infant, in whom pulmonary vascular resistance may be low. In the premature baby with respiratory distress syndrome, the pulmonary vascular resistance is, however, high, and continues to be so if the newborn is placed on a ventilator with high peak expiratory (PEEP) values. While a patent ductus does not create a significant volume overload in such infants, it will do so if it remains patent as soon as the lung disease improves and the PEEP values are decreased in preparation for weaning from the ventilator. Both events allow the pulmonary vascular resistance to decrease to the extent that a significant left-to-right shunt occurs across the patent ductus as soon as positive pressure ventilation is discontinued. In many instances, positive pressure ventilation cannot be discontinued, because as soon as one attempts to do so, the ductus starts shunting from left-to-right, resulting in significant volume overload to the left heart, manifested by lung edema, respiratory distress, and CO_2 retention. Conversely, a significant patent ductus arteriosus must be suspected every time there is failure to wean a newborn from the ventilator.

Diagnostic Methods

In the past, prenatal diagnosis of congenital problems was difficult, if not impossible. Recent procedural and technical advances, particularly in the areas of genetics and imaging [8–10], have enabled investigators to diagnose accurately many congenital diseases, cardiac disease included, prior to birth. Recent advances in radiology [11,12] have resulted in accurate and less invasive methods for the diagnosis and follow-up of congenital heart disease in the newborn. Such capabilities have changed the way infants with heart disease are managed nowadays and have had a profound impact on prognosis.

Regardless of the methods utilized in prenatal and postnatal diagnosis, all approaches must start with a reasonable index of suspicion. Diagnostic assessments for cardiac disease have been recommended in four groups of patients.

1. Family history of congenital heart disease. The incidence of congenital heart disease is about 1%. This increases to 4% with a positive family history and to 14% if the mother has congenital heart disease [13].
2. Maternal conditions such as age, diabetes, hyperinsulinism, isoimmunization, and connective tissue disease are associated with an increased risk for the fetal development of cardiac disease such as chromosomal anomalies associated with heart disease, congenital defects, myocardial and septal hypertrophy, intrauterine congestive heart failure, and heart blocks [14–17].
3. Pregnant women who have been exposed to teratogens during critical periods of fetal development. The teratogenic effects of viral infections such as rubella and drugs such as phenytoin, alcohol, cithium, hydralazines, beta-blockers, and prostaglandin inhibitors are well documented.

4. Pregnancies associated with macrosomia, intrauterine growth retardation, polyhydramnios, oligohydramnios, abnormal studies after amniocentesis, and abnormal fetal heart rate, whether tachycardia or bradycardia, are associated with a risk of a cardiac defect in 30 to 50% of newborns [18].

After birth, cardiac disease must be suspected in any newborn with respiratory distress and/or persistent cyanosis in the absence of significant lung disease; with evidence of congestive heart failure, abnormal cardiac shadow on the chest x-ray, abnormal cardiac rhythm, or heart murmur no matter how insignificant it may sound; or with respiratory distress syndrome who cannot be weaned from positive pressure ventilation. Cardiac disease must also be suspected and ruled out in all infants with dysmorphic features suggestive of a chromosomal problem, especially the trisomies.

Prenatal Diagnosis

The prenatal diagnosis of fetal malformations centers around two major methods. The first is chemical, hormonal, pathologic, genetic analysis of amniotic fluid or chorionic villi obtained by amniocentesis or chorionic villus sampling as early as 16 weeks of gestation [8,9]. This is not without risk, and with regard to congenital heart disease the yield has been minimal unless the genetic analysis reveals a chromosomal abnormality, in which case the incidence of cardiac disease is greatly increased. Conventional monitoring of the fetal heart beat in an attempt to define clinically significant abnormalities was proven to be unsatisfactory in earlier studies [19].

The use of ultrasound to study the fetus is the second major method utilized in prenatal diagnosis. While ultrasonography and two-dimensional fetal echocardiography were introduced a long time ago, the results have not been satisfactory, due mainly to technical problems. Recent advances in technology and the introduction of extremely high-resolution ultrasound and Doppler techniques, coupled with improved skills, have made it possible now to examine the human fetus noninvasively and assess the cardiac anatomy, rhythm, and function fairly and accurately [20,21].

EQUIPMENT AND TECHNIQUE

Equipment and methods used to perform fetal echocardiography and Doppler studies have been described [22]. Most commercially available two-dimensional echocardiographic and Doppler systems may be used. Although 3.5 and 5 MHz transducers have been used, it appears that a 5-MHz transducer is most suitable in the majority. Food and Drug Administration-imposed limitations on the used accoustic frequencies, and other guidelines, must be observed.

The two-dimensional imaging scan is performed to obtain four basic views:

Four chamber view
Short axis view
Long axis view and
View to visualize the great vessels

This is followed by a pulsed Doppler study to obtain Doppler flow velocity tracings. The study may be performed simultaneously with an abdominal fetal electrocardiogram.

The four-chamber view of the two-dimensional image scan is obtained in a transverse plane perpendicular to the fetal spine. The ventricle closest to the spine is the left ventricle; the right ventricle is closest to the fetal chest wall. The heart occupies one third of the chest. In this view, the patent foramen ovale pulmonary veins and the mitral and tricuspid valves will be visualized. Fractional shortening measurements can be obtained with an M-mode tracing performed in a plane perpendicular to the ventricular septum. Rhythm strips are obtained simultaneously.

The four-chamber view is used for screening, because it identifies most of the cardiac malformations.

The short-axis view is obtained by directing the transducer cephalad. The pulmonary artery is visualized with the right pulmonary artery separating from the pulmonary trunk and the ductus as an extension of the pulmonary trunk into the descending aorta, which lies near the fetal spine.

The long-axis view is obtained in a plane parallel to the fetal spine. The aorta is seen exiting the left ventricle. Anterior to the aorta is the main pulmonary artery, and posterior to the aorta is the superior vena cava. The aortic arch is identified by the carotid vessels. It is narrower, higher in the fetal body, and more posterior than the arch formed by the main pulmonary artery and the ductus as it enters the descending aorta.

Maximal Doppler flow velocities are obtained across and proximal to the valves. Flow velocities are obtained parallel to the direction of blood flow and compared with those obtained from normal fetuses (Table 21.2).

The calculated volume flow of the right ventricle is about 307 ± 30 ml/kg/min and of the left ventricle is 232 ± 25 ml/kg/min. Such studies and measurements of fractional shortening of the ventricles, when performed during an episode of fetal tachyarrhythmia, identify significant decrease of the fetal cardiac output during such episodes.

TABLE 21.2. Mean Doppler flow velocities in normal fetuses.

	Maximum velocity (cm/sec)	Mean velocity (cm/sec)	Area (cm^2)
Tricuspid valve	51.0 ± 1.2	11.8 ± 0.4	0.26–0.74
Mitral valve	47.0 ± 1.1	11.2 ± 0.3	0.25–0.62
Pulmonary artery	58.5 ± 3.6	18.0 ± 2.0	0.47
Aorta	71.9 ± 4.0	18.8 ± 2.1	0.35

Postnatal Diagnosis

Until recently, only invasive diagnostic techniques such as cardiac catheterization and angiography were accurate enough to yield a definitive anatomic diagnosis of congenital cardiac malformations. Improved technology in echocardiography has made possible performance of detailed and accurate studies, thus delaying or eliminating the need to perform high-risk procedures on critically ill neonates. Color flow mapping with Doppler is the latest of those advances [23]. Magnetic resonance imaging and ultrafast computed tomography (CT) are two other methods currently used to study infants and children with cardiac disease, again making it possible to avoid or delay the use of higher risk diagnostic procedures.

Magnetic resonance imaging is a high-resolution tomographic imaging technique that does not utilize ionizing radiation or contrast media. It is based on the principle that hydrogen protons, widely distributed in body tissues, can be made to align with the application of a magnetic field. Low-energy radio waves, when applied, cause the aligned protons to resonate and generate low-frequency signals, which can be encoded to obtain images.

Cardiac imaging using magnetic resonance is based on the principle that blood flow is too rapid to produce radiofrequencies of significant amplitude, and hence it appears as dark areas on the obtained image, allowing the visualization of the cardiac chambers and structures. Image decay because of motion can be prevented by gating signal acquisition to the R wave of the electrocardiogram. Most pediatric investigative procedures were performed using the spin-echo multislice technique, 0.6 Tulsa superconducting magnet, and a resonance frequency of 25.4 MHz. Scanning is done in multiple planes including transverse, sagittal, and oblique. The ability to acquire multiplane images is a distinct advantage over CT scans, in which images can be obtained in the transverse plane only. Initial investigations revealed that it adequately visualized atrial septal defects, tetralogy of Fallot, and tricuspid atresia. It proved to be superior to two-dimensional echocardiology for the visualization of coarctation of the aorta, the aortic arch, and the arch vessels when images were obtained in the sagittal plane and 60° left anterior oblique position. It cannot be used in patients with arrhythmias, however, since it cannot be gated, nor in patients with pacemakers or metallic surgical clips.

In Doppler color imaging, the Doppler processor color encodes velocities determined by an autocorrelation solution of the Doppler-shifted frequencies so that blood flow directed toward the transducer is shown as red-orange and flow directed away from the transducer as blue. With turbulent blood flow, the system adds mixtures of green. The system then superimposes these velocity images on the gray-scale two-dimensional ultrasound images. The images can be stored on video. Hardcopies can be made as polaroid color prints. In the preterm infant with patent ductus arteriosus, Doppler color flow mapping has already been shown to be superior to conventional Doppler, especially when the ductus is constricted, allows right-to-left shunting, or is associated with additional intracardiac defects. Its use in other types of cardiac disease is under investigation.

Recent technologic advances in computed tomography resulted in the development of ultrafast CT imaging systems. Prolonged scan acquisition times required for imaging have limited the use of conventional CT in cardiac disease. Ultrafast CT scanners, however, are able to image at ultrafast scanning speeds (50 ms/slice). Coupled with peripheral rather than central contrast material injections, its superior spatial resolution and three-dimensional image capability make ultrafast CT imaging a valuable addition to the available diagnostic methods.

Experience in the utilization of ultrafast CT scanning in congenital heart disease is very limited. Initial reports indicate that it can be used fairly safely and accurately [11]. There is also evidence that it may even be superior to conventional cardiac catheterization and angiography in providing anatomic detail in some groups of patients, such as those with pulmonary venous obstruction and postmustard surgical procedures for transposition of the great arteries (T. Husayni, personal communication).

REFERENCES

1. Rose V: A possible increase in the incidence of congenital heart disease among the offspring of affected parents. *J Am Cardiol* **6**:376–382, 1985.
2. Lingman G, Lundstrom MR, Morsal K, et al: Fetal cardiac arrhythmias: Clinical outcome of 113 cases. *Acta Obstet Gynecol Scand* **65**:263–267, 1986.
3. Azancot A, Caudell TP, Allen HD, et al: Analysis of ventricular shape by echocardiography in normal fetuses, newborns and infants. *Circulation* **68**:1201–1211, 1983.
4. Kleinman CS, Donnerstein RL: Ultrasonic assessment of cardiac function in the intact human fetus. *J Am Coll Cardiol* **5**:845–945, 848–948, 1985.
5. Rudolf AM: Distribution and regulation of blood flow in the fetal and neonatal lamb. *Circ Res* **57**:811–821, 1985.
6. Rudolph AM: Fetal circulation and cardiovascular adjustments after birth. In Rudolph AM (Ed): *Pediatrics*. 17th ed. Norwalk, CT: Appleton-Century-Crofts, 1982, pp. 1231–1235.
7. Kenny JF, Plappert T, Doubilet P, et al: Changes in intracardiac blood flow, velocities and right/left ventricular stroke volumes with gestational age in the normal newborn fetus: A prospective Doppler echocardiographic study. *Circulation* **74**:1208–1216, 1986.
8. Hogge AW, Schonberg AS, Golbus SM, et al: Chorionic villus sampling: Experience of the first 1000 cases. *Am J Obstet/Gynecol* **154**:1249–1252, 1986.
9. Nicolaides HK, Gosden MC, Rodeck HC, et al: Rapid karyotyping in nonlethal fetal malformations. *Lancet* **1**:283–287, 1986.
10. Allan DL, Crawford CD, Chita KS, et al: Prenatal screening in congenital heart disease. *Br Med J* **292**:1717–1719, 1986.

11. Lipton MJ, Higgins CB, Farmer D, et al: Cardiac imaging with a high speed cine CT scanner. *Radiology* **52**:579, 1984.
12. Boxer RA, Sharanjeef S, Jacarta AM, et al: Cardiac magnetic resonance imaging in children with congenital heart disease. *J Pediatr* **109**:460–464, 1986.
13. Whittemore R, Hobbins JC, Engle MA, et al: Pregnancy and its outcome in women with and without surgical treatment of congenital heart disease. *Am J Cardiol* **50**:641–651, 1982.
14. Nora JJ: Etiologic aspects of heart diseases. In Moss JA, Adams HF, Emmanouilidis CG (Eds): *Heart Diseases in Infants,* Baltimore, MD: Williams & Wilkins, 1983, pp. 2–10.
15. Goodwin JF, Oakley CM: The cardiomyopathies. *Br Heart J* **34**:545, 1972.
16. Rightmire DA, Nicolaides KH, Rodeck CH, et al: Fetal blood velocities in RH isoimmunization: Relationship to gestational age and to fetal hematocrit. *Obstet/Gynecol* **68**:233–236, 1986.
17. McCue CM, Mantakas ME, Tingelstad JB, et al: Congenital heart block in newborns of mothers with connective tissue disease. *Circulation* **56**:82–90, 1977.
18. Stewart PA, Tonge HM, Wladimiroff JW, et al: Arrhythmia and structural abnormalities of the fetal heart. *Br Heart J* **50**:550–554, 1983.
19. Beall NH, Paul RH: Artifacts, blocks and arrhythmias confusing nonclassical heart rate changes. *Clin Obstet/Gynecol* **29**:83–94, 1986.
20. Reed LK: Fetal and neonatal cardiac assessment with Doppler. *Sem Perinatol* **11**:347–356, 1987.
21. Lingman G, Morsal K: Fetal cardiac arrhythmias: Doppler assessment. *Sem Perinatol* **11**:357–381, 1987.
22. Allan LD: *Manual of Fetal Echocardiography.* Boston: MTP Press, 1986.
23. Swensson RE, Valdez-Cruz LM, Sahn DJ, et al: Real-time Dopper color flow mapping for detection of patent ductus arteriosus. *J Am Coll Cardiol* **8**:1105–1112, 1986.

Index

FSC
www.fsc.org
MIX
Papier aus verantwortungsvollen Quellen
Paper from responsible sources
FSC® C105338